THE DOMESTIC ANIMAL/WILDLIFE INTERFACE

ISSUES FOR DISEASE CONTROL, CONSERVATION, SUSTAINABLE FOOD PRODUCTION, AND EMERGING DISEASES

ANNALS OF THE NEW YORK ACADEMY OF SCIENCES

Volume 969

THE DOMESTIC ANIMAL/WILDLIFE INTERFACE

ISSUES FOR DISEASE CONTROL, CONSERVATION, SUSTAINABLE FOOD PRODUCTION, AND EMERGING DISEASES

Edited by E. Paul J. Gibbs and Bob H. Bokma

The New York Academy of Sciences
New York, New York
2002

Library of Congress Cataloging-in-Publication Data

The domestic animal/wildlife interface issues for disease control, conservation, sustainable food production, and emerging diseases / edited by E. Paul J. Gibbs and Bob H. Bokma.
    p. ; cm. — (Annals of the New York Academy of Sciences ; v. 969)
Includes bibliographical references and index.
    ISBN 1-57331-438-2 (cloth : alk. paper) — ISBN 1-57331-439-0 (paper : alk. paper)
    1. Animals as carriers of disease—Congresses. 2. Livestock—Diseases—Congresses. 3. Wildlife diseases—Congresses. 4. Communicable diseases in animals—Congresses.

    [DNLM: 1. Animal diseases—prevention & control—Congresses. 2. Animal Diseases—transmission—Congresses. 3. Animals, Domestic—Congresses. 4. Animals, Wild—Congresses. 5. Communicable Diseases, Emerging—veterinary—Congresses. SF 740 D668 2002] I. Gibbs, E. P. J. (E. Paul J.) II. Bokma, Bob H. III. Series.
    Q11 . N5 v. 969
    [SF740]
    500 s—dc21
    636.089'443—dc21   2002013891

GYAT / PCP
Printed in the United States of America
ISBN 1-57331-438-2 (cloth)
ISBN 1-57331-439-0 (paper)
ISSN 0077-8923

ANNALS OF THE NEW YORK ACADEMY OF SCIENCES
Volume 969
October 2002

THE DOMESTIC ANIMAL/WILDLIFE INTERFACE

ISSUES FOR DISEASE CONTROL, CONSERVATION, SUSTAINABLE FOOD PRODUCTION, AND EMERGING DISEASES

Editors
E. PAUL J. GIBBS AND BOB H. BOKMA

Scientific Reviewers
EDMOUR F. BLOUIN, MICHAEL J. BURRIDGE, EMMANUEL CAMUS,
SIDNEY EWING, WILL L. GOFF, WILLIAM KARESH, KATHERINE M. KOCAN,
SUMAN MAHAN, ANITA MICHEL, GARY R. MULLINS, BANIE PENZHORN,
JEREMIAH T. SALIKI, AND OLIVIER A.E. SPARAGANO

Conference Organizers

Society for Tropical Veterinary Medicine
BOB H. BOKMA, DANIËL T. DE WAAL, E. PAUL J. GIBBS
PATRICIA CONRAD, EDMOUR F. BLOUIN, THOMAS E. WALTON,
AND EMMANUEL CAMUS

Wildlife Diseases Association
DAVID JESSUP, EMILY LANE, TONIE E. ROCKE, AND JONNA MAZET
Assisted by Sandra Collier and staff of EventDynamics

This volume is the result of a conference and workshop series entitled **Wildlife and Livestock, Disease and Sustainability: What Makes Sense?** held 22–27 July 2001 in Pilanesberg National Park, South Africa.

CONTENTS

Bacteria

The Society for Tropical Veterinary Medicine and the Wildlife Diseases Association would like to thank the following sponsors for their valuable contribution to the success of the conference:

- BAYER
- MERIAL ANIMAL HEALTH
- NOVARTIS
- PFIZER
- UNITED STATES DEPARTMENT OF AGRICULTURE
  AGRICULTURAL RESEARCH SERVICE
  ANIMAL AND PLANT HEALTH INSPECTION SERVICE
  COOPERATIVE STATE RESEARCH, EDUCATION AND
  EXTENSION SERVICE
- THE WELLCOME TRUST

Introduction

E. PAUL J. GIBBS[a] AND BOB H. BOKMA

[a]College of Veterinary Medicine, University of Florida, Gainesville, Florida 32611, USA

[b]National Center for Import and Export, Veterinary Services, Animal and Plant Health Inspection Service, Riverdale, Maryland 20737, USA

The previous meeting of the Society for Tropical Veterinary Medicine in Key West in 1999 examined the *Control and Prevention of Tropical Animal Diseases in the Context of the New World Order* (the proceedings of which were published as Volume 916 of the *Annals of the New York Academy of Sciences*). During this meeting we recognized that the respective interests of wildlife and animal agriculture are, at times, in conflict and yet both have clear financial, biological, social, and even spiritual value. The STVM considered further examination of the topic to be important and an excellent theme around which to build the 2001 conference in South Africa. To strengthen the scientific discussion, we invited the Wildlife Diseases Association to celebrate their 50th Anniversary by joining us in South Africa at a conference focused on *The Domestic Animal/Wildlife Interface: Issues for Disease Control, Conservation, Sustainable Food Production, and Emerging Diseases.* We were pleased that they accepted our invitation.

Within this context, the papers that were submitted for publication in the proceedings are arranged in the following sections/subsections:

- The importance of disease in wildlife and domestic livestock and its relationship to issues of conservation and sustainability;
- Approaches to disease control;
    - *(i)* diagnostics;
    - *(ii)* vaccines, immunology, and genomics;
    - *(iii)* epidemiology, surveillance, and disease management; and
- General—this section includes several papers describing emerging diseases, reproductive behavior, and restoration programs involving wildlife.

At the conclusion of the conference, participants agreed that the importance of the wildlife/domestic animal interface and the need for cross-disciplinary science were not sufficiently recognized by those organizations (governments, international agencies and non-governmental organizations [NGOs]) that support the concept of sustainability. To draw attention to this concern, a resolution was passed by the joint membership present at the conference and submitted to government departments and organizations around the world. This resolution, which has become known as the Pilanesberg Resolution, is presented as Appendix 1.

We hope that you will enjoy reading these proceedings.

Ann. N.Y. Acad. Sci. 969: xiii–xiv (2002). © 2002 New York Academy of Sciences.

Once again, the STVM is indebted to the staff of the New York Academy of Sciences, particularly Joyce Hitchcock, Associate Editor, for editorial assistance and patience.

Sustainability

From Fringe to Mainstream

GARY R. MULLINS

United States Agency for International Development, Gaborone, Botswana

Five years ago, discussions regarding "sustainability" revolved around a seemingly never-ending, academic debate regarding the meaning of the term. Although equally supportive of the concept, proponents were divided by discipline over minutiae of the details of the meaning of sustainability. Should it be "sustainable development," or "sustainable economy," or "sustainable use"? In reflecting on my own definition of sustainability, I am always reminded of what the U.S. Supreme Court Justice Learned Hand had to say about the definition of "obscene" material: "While it may not be easy to arrive at a single, agreed definition, most people know it when they see it." For me, sustainability is a lot like that, and it may be as well for many of you. But for those who are not satisfied with such an offering, I would provide one of the more generally accepted definitions of sustainable development, as put forward by the World Commission on Environment and Development: sustainable development is that which "meets the needs of the present without compromising the ability of future generations to meet their own needs."

Fortunately, the debate over the meaning of sustainability has largely been resolved, perhaps as much due to fatigue than finding a superior wording, and the work of determining how to realize sustainable results was begun in earnest. Why else this sharpening of focus? I would also venture that it is because the world has at last encountered many environmental limitations that in the past appeared distantly on the horizon.

In his book, *The Economics of Biodiversity Conservation in Sub-Saharan Africa: Mending the Arc* (1999), Charles Perrins observes four processes underlying biodiversity loss in Sub-Saharan Africa:

(1) the destruction and fragmentation of habitat associated with the expansion of mining, forestry, and agriculture;
(2) the degradation and arable and grazing lands;
(3) the controlled or uncontrolled introduction of species, and he particularly notes imports supporting agriculture and fisheries, and;
(4) the harvesting and hunting of individual wild species, taking special note of hunting to protect crops and livestock.

Address for correspondence: Gary R. Mullins, Ph.D., Team Leader, Agriculture and Natural Resource Management, c/o USAID/RCSA, Department of State, 2170 Gaborone Place, Washington, DC 20521-2170. Voice: +267-324-449 ext. 399; fax: +267-324-404.
  gmullins@usaid.gov

Ann. N.Y. Acad. Sci. 969: 1–3 (2002). © 2002 New York Academy of Sciences.

All of these are closely related with livestock and wildlife and their sustainable management and have disease risk and control implications.

More recently, the IUCN-conducted, Future Harvest–sponsored study *Common Ground, Common Future* (2001) carried out by researchers Jeffrey McNeely and Sara Scherr, compiles promising evidence that conservation of biodiversity and agricultural production **can** be pursued on the same land, netting positive results for both. *Common Ground, Common Future* documents dozens of such cases in different ecosystems around the world, choosing to characterize them using the newly coined term "ecoagriculture." Whether this will become yet another overused piece of jargon is still to be seen, but there is substance to the successful cases of biodiversity coexistent with agriculture identified in McNeely and Scherr's report.

From these case studies, the authors distill six key ecoagricultural strategies that can help farmers grow the food they need without destroying wild species habitats:

(1) reduce habitat destruction by increasing agricultural productivity on lands already being farmed;
(2) enhance wildlife habitat on farms and establish farmland corridors that link uncultivated spaces;
(3) establish protected areas near farming areas;
(4) mimic natural habitats by integrating productive perennial plants;
(5) use farming methods that reduce pollution, and;
(6) modify resource management practices to enhance habitat quality in and around farmlands.

Some of these strategies may, at first blush, seem remote from our own areas of interest. But on closer inspection, one finds intrinsic linkages that are very relevant to the direction and the way we proceed with our future work.

What is this relevance? To me, it is the reason that we, the members of STVM and WDA have come together here in Pilanesberg, a place once under exclusive livestock and crop production—in fact, in some areas of the park, if you look closely enough, you can still see the crop furrows—but that now sustains substantial biodiversity of wild species.

We are here not only to share our scientific discoveries, but to determine how we can use these discoveries to promote the sustainable use of both livestock and wildlife. It is very important, in my estimation, that we spend this precious time together focused on the future and asking ourselves: How can we work together? By what means can we collaborate to make progress on this front?

I think we must be results oriented, results in the sense of delivering practicable strategies for managing livestock and wildlife together. This will entail not only the essential component of disease control. As you can see in the model of Pilanesberg, our strategies will necessarily also include economic, ecological, and social elements. I hope this idea does not sound heretical—I simply view an integrated approach as imperative if we are to arrive at practicable and sustainable solutions.

One of the most interesting aspects of the McNeely/Scherr study was their statement that, in almost all of their case studies, the successful, simultaneous achievement of biodiversity conservation and increased agricultural production was serendipitous. It was unintended, it happened by chance! One must then ask oneself: How many more systems could be designed, how much more could be achieved were we to actually work towards the goal of successful eco-agriculture?

I said earlier that I believe the idea of sustainability has now gained wide accep-
tance in scientific circles because it is recognized that we have reached many natural
limits. I see this as a very positive development; however, I do not see or nor do I
hear enough discussion about sustainability among the general public. Indeed,
across the globe the focus is still on economic growth, expanding markets, consumption. It is a failure on the part of the leadership of scientific organizations such as
ours to guide the public into a new mentality, one that recognizes humankind's reliance on natural resources and seeks to live within its limits, guided by nature's en-
dowment, not by the level of one's income.

Pie in the sky? Twenty-five, even 10 years ago, perhaps it was an idea whose time
had not yet come. But in the 21st century, there is little choice.

The responsibility for creating this new mentality does not rest solely with political leaders. We, as animal health professionals, as scientists and applied practitioners of biodiversity conservation also have a responsibility to work towards bringing
the idea of sustainability from the fringe to the mainstream. What is the way forward? I think that the first step is to rethink and reorganize our collaborative activities to reflect achieving sustainable livestock/wildlife management systems.
Secondly, our collaborative partners in future must include not only other scientific
disciplines but also the communities that ultimately will employ and be responsible
for the day-to-day management of the animal resources. And, thirdly, we must network among ourselves and with communities in different sites in different ecological
zones in order to increase the probability of finding practicable solutions. When we
have generated favorable results, as I'm certain we can, it will make promotion of
sustainable livestock/wildlife systems significantly easier. Indeed, I think society
will then regard livestock and wildlife not as threatening to one another, as is often
the case today, but as sensibly coexisting.

This is the time and this is the place to begin new collaboration. I encourage you
all to make the most of this opportunity over the next few days.

A Review of Mutual Transmission of Important Infectious Diseases between Livestock and Wildlife in Europe

K. FRÖLICH, S. THIEDE, T. KOZIKOWSKI, AND W. JAKOB

Institute for Zoo Biology and Wildlife Research, Berlin, Germany

ABSTRACT: Oral vaccination of red foxes against rabies has been practiced in Europe since 1978 and has succeeded in greatly reducing the occurrence of this disease in foxes: this is an example of coordinated activity against a disease that affects both wild and domestic animals as well as humans. Some examples of diseases that affect both domestic and wild animals in Europe are: classical swine fever (hog cholera) in wild boars and domestic swine; myxomatosis and rabbit hemorrhagic disease in domestic and wild rabbits; bovine viral diarrhea (BVD) in cattle and roe deer; contagious ecthyma in domestic sheep and goats and also in, e.g., chamois, muskox, and reindeer; *Mycobacterium bovis* in cattle, wild boars, badgers, and deer; and brucellosis in a broad range of livestock and wildlife in all European countries. In addition, serological surveys performed in different free-ranging ungulate species revealed the presence of alphaherpesviruses related to bovine herpesvirus-1 in 7 European countries; and a study of malignant catarrhal fever in deer in Germany might indicate that in this case sheep are the main reservoir species. Although many data on infectious diseases are available in various European countries, there is more need for systematic surveillance and coordinated research.

KEYWORDS: wildlife; livestock; infectious diseases; two-way transmission; Europe

INTRODUCTION

Beginning in the early 1980s and especially in the last decade, wildlife issues have been more intensely investigated within Europe. In 1999, a European network on wildlife as reservoirs of pathogens was created as part of the FAIR 6 program concerted action (CT98-4361). The network learned that Denmark, Finland, France, Norway, and Sweden have instituted general surveillance programs. The remaining European nations rely upon informal information gathering networks composed of wildlife institutes, veterinary and medical research laboratories, veterinary universities, and volunteers.[1]

Here we focus on the most relevant diseases in free-living animals within Europe with respect to potential transmission between livestock and wildlife.

Address for correspondence: PD Dr. Dr. K. Frölich, Institute for Zoo Biology and Wildlife Research, Berlin, Germany.
froelich@izw-berlin.de

Ann. N.Y. Acad. Sci. 969: 4–13 (2002). © 2002 New York Academy of Sciences.

VIRAL DISEASES IN UNGULATES

Bovine Viral Diarrhea/Mucosal Disease (BVD/MD)

Bovine viral diarrhea virus (BVDV) belongs to the genus *Pestivirus* within the family Flaviviridae and is a major pathogen of cattle with worldwide economic impact. Primary clinical signs in wild ruminants are erosion and ulceration of the oral mucosa, hemorrhagic enteritis, interdigital ulceration, and general physical impairment. Serological surveys and virus isolation in free-ranging populations have been successfully conducted in various species from several European countries.[2] The natural mode of transmission of BVDV to wild ungulates is still not clear. Similarly, it is not known whether persistent BVDV infections occur in wild ruminant species as they do in domestic ruminants, but there are, however, some indications that this might happen.[2] Neumann *et al.*[3] and Kocan *et al.*[4] assume a causal relationship between the massive spread of BVDV in cattle and its occurrence in deer. In contrast, Weber *et al.*,[5] Pastoret *et al.*,[6] Lieberman *et al.*,[7] and Frölich[8] postulate an independent infection process in wild ruminants. Frölich[8] found no significant difference in antibody prevalence among deer in habitats with high, intermediate, and low cattle population densities. The sequence analysis of the BVDV isolated from roe deer (*Capreolus capreolus*)[9] showed a unique position of this roe deer strain within the BVDV group I. This study indicated that distinct BVDV-strains might circulate in free-ranging roe deer populations in Germany and that virus transmission in these areas is independent of domestic livestock.[10]

Alphaherpesvirus Infections

Serological surveys performed in different ruminant species revealed the presence of alphaherpesviruses related to bovine herpesvirus-1 (BHV-1). Such viruses include BHV-1, the herpesvirus of red deer (*Cervus elaphus*) (HVC-1), the rangifer herpesvirus (RanHV-1) and the caprine herpesvirus-1 (CapHV-1). The clinical signs associated with these herpesvirus infections in ruminants include conjunctivitis, lacrimation, corneal lesions, and a serous or purulent nasal discharge.[11,12] Serological surveys in free-ranging populations have been successfully conducted in many wild ungulate species from Europe.[11,13] The mode of infection in free-ranging ungulates is still unknown. In Germany, no association was found between cattle density and antibody prevalence against alphaherpesviruses in deer. In these deer populations, contact with cattle is obviously not essential for viral transmission.[13] Nettleton *et al.*[14] and Kokles[15] also assume that herpesviruses of free-ranging deer have not posed a threat to livestock[16] and stated that there may have been a separate parallel evolution of viruses in both wild and domestic ruminants. Weber *et al.*[17] and Lawman *et al.*,[18] however, do assume two-way transmissions between domestic and wild hosts.

Malignant Catarrhal Fever (MCF)

MCF affects many species of wild ruminants; however, there is great interspecies variation in susceptibility to infection.[19–21] The two major epizootiological entities of the disease are wildebeest-associated (WA) and sheep-associated (SA) MCF.[19] The disease tends to be peracute or acute.[21] Typically, affected animals show temperatures above 40°C and, in some cases, dysentery develops and death can occur within 12h. In other cases the disease runs a longer course; lymph nodes are enlarged, while initially serous ocular and nasal secretions become mucopurulent. In contrast to many reports in captive ruminants only two cases of MCF in free-ranging European ruminants have been documented so far. First, the disease was diagnosed by histopathology in two free-ranging moose (*Alces alces*) from Sweden showing CNS symptoms.[22] Second, Frölich *et al.*[23] found seropositive reactors in free-ranging fallow deer (*Cervus dama*). The cause of cervid MCF in most cases is thought to be a virus carried by clinically normal sheep.[21,23,24] The existence of only two reports of the disease or exposure to MCFV in free-ranging deer in Europe may reflect a lack of surveillance and awareness of the disease in wild cervids in Europe.

Classical Swine Fever (CSF, Hog Cholera)

CSF is a highly contagious disease that affects all *Suidae*. The clinical picture varies from acute forms with predominantly hemorrhagic and septicemic signs to subacute and chronic forms accompanied by inflammation of the respiratory and digestive tracts. Postmortem lesions are characterized by petechial hemorrhages on serosal surfaces and in the renal cortex. Chronically infected individuals may show "button ulcers" up to 10 mm in diameter in the mucosa of the large intestine. Young animals which recover are permanently stunted.[25,26] CSF affects wild boars (*Sus scrofa*) and domestic pigs in several parts of Europe. Mutual transmission between pigs and wild boars mainly occurs by ingestion of virus-contaminated food or water. Since the use of CSF vaccines in domestic pigs is banned within the EU, the disease can only be controlled by culling. Additionally, a targeted vaccination of wild boars has been performed. Presently, CSF officially occurs in wild boars in six European countries: Germany, Italy, Austria, France, Slovakia and the Czech Republic.

Aujeszky's Disease (AK)

The causative virus of AK is suid herpesvirus 1, also known as pseudorabies virus (PrV). Although many domestic animal species are susceptible to infections by pseudorabies virus (PrV), pigs are considered the main host reservoir. Clinical signs include a brief course of hyperexcitability, ataxia, coma, and progressive paralysis. The disease is relatively mild in adult animals, causing heavy mortality only in the young.[25] Limited data exist on natural infection in wildlife in Europe. In eastern Germany, 8.9% of wild boar samples were seropositive in 1991–1994.[27] On the basis of epidemiological analysis, the authors concluded that PrV infections occurred in wild boar populations of the examined region for a number of years with increasing prevalence. Interestingly, AK was eradicated in domestic pigs in this area in 1985. Four strains of PrV were isolated from endemic areas. Molecular biological analysis showed considerable differences from PrV-strains obtained from domestic animals. Thus, infections in the wild boar populations appear to be endemic without affecting the domestic pig population.[27]

VIRAL DISEASES IN LAGOMORPHS

Rabbit Hemorrhagic Disease (RHD)

RHD is caused by a calicivirus, which is distinct from the calicivirus implicated in European brown hare syndrome.[28] Experimental data show that mainly lagomorphs are susceptible to RHDV, although other mammals, such as carnivores, may carry and shed the virus.[29] The most typical pathological findings include degenerative and necrotic lesions in the liver and hemorrhages in different organs. The main mode of viral transmission is oral, but infection may be spread through conjunctival and respiratory routes or by skin trauma.[30,31]

The first outbreak of RHD occurred in 1984 in China in a shipment of angora rabbits from Germany. Since that time, the virus has spread throughout Europe and to localities throughout the world including Mexico, Australia, New Zealand, and South Korea. The high mortality rate (40–90%) of RHD, in combination with myxomatosis, has led to a considerable decrease in local wild European rabbit (*Oryctolagus cuniculus*) populations. Interestingly, analyses of gene sequence of RHDV isolates from domestic and wild rabbits in Spain and Austria suggest that RHDV has spread from the wild to the domestic rabbit populations.[28]

Myxomatosis

The myxoma virus is a poxvirus of the genus *Leporipoxvirus*.[32] The virus evolved in North and South American rabbits (*Sylvilagus bachmani* and *S. braziliensis*) and has a non-pathogenic relationship with its natural host.[33] In the European rabbit, however, myxomatosis causes high mortality rates. It is characterized by swelling of the head and cutaneous mucoid tumors.[32] Additionally, the virus may cause severe immunosuppression accompanied by supervening bacterial infections of the respiratory tract.[33] The virus can be transmitted directly or indirectly by arthropod vectors and the virulence appears to be temperature dependent.[32,33] Myxomatosis has been endemic throughout Europe since the 1950s.[32] A combined vaccine against myxomatosis and RHD is currently being developed.[34]

European Brown Hare Syndrome (EBHS)

In 1989, Lavazza and Vecchi[35] found viral particles in European brown hares (*Lepus europaeus*) that had died from EBHS by negative staining immune electron microscopy of the liver. The causative agent of EBHS was classified as a calicivirus, which is distinct from the calicivirus implicated in RHD. The clinical and pathological findings of EBHS and RHD are remarkably similar.[36] EBHS has been demonstrated in European brown hares and mountain hares (*Lepus timidus*), and has been reported in many European countries.[37] EBHS may be one of the causes for increased mortality in hare populations in Europe over the past years. However, due to differences in (1) the distribution of the disease and (2) the variability of its virulence, the effects of EBHSV on hare populations differ considerably in various parts of Europe.

VIRAL DISEASES IN CARNIVORES

Rabies

Rabies is caused by a *Lyssavirus* of the family Rhabdoviridae. There are seven distinct lineages within the genus *Lyssavirus*: true rabies virus (serotype I), Lagos bat virus (serotype II), Mokola rhabdovirus (serotpe III), Duvennago rhabdovirus (serotype IV), European bat lyssavirus I and II (serotypes V and VI), and Australian bat virus (serotype VII). The rabies virus causes an acute infectious disease of the CNS.[38] The two primary reservoirs of rabies in Europe are terrestrial carnivores and insectivorous bats. In western Europe the main vector species is the red fox (*Vulpes vulpes*). Additional vectors include the arctic fox (*Alopex lagopus*) in circumpolar regions, racoon dogs (*Nyctereutes procyanoides*) in eastern Europe, bats in northern Europe, and domestic dogs in Turkey.[38] Since the introduction of oral immunization vaccine bait in 1978, a combination of culling and vaccination have been used to control the rabies epidemic in carnivores.[39] In the past, countries that have brought their rabies epidemics under control have seen a re-emergence of the disease because neighboring countries had not developed adequate rabies vaccination programs.[39] Today, Switzerland, Scandinavia and the EU members UK, Italy, Portugal, Greece, Iceland, Luxembourg, Malta, and Cyprus are rabies free. The remaining European nations are investing significant resources to halt the spread of rabies.[40]

BACTERIAL INFECTIONS

Tuberculosis

Tuberculosis is primarily a respiratory disease and transmission is mainly air-borne. *Mycobacterium bovis*, the etiologic agent of bovine-type tuberculosis, has an exceptionally wide host range.[41] Presently, Switzerland and the following EU-member states are officially bovine tuberculosis free: Austria, Denmark, Germany, Luxembourg, Finland, the Netherlands, Sweden, and parts of Italy. Less than 1% of the cattle herds in Belgium, France, Portugal, UK, and Italy are infected, whereas in the other EU states more than 1% are infected.[42] Bovine tuberculosis in wildlife is still periodically reported from Spain, Italy, and the UK. Wildlife species, such as badgers (*Meles meles*) in the UK, seem to act as maintenance hosts for *M. bovis* and contribute to spread and persistence of tuberculosis in associated cattle popula-tions.[43,44] A study from Ireland provided evidence that a badger-control program was effective in reducing the risk of a trade restriction to cattle herds.[45] Costello *et al.*[46] showed that the same range and geographic distribution of strains were found for the majority of isolates from cattle, badgers, and deer. This suggests that trans-mission of infection among these species is a factor in the epidemiology of *M. bovis* infection in Ireland. In Italy, an epidemiological survey for the monitoring of bovine tuberculosis showed the presence of a common *M. bovis* genotype in both cattle and wild boars, confirming the possibility of interspecies transmission.[47]

Paratuberculosis

Mycobacterium avium subspecies *paratuberculosis* is the etiologic agent of paratuberculosis (Johne's disease), a chronic enteritis in ruminants that causes enormous economic losses worldwide. *M. paratuberculosis* affects a wide range of domestic and wild species.[48] Ferroglio *et al.*[49] and Nebbia *et al.*[50] reported on *M. paratuberculosis* infections in free-ranging Alpine ibex *(Capra ibex)* and red deer from Italy. Susceptibility of *Caprinae* to *M. paratuberculosis* of bovine origin has also been demonstrated by Thoresen and Olsaker.[51] Nebbia *et al.*[50] found paratuberculosis in red deer in the western Alps (Italy). Generally, young red deer show a sudden onset, with rapid loss in body condition and diarrhea. Adults rarely develop clinical signs, although they may be seropositive and show pathological lesions. Sixty-seven percent of wild rabbits in Scotland were infected with *M. paratuberculosis*. Molecular genetic typing techniques could not discriminate between selected rabbit and cattle isolates from the same or different farms, suggesting that the same strain may infect and cause disease in both species and that interspecies transmission may occur.[52]

Brucellosis

The etiologic agents, *Brucella abortus*, *B. melitensis*, and *B. suis*, are highly pathogenic for domestic and wild animal species and for humans. *Brucella abortus* biotype 1 was isolated from chamois (*Rupicapra rupicapra*) in Italy, in an area where an infected cattle herd had been grazed illegally.[53,54] Systemic brucellosis caused by *Brucella melitensis* biotype 3[55] was also identified in a chamois from France and in an alpine ibex from Gran Paradiso National Park (Italy), where *B. melitensis* biotype 2 was isolated.[56] *B. suis* is the etiologic agent of brucellosis in domestic pigs, wild boars, and European brown hares. Infection can be transmitted among these species and to humans.[57] *Brucella suis* biotype 2 has been isolated from hares in Austria and in Italy,[58,59] and serologic surveys also showed *B. suis* to be endemic in wild boars and European brown hares from Poland.[60] Since 1998, the EU-members Austria, Denmark, Finland, Germany, UK, Luxembourg, Sweden, the Netherlands, and parts of Italy have acquired an officially bovine brucellosis-free status (*B. abortus*). Nine EU states were declared officially free of ovine and caprine brucellosis (*B. melitensis*): Belgium, Denmark, Finland, Germany, UK, Ireland, Luxembourg, Sweden, and the Netherlands.[42]

Tularemia

Tularemia is a zoonotic disease caused by *Francisella tularensis*. Tularemia has been reported in more than 250 species. In Europe, tularemia is most frequently seen in hares, although they are probably not a reservoir for this pathogen.[61] In a serological survey of different domestic and wild animal species, Mörner and Sandstedt[62] showed that Scandinavian beavers (*Castor fiber*) play an important role in the epizootiology, while cattle and moose do not seem to be susceptible. In Sweden, tularemia mainly occurs in the highly susceptible Mountain hare with severe pathological findings such as focal coagulative necrosis in liver, spleen, and bone marrow as well as hemorrhagic enteritis, including typhlitis.[63] Tularemia was also diagnosed in foxes and European brown hares from Austria.[64] Monitoring of ticks like *Dermacentor reticulatus* for *F. tularensis* may be a valuable contribution to the surveillance of tularemia in Europe.[65]

Infectious Keratoconjunctivitis (IKC)

IKC, caused by *Mycoplasma conjunctivae*, is a highly contagious ocular infection. In the European Alps, IKC is of particular interest for both domestic and wild *Caprinae*. Blind chamois and ibex face particularly treacherous circumstances in steep rocky areas, and the mortality rate can attain 30%. Flies are considered as possible vectors for interspecies transmission of *M. conjunctivae*. Spill-over from sheep living in close proximity to wildlife during summer may be the origin of point source epidemics in wild *Caprinae*. IKC, however, is not self-maintained in wildlife.[66]

CONCLUSIONS

Only single investigations have been performed regarding mutual transmission of pathogens between livestock and wildlife in Europe. Therefore, the modes of transmission for most infectious diseases in wildlife have not been fully elucidated. Moreover, the ecological impact for most of the diseases in wildlife is still unknown. These limited findings may reflect a lack of adequate surveillance of infectious diseases in European wildlife.

REFERENCES

1. ARTOIS, M., P. AZNARTE, V. BRIONES, *et al.* 2000. Surveillance and monitoring of wildlife diseases in Europe. 1st Workshop of the European Wildlife Diseases Network. Madrid, June 18–19.
2. VAN CAMPEN, H., K. FRÖLICH & M. HOFMANN. 2001. Pestivirus Infections. *In* Infectious Diseases of Wild Mammals. E. S. Williams & I. K. Barker, Eds.: 232–244. Iowa State University Press. Ames, Iowa.
3. NEUMANN, W., J. BUITKAMP, G. BECHMANN & W. PLÖGER. 1980. BVD/MD Infektion bei einem Damhirsch. Dtsch. Tierärztl. Wochenschr. **87:** 94.
4. KOCAN, A., A.W. FRANZMANN, K.A. WALDRUP & G.J. KUBAT. 1986. Serological studies of selected infectious diseases of moose (*Alces alces*) from Alaska. J. Wildl. Dis. **22:** 418–511.
5. WEBER, A., K.P. HÜRTER & C. COMMICAU. 1982. Über das Vorkommen des Virus diarrhoe/Mucosal Disease-Virus bei Cerviden in Rheinland-Pfalz. Dtsch. Tierärztl. Wochenschr. **89:** 1–3.
6. PASTORET, P.P., E. THIRY, B. BROCHIER, *et al.* 1988. Diseases of wild animals transmissible to domestic animals. Rev. Sci. Tech. Off. Int. Epizoot. **7:** 705–736.
7. LIEBERMANN, H., D. TABBAA, J. DEDEK, *et al.* 1989. Serologische Untersuchungen auf ausgewählte Virusinfektionen bei Wildwiederkäuern in der DDR. Monh. Vet. Med. **44:** 380–382.
8. FRÖLICH, K. 1995. Bovine virus diarrhea and mucosal disease in free-ranging and captive deer (Cervidae) in Germany. J. Wildl. Dis. **31:** 247–250.
9. FRÖLICH, K. & M. HOFMANN. 1995. Isolation of bovine viral diarrhea virus-like pestiviruses from roe deer (*Capreolus capreolus*). J. Wildl. Dis. **31:** 243–246.
10. FISCHER, S., E. WEILAND & K. FRÖLICH. 1998. Characterization of bovine viral diarrhea virus isolated from roe deer in Germany. J. Wildl. Dis. **34:** 47–55.

11. NETTLETON, P.F., J.A. SINCLAIR, J.A. HERRING, *et al.* 1986. Prevalence of herpesvirus infection in British red deer and investigations of further disease outbreaks. Vet. Rec. **118:** 267–270.
12. REID, H.W., D. BUXTON, I. POW & J. FINLAYSON. 1986. Malignant catarrhal fever: experimental transmission of the "sheep-associated" form of the disease from cattle, deer, rabbits and hamsters. Res. Vet. Sci. **41:** 76–81.
13. FRÖLICH, K. 1996. Seroepizootiologic investigations of herpesviruses in free-ranging and captive deer (Cervidae) in Germany. J. Zoo Wildl. Med. **27:** 241–247.
14. NETTLETON, P.F., E. THIRY, H. REID & P.P. PASTORET. 1988. Herpesvirus infections in Cervidae. Rev. Sci. Tech. Off. Int. Epizoot. **7:** 977–988.
15. KOKLES, R. 1977. Untersuchungen zum Nachweis von IBR/IPV-Antikörpern bei verschiedenen Haus- und Wildtieren sowie beim Menschen. Monh. Vet. Med. **32:** 170–171.
16. BARADEL, J.M., J. BARRAT, J. BLANCHOU, *et al.* 1988. Results of a serological survey of wild mammals in France. Rev. Sci. Tech. Off. Int. Epizoot. **7:** 873–883.
17. WEBER, A., J. PAULSEN & H. KRAUSS. 1978. Seroepidemiologische Untersuchungen zum Vorkommen von Infektionskrankheiten bei einheimischem Schalenwild. Prakt. Tierarzt **59:** 353–358.
18. LAWMAN, M.J., D. EVANS, E.P.J. GIBBS, *et al.* 1978. A preliminary survey of British deer for antibody to some virus diseases of farm animals. Br. Vet. J. **134:** 85–91.
19. REID, H.W. 1992. The biology of a fatal herpesvirus infection of deer (malignant catarrhal fever). *In* The Biology of Deer. R. D. Brown, Ed.: 93–100. Springer Verlag. New York.
20. MACKINTOSH, C. 1993. Importance of infectious diseases of New Zealand farmed deer. Surveillance **20:** 24–26.
21. BUXTON, D. 1988. The diagnosis of malignant catarrhal fever in deer. *In* The Management and Health of Farmed Deer. H. W. Reid, Ed.: 159–167. Kluwer Academic Publishers. Dordrecht, Holland.
22. WARSAME, I.Y. & M. STEEN. 1989. Malignant catarrhal fever in wild Swedish moose (*Alces alces* L.). Rangifer **9:** 51–57.
23. FRÖLICH, K., H. LI & U. MÜLLER-DOBLIES. 1998. Serosurvey for antibodies to malignant catarrhal fever-associated viruses in free-living and captive cervids in Germany. J. Wildl. Dis. **34:** 777–782.
24. TOMKINS, N.W., N.N. JONSSON, M.P. YOUNG, *et al.* 1997. An outbreak of malignant catarrhal fever in young rusa deer (*Cervus tunorensis*). Aust. Vet. J. **75:** 722–723.
25. WALLACH, J.D. & W.J. BOEVER. 1983. Diseases of Exotic Animals. W.B. Saunders Co. Philadelphia, pp. 269–642.
26. DEDEK, J. & TH. STEINECK. 1994. Wildhygiene. Fischer-Verlag. Jena, Germany, pp. 17–19.
27. MÜLLER, T., D. JUNGHANS, R. ZELLMER, *et al.* 1996. Occurrence of pseudorabies virus (Aujeszky's disease) infections in European wild boar in eastern Germany. *In* European Section Wildlife Diseases Association, Vol. **2:** 21. Second European Conference, Wroclaw, Poland.
28. NOWOTNY, N., C.R. BASCUNANA, A. BALLAGI-PORDANY, *et al.* 1997. Phylogenetic analysis of rabbit haemorrhagic disease and European brown hare syndrome viruses by comparison of sequences from the capsid protein gene. Arch. Virol. **142:** 657–673.
29. FRÖLICH, K., F. KLIMA & J. DEDEK. 1998. Antibodies against rabbit hemorrhagic disease in free-ranging red foxes in Germany. J. Wildl. Dis. **34:** 436–442.
30. MARCATO, P.S., G. VECCHI, M. GALEOTTI, *et al.* 1991. Clinical and pathological features of viral haemorrhagic disease of rabbits and the European brown hare syndrome. Rev. Sci. Tech. Off. Int. Epiz. **10:** 371–392.
31. VILLAFUERTE, R., C. CALVETE, C. GORTAZAR & S. MORENO. 1994. First epizootic of rabbit hemorrhagic disease in free-living populations of *Oryctolagus cuniculus* at Donana National Park, Spain. J. Wildl. Dis. **30:** 176–179.
32. KERR, P.J. & S.M. BEST. 1998. Myxoma virus in rabbits. Rev. Sci. Tech. Off. Int. Epizoot. **17:** 256–268.
33. NASH, P., J. BARRETT, J.X. CAO, *et al.* 1999. Immunomodulation by viruses: the myxoma virus story. Immunol. Rev. **168:** 103–120.

34. TORRES, J.M., M.A. RAMIREZ, M. MORALES, *et al.* 2000. Safety evaluation of a recombinant myxoma-RHD virus inducing horizontal transmissible protection against myxomatosis and rabbit haemorrhagic disease. Vaccine **19:** 174–182.
35. LAVAZZA, A. & G. VECCHI. 1989. Osservazioni su alcuni episodi di mortalità nelle lepri. Evidenziazione al microscopio elettronico di una particella virale. Nota preliminare. Selezione Vet. **30:** 461–467.
36. OHLINGER, V.F. & H.J. THIEL. 1991. Identification of the viral hemorrhagic disease virus of rabbits as a calicivirus. Rev. Sci. Tech. Off. Int. Epizoot. **10:** 311–323.
37. FRÖLICH, K., G. HAERER, L. BACCIARINI, *et al.* 2001. Survey for European brown hare syndrome (EBHS) in free-ranging European brown hares (*Lepus europaeus*) and mountain hares (*Lepus timidus*) from Switzerland. J. Wildl. Dis. **37:** 803–807.
38. RUPPRECHT, C.E., K. STÖHR & C. MEREDITH. 2001. Rabies. *In* Infectious Diseases of Wild Mammals. E.S. Williams & I.K. Barker, Eds.: 3–26. Iowa State University Press. Ames, IA.
39. BREITENMOSER, U., T. KAPHEGYI, A. KAPPELER & R. ZANONI. 1995. Significance of young foxes for the persistence of rabies in northwestern Switzerland. Proc. Congress Eur. Soc. Vet. Virol. **3:** 391–396.
40. Anonymous. 2001. Handistatus II: prototype; Europe/rabies; multiannual animal disease status. OIE, www.oie.int/hs2.
41. MORRIS, R.S., D.U. PFEIFFER & R. JACKSON. 1994. The epidemiology of *Mycobacterium bovis* infections. Vet. Microbiol. **40:** 153–177.
42. ANONYMOUS. 1998. Community Reference Laboratory on the Epidemiology of Zoonoses, BgVV, 1998. Trends and sources of zoonotic agents in animals, feedstuff, food and man in the European Union in 1998. Document No. SANCO/409/2000–Rev. 2 of the European Commission, Part 1.
43. DELAHAY, R.J., L.M. ROGERS, G.C. SMITH, *et al.* 1998. The transmission of bovine tuberculosis in badgers (*Meles meles*) and domestic cattle in England. Gibier Faune Sauv. **15:** 805–814.
44. GORMLEY, E. & J.D. COLLINS. 2000. The development of wildlife control strategies for eradication of tuberculosis in cattle in Ireland. Tuber. Lung. Dis. **80:** 229–236.
45. MAIRTIN, D.O., D.H. WILLIAMS, L. DOLAN, *et al.* 1998. The influence of selected herd factors and a badger-intervention tuberculosis-control programme on the risk of a herd-level trade restriction to a bovine population in Ireland. Prev. Vet. Med. **35:** 79–90.
46. COSTELLO, E., D. O'GRADY, O. FLYNN, *et al.* 1999. Study of restriction fragment length polymorphism analysis and spoligotyping for epidemiological investigation of *Mycobacterium bovis* infection. J. Clin. Microbiol. **37:** 3217–3222.
47. SERRAINO, A., G. MARCHETTI, V. SANGUINETTI, *et al.* 1999. Monitoring of transmission of tuberculosis between wild boars and cattle: genotypical analysis of strains by molecular epidemiology techniques. J. Clin. Microbiol. **37:** 2766–2771.
48. CLARKE, C.J. 1997. The pathology and pathogenesis of paratuberculosis in ruminants and other species. J. Comp. Path. **116:** 217–261.
49. FERROGLIO, E., P. NEBBIA, P. ROBINO, *et al.* 2000b. *Mycobacterium paratuberculosis* infection in two free-ranging Alpine ibex. Rev. Sci. Tech. Off. Int. Epizoot. **19:** 859–862.
50. NEBBIA, P., P. ROBINO, E. FERROGLIO, *et al.* 2000. Paratuberculosis in red deer (*Cervus elaphus hippelaphus*) in the western Alps. Vet. Res. Commun. **24:** 435–443.
51. THORESEN, O.F. & I. OLSAKER. 1994. Distribution and hybridization patterns of the insertion element IS900 in clinical isolates of *M. paratuberculosis*. Vet. Microbiol. **40:** 293.
52. GREIG, A., K. STEVENSON, D. HENDERSON, *et al.* 1999. Epidemiological study of paratuberculosis in wild rabbits in Scotland. J. Clin. Microbiol. **37:** 1746–1751.
53. FERROGLIO, E., L. ROSSI, S. GENNERO & F. TOLARI. 2000a. Brucellosis in Alpine chamois (*Rupicapra rupicapra*). Presented at the 4th meeting of the European Wildlife Disease Association. Zaragoza, Spain, September 20–23.
54. FERROGLIO, E., L. ROSSI & S. GENNERO. 2000c. Lung-tissue extract as an alternative to serum for surveillance for brucellosis in chamois. Prev. Vet. Med. **43:** 117–122.
55. GARIN-BASTUJI, B., J. OUDAR, Y. RICHARD & J. GASTELLU. 1990. Isolation of *Brucella melitensis* Biovar 3 from a chamois (*Rupicapra rupicapra*) in the southern French Alps. J. Wildl. Dis. **26:** 116–118.

56. FERROGLIO, E., F. TOLARI, E. BOLLO & B. BASSANO. 1998. Isolation of *Brucella melitensis* from Alpine ibex. J. Wildl. Dis. **34:** 400–402.
57. DEDEK, J. 1994. Brucellose. *In* Wildhygiene. J. Dedek & Th. Steineck, Eds.: 48–51. Gustav Fischer Verlag. Jena, Germany.
58. STEINECK, TH. & K. HACKLÄNDER. 2000. How healthy are "healthy" brown hares (*Lepus europaeus*)? Presented at the 4th meeting of the European Wildlife Disease Association. Zaragoza, Spain, September 20–23.
59. QUARANTA, V., R. FARINA, A. POLLI, *et al.* 1995. Sulla presenza di *Brucella suis* Biovar 2 nella lepre in Italia. Sel. Vet. **36:** 953–958.
60. SZULOWSKI, K., J. PILASZEK & W. IWANIAK. 1999. Preliminary investigations into the prevalence of brucellosis in wild boars in Poland. Zycie Wet. **74:** 399–401.
61. MÖRNER, T. 1992. The ecology of tularaemia. Rev. Sci. Tech. Off. Int. Epizoot. **11:** 1123–1130.
62. MÖRNER, T. & K. SANDSTEDT. 1983. A serological survey of antibodies against *Francisella tularensis* in some Swedish mammals. Nord. Vet. Med. **35:** 82–85.
63. MÖRNER, T., G. SANDSTRÖM, R. MATTSSON & P.-O. NILSSON. 1988. Infections with *Francisella tularensis* Biovar *palaearctica* in hares (*Lepus timidus, Lepus europaeus*) from Sweden. J. Wildl. Dis. **24:** 422–433.
64. HÖFLECHNER-PÖLTL, A., E. HOFER, M. AWAD-MASALMEH, *et al.* 2000. Tularämie und Brucellose bei Feldhasen und Füchsen in Österreich. Tierärztl. Umsch. **55:** 264–268.
65. HUBALEK, Z., W. SIXL & J. HALOUZKA. 1998. *Francisella tularensis* in *Dermacentor reticulatus* ticks from the Czech Republic and Austria. Wien. Klin. Wochenschr. **110:** 909–910.
66. GIACOMETTI, M., J. FREY, M. EL ABDO, *et al.* 2000. Infectious keratoconjunctivitis. Schw. Arch. Tierheilk. **142:** 235–240.

Yankey's Dilemma

Conservation versus the People of Ghana

MICHAEL MURPHREE

Ecologist, Mount Pleasant, Harare, Zimbabwe

ABSTRACT: The past 20 years have seen a shift in conservation approaches to realize the importance of people in conservation and wildlife management (CWM). To this extent, in most conservation circles the concept of community involvement is no longer debated. The following factors have influenced the growth of CWM, especially in Africa: (i) recent developments in postcolonial governments have made them unable to manage and control the use of natural resources in the restrictive manner mandated by the legislation of the colonial past still in place; (ii) successes, particularly in southern Africa, of approaches that involved devolution of greater access rights and responsibilities to communities have led to these approaches being used by other countries; (iii) donor agencies, encouraged by the success of these approaches, have allocated more of their resources to community-based projects; and (iv) changes in international perceptions have been heavily influenced by the growing voice of the "South" in international fora. While there has been some success, there have also been failures. In Ghana, there has been considerable effort to develop programs that incorporate community aspirations into specific objectives; one inherent problem with these programs—not exclusive to Ghana—is the tendency for conservation programs to try to fit community aspirations into conservation objectives as opposed to finding ways of using conservation to help fulfill community aspirations. When community-based programs fail to recognize this, they are generally unable to deliver on their expected outputs. Some critics have used this to dismiss the community approach, which poses a dangerous reversion to a paradigm that has significantly failed in Africa, and much of the developing world, especially in regard to wildlife outside of protected areas.

KEYWORDS: conservation; wildlife management; community-based programs; Ghana

BACKGROUND

This paper is based on the experiences of the Protected Areas Development Programme of the Ghana Wildlife Division. This program seeks to develop Ghana's protected area network, focusing on three protected areas in Ghana's Western Region for which park plans have been prepared. As a component of this program the issue of wildlife and people living outside of the park has been addressed, and in the

Address for correspondence: Michael Murphree, Ecologist, P.O. Box MP 4, Mount Pleasant, Harare, Zimbabwe.
murphree@africaonline.co.zw

Ann. N.Y. Acad. Sci. 969: 14–19 (2002). © 2002 New York Academy of Sciences.

course of this work Ghana has started a pilot program in two communities that serve as the inspiration for this paper.

YANKEY'S STORY

One hot and humid afternoon four men sat in a rickety old shelter in a small village on the edge of one of the last remnants of rainforest in the Western Region of Ghana. The sweet smell of fresh palm wine mixed with the smoke of the cooking fire drifted through the village. Sweating in the humidity and longing for a comfortable chair the consultant sat with his two Ghanaian colleagues from the Wildlife Division and a village elder or "head of family" Abusuapayin Yankey. Their mission was part of a four-year, EU-funded parks and protected areas development program. For Yankey, he had seen in four years teams of consultants come and go, they took up his time and never delivered on what he really wanted. He was convinced that they really had no interest in what he and his people needed—from his perspective they just wanted more land for the national park and to stop his people from using the animals. Almost frustrated he narrowed his eyes, held up is callused hands, and said to the consultant: "You see, the problem is this; our brothers on the coast are free! For they can take their nets, get into their boats and harvest the resources of the sea without restriction. But for us forest communities we are denied the riches of the forest. We are told that these belong to the government and the world. This is unfair." The consultant smiled—the old man had a point. As a consultant it was his mission to advise the Ghanaians on options that would ensure the conservation of natural resources while devolving the authority to manage those resources to communities such as Yankey's. What amazed the consultant was that the wildlife resources that the communities sought to use were not the rare and endangered but fast-breeding rodents and small ungulates that thrive on the secondary growth associated with the small-scale farms of Ghana's Western Region. The evidence seen by the consultant on his brief stay in the area was how thirty years of conservation had failed to meet the aims of both community and conservation. For Yankey his dilemma was: obey the law and see the resources on his land squandered by the state and others, or break the law and face arrest for using natural resources on his own land. Yes, it is unfair. In this instance Yankey can relate to an 18th-century English rhyme that states:

> The law doth punish man or woman,
> That steals the goose from off the common,
> But lets the greater felon loose,
> That steals the common from the goose.

HE WHO LIVES WITH THE GOOSE COOKS IT!

Land tenure in Ghana is a complicated arrangement of land ownership and rights of access. In the Western Region, land is not communally held but regulated under a traditional tenure system of "stool lands." Individual farms in the region are either owned or leased. The use of natural resources, however, falls under state control and this applies to both valuable timber resources and wildlife. This distortion in the tenure status of land vs. natural resources in Ghana has therefore "devalued" natural resources and negated their sustainable use in favor of conventional agricultural and livestock production where tenure and use are securely held by the landholder. Land is a valuable commodity, but virgin land with abundant natural resources is worth a fraction of cultivated land—as the prospective buyer would first have to rid the land of trees and wildlife before it could be considered a productive unit. Natural resources are thus exploited in a manner of "maximum possible" off-take, and for wildlife this has resulted in a decline of many species, especially those that are habitat sensitive. The exceptions in this trend are the fast breeding rodents and small ungulates that constitute the principal species in the "bushmeat" market. Current research is showing that densities of these species actually increases in the secondary growth associated with farming. For the farmer, wildlife are pests that compete with his agriculture. However, the Wildlife Act technically restricts the use of these animals and the farmer can only kill these pests with a permit. In reality, though, the use and trade of these animals is extensive throughout Ghana. In addition to state control, a recent and growing move by international conservation groups to stop the bushmeat trade and "save wildlife" will only further alienate wildlife from the landholder and increase the pressure to remove the competition to agricultural production. In this case, wildlife will further decline into habitat islands mostly represented by state-protected areas. For the reality is, that it is only he who lives with the goose who will cook it or look after it!

The alternative scenario is to enable wildlife to compete as a viable land-use option and for the landholder to decide on consumptive or nonconsumptive uses as the market dictates. The central key is resource tenure for the landholder, but this requires a devolutionary process that most conservation organizations and governments consider a gamble far to risky to take. State and nongovernment organizations have therefore sought a more collaborative arrangement where decision-making is retained at the center while percentage benefits are distributed to the "community." The idea is to have the community "buy into" conservation. This type of program is very prevalent in Africa, resulting in a multitude of "community-based" wildlife program. Unfortunately, in most cases these ultimately fall short of their objectives because real decision-making is not done at the level of the landholder or community. The problem, to return to the goose analogy, is that someone else makes the decision on when and how to cook the goose.

There are, however, examples of the state truly devolving its authority. In Zimbabwe, the state devolved its authority for wildlife to private landowners resulting in wildlife becoming a viable land-use option and creating a multimillion dollar industry on private land based on the consumptive and nonconsumptive use of wildlife. In Ghana, the bushmeat trade is currently valued at over 200 million dollars per year, a figure that is well in excess of Zimbabwe's wildlife industry and in a legal environment that does not cater for wildlife production by Ghanaian farmers. If anything the current legal environment seeks to restrict the production of bushmeat through a complicated licensing system on both production and trade.

If the answer to securing wildlife and natural resources is dependent on the devolution of tenure authority to the landholder, why has this not been done more often and where is the problem? In Ghana the issue is scale. Unlike the commercial farmer in Zimbabwe (despite recent dramatic changes) farms are small production units with shared wildlife resources. Social organization is also far less individualistic, and it is here that the concept of "community" comes in. For the state this is important, for even though it recognizes the need to devolve authority it is looking for something to devolve authority to. The state seeks accountability should "things go wrong." Even though Mr. Yankey's dilemma is recognized by many in Ghana—including some in positions of authority—the risk for them and the problem of devolution centers on three fundamental questions:

- What is a community?
- How does a community regulate and control wildlife use?
- How does the State benefit?

To answer these questions, the Ghanaians are experimenting with what they call Community Resource Management Areas or CREMA's.

WHAT IS A COMMUNITY?

The first point is that there is no set definition of what constitutes a community. The community in this Ghanaian case is a functional arrangement between individuals or groups of individuals often linked through extended families. The traditional authority structure may serve as a focus for the linkage, but the greater strength comes from daily interactions between people living in close proximity to each other and dependent on each other for various needs. The CREMA program recognized that the community is internally defined and that external preconceptions of community structure rarely fit local realities. To define the community, the CREMA looked at how people make simple decisions or resolve conflicts. In doing this it was found that there were several layers of decision-making depending on the importance of the issue and the number of people involved.

HOW DOES A COMMUNITY REGULATE AND CONTROL WILDLIFE?

Currently communities do not regulate or control the use of wildlife, as there is no incentive for them to do so. However, this does not mean that they do not have the mechanisms to control or regulate wildlife use. In Ghana, farm produce is regularly traded at weekly local markets. There are several instances where communities establish their own rules regarding the supply of produce that may be sold in the market place to ensure that the market is not over supplied and prices are maintained. The community develops the control mechanisim because there is an incentive to maintain a price that matches input costs and effort. These same mechanisms can be employed to the production and use of wildlife as long as the same incentive can be given to wildlife as a product.

The CREMA approach in Ghana builds on this by developing a production and marketing agreement based on the community decision-making process. This agreement is the CREMA constitution, and it clearly states the rules and conditions under which wildlife may be used and traded in the market. It defines access rights and the means by which the community will enforce conformity to the rules that it makes.

HOW DOES THE STATE BENEFIT?

For the state, the costs of conservation are high, especially if areas outside of protected areas are included. The CREMA program in Ghana was initiated because of a need to secure the boundaries of a protected area. By devolving authority for wildlife management to neighboring communities and creating an incentive for conservation, the state is able to:

- increase the level of protection of the protected area through the creation of a reciprocal relationships with neighboring communities; and

- provide the opportunity to formalize and develop a sustainable bushmeat market that is currently worth over 200 million dollars.

ESTABLISHING THE PRINCIPLES

In developing the CREMA program in Ghana, one of the foundations was developing a set of guiding principles. These principles were then incorporated into a draft policy for the management of wildlife outside of protected areas. The principles were based on principles earlier defined in southern Africa but adapted to Ghanaian conditions. They are critical and show the level of commitment being made by the Ghanaian government:

(1) Effective management of wildlife is best achieved by giving it focused value for those who live with it.

(2) Those who live with and bear the cost of wildlife must be the primary beneficiaries of its management.

(3) The control of access and benefit from wildlife, whether by the individual or collectively, must be determined by those who live with the resource.

(4) Wildlife should be recognized in its own right as an integral and viable component of national land use policy.

(5) Wildlife is a unique natural resource offering various opportunities for sustainable rural development and economic utilization.

(6) To create the incentive for sustainable wildlife management at the community level, the authority to manage and benefit from wildlife must be devolved to an appropriate representative community institution.

(7) The role of traditional authorities, traditional knowledge and other cultural aspects in wildlife management must be recognized and encouraged. Such appropriate traditional institutions, knowledge and forms of management should be enhanced and incorporated into national strategies and wildlife management techniques.

(8) The role of women is central to achieving sustainable wildlife use. Women must be integrated into the development and implementation of wildlife management programs at all levels.

(9) The role of the Wildlife Division as the national authority for wildlife must be recognized, and it must be accepted that in certain cases it may control levels or modes of use even where authority is devolved, if it is in the national interest to do so.

CONCLUSION

For Mr. Yankey, his dilemma may not yet be over. But his community now has a government that is willing to listen, the community has now established a constitution, defined its rules and regulations, and demarcated its boundaries. For him, the opportunity to incorporate wildlife into his farming practices and benefit from the resources of the forest as his brothers benefit from the resources of the sea is near.

Multiple Species Production Systems

Reversing Underdevelopment and Nonsustainability in Latin America

MARCELA UHART[a,b] AND FERNANDO MILANO[b]

[a]Field Veterinary Program, Wildlife Conservation Society, , Buenos Aires, Argentina

[b]Area Recursos Naturales y Sustentabilidad, Facultad de Ciencias Veterinarias, Universidad Nacional del Centro, Tandil, Argentina

ABSTRACT: Latin America (LA) is suffering the environmental consequences of worldwide increased productivity and agricultural expansion as well as strong economic restrictions. To survive, LA landowners must turn to higher income products and/or increase productivity. Alternatives are few. But while intensification relies on unaffordable and nonsustainable subsidies, diversification is solely dependent on improved management of available resources. Diversified, multiple-species production systems (MSPS) add wildlife use to traditional production systems, promoting economic and ecological stability. We present examples of MSPS in Latin America. Although results are technically encouraging, their future sustainability is threatened by: i) local subvaluation of wildlife and ii) restricted international markets.

KEYWORDS: multiple-species production systems; sustainability; wildlife use; Latin America; development

INTRODUCTION

During the last century, humans have increased productivity per unit area worldwide, and agriculture has significantly expanded. This change has been at the expense of biodiversity and ecological stability, the addition of energy subsidies, important nutrient losses, and high levels of contamination. Latin America has followed the same trend, but in contrast to more developed countries, it has also suffered from external debt and unfavorable terms of trade and protectionism. Thus, environmental degradation and poverty become both cause and effect, in a dreadful cycle.

To counteract this situation, Latin American landowners are forced to turn to higher income products and/or, once again, increase production scale. However, intensification relies on input technologies that result in further ecosystem degradation and economic, agrochemical, and climatic dependence. An alternative is to increase productivity by means of "processes technologies," based on systems management

Address for correspondence: Dr. Marcela Uhart, Field Veterinary Program, Wildlife Conservation Society, 14 de julio 430, (7000) Tandil, Buenos Aires, Argentina.
muhart@satlink.com

Ann. N.Y. Acad. Sci. 969: 20–23 (2002). © 2002 New York Academy of Sciences.

and diversification of production using natural resources. Diversified production systems or "multiple-species production systems" (MSPS) include the combined use of grasslands, livestock, wildlife, fisheries and forests.[1] Productive activities may be consumptive (i.e., commercialization of products) or nonconsumptive (i.e., tourism). Considering the biodiversity richness upon which they depend and the broad range of goods and services they can provide, these systems promote economic and ecological stability, two qualities that make them models for sustainable use on private lands.[2] Further development of these systems should prioritize analysis of dietary overlap and disease transmission between species included in the model.

In Latin America, some MSPS have become well established: caiman and capybara in Venezuela, vicuña in Peru, green iguanas in Panama, and peccaries in Brazil, to mention just a few.[3] Ecotourism is also growing, and several ranchers are offering tourist services for wildlife watching.

MULTIPLE SPECIES PRODUCTION SYSTEMS: EXAMPLES IN ARGENTINA

The main ecoregions in Argentina are currently under heavy productivity pressure. MSPS alternatives are discussed for the Pampas, Patagonia, and the Chaco.

In the Pampas grasslands, areas with low agricultural potential are used for cattle production based on native vegetation and pastures. In this environment, wild rhea or American ostrich (*Rhea americana*) appear as potential alternatives to increase productivity. Their feathers and skins have been historically commercialized in local and foreign markets and their meat could soon be added. Rhea are unable to jump over cattle fences and become tame with appropriate handling. Their diet is complementary to that of cattle (overlap near 50–60%), which further encourages rhea and cattle combined grazing systems.

The Patagonia Steppe is an arid and semiarid plain, covered by shrubs and grasses. It has been severely eroded by large numbers of sheep introduced in the late 19th century for wool and meat production. Guanaco (*Lama guanicoe*) are native camelids traditionally regarded by landowners as a source of disease and food competition with sheep. However, as a result of high prices for their wool ($100/kg), considered similar to vicuña wool, they are beginning to be considered as resources. Experimental, semicaptive breeding programs based on wild-captured newborns, which are tamed by continuous human contact and supplemental feeding, are being implemented for the use of this species. Traditional sheep fencing has to be modified, adding significantly to start-up costs. Darwin's rhea (*Pterocnemia pennata*) is also managed for MSPS in Patagonia.

The Chaco is a vast plain extending over Bolivia, Paraguay, Brazil, and Argentina, which is covered by grasslands, tropical dry forests, and extensive wetlands. It is home for the two caiman species found in Argentina, *Caiman yacare* and *C. latirostris*. Caiman "ranching" is starting at five farms in Argentina based on the harvest of wild caiman nests and the captive-breeding of juveniles. Considering the current low demand for their skins (which has fallen from 10 million to one million in the last 50 years) and low international prices, initial infrastructure costs appear as limiting factors for this alternative. MSPS in the Chaco also include the use of tegu lizards (*Tupinambis* sp.) and the capybara (*Hydrochaerus hidrochaeris*) with good results.

A different MSPS for the Chaco is based on the harvest of blue-fronted Amazon parrots (*Amazona aestiva*) for the "pet" market. A recently established governmental MSPS includes the creation of protected areas with funds collected from parrot sales, education against systematic destruction of nest-trees, and harvest control. This project actively involves local aboriginal communities, whose income is increased ten-fold by eliminating middlemen in the parrot commercialization process.

DISCUSSION

Many Latin Americans are descendants of European immigrants, who have adopted cattle, pork, and poultry as dietary protein sources. Inherited European farming practices did not consider the use of native species as alternatives to livestock production. Instead, wildlife was perceived as a problem for animal farming and agriculture. These cultural concepts lead to a general disregard for wildlife as valuable and useful resources, low demand for their products, and lack of active conservation initiatives. For the rest of the world, the perception of wildlife has changed significantly in the last century: wildlife has been hunted for food, considered defenseless against human environmental impact, assigned "animal rights," and recently regarded as valuable "resources" that can and must be used for the survival of humanity. This diversity of concepts has affected wildlife-product markets and still divides modern consumer society. Thus, it is urgent to build public awareness about the ecological importance and productive aspects of wildlife.[4]

In addition, most wildlife use initiatives are based on intensive and semi-intensive management. While these might be efficient in terms of productivity, they do not support basic sustainability concepts: a) they have limited impact on habitat conservation, b) they disregard intrinsic species advantages and depend on external input, and c) they increase the risk of disease transmission. Health concerns in MSPS must be addressed. Systems which combine wildlife use with traditional livestock would benefit from the selection of zoologically distant species to reduce disease transmission risks.

To sustain international and local market prices and consequent high profitability, wildlife production must be managed. However, this is easier said than done. A careful balance between quantities, qualities, prices, and demand for the natural goods produced is needed to ensure the sustainability and conservation of resources.

CONCLUSION

MSPS represent excellent options to traditional animal production systems. Nevertheless, the combination of limited foreign markets and low local demand for nontraditional products hinders their development. As a result, when production is increased to compensate for low profits, a new fall in prices occurs. Development of sustainable alternatives can only succeed if higher prices compensate for lower productivity. To meet this objective, a radical change must take place in world policies for food production. We need to work toward the creation of a new "consumer" profile that assigns a higher inherent (and thus economic) value to nature. Latin America can still provide high quality goods from untouched environments, generating additional revenue from its natural beauties or from organic products. Based on our natural riches we can still change our trademark from "underdeveloped" to "sustainably developed."

REFERENCES

1. BUCHER, E.H. 1989. Conservación y desarrollo en el neotrópico: en búsqueda de alternativas. Vida Silvestre Neotrop. **2** (1): 3–6.
2. LUXMORE, R. & T.M. SWANSON. 1992. Wildlife and wildland utilization and conservation. *In* Economics for the Wilds: Wildlife, Wildlands, Diversity and Development. T.M. Swanson & E.B. Barbier, Eds.: 171–194. Earthscan Publications, Ltd. London.
3. ROBINSON, J.G. & K.H. REDFORD, Eds. 1991. Neotropical wildlife use and conservation. University of Chicago Press. Chicago, IL, 520 pp.
4. CHARDONNET, PH., B. DES CLERS, J. FISCHER, *et al.* 2002. The value of wildlife. Rev. Sci. Tech. Off. Epizoot. **21** (1): 15–51.

Wildlife and Pastoral Society—Shifting Paradigms in Disease Control

RICHARD KOCK, BIDJEH KEBKIBA, RISTO HEINONEN, AND BERHANU BEDANE

Epidemiology Unit, OAU IBAR – PACE, Nairobi, Kenya

ABSTRACT: The dramatic changes in the human and animal populations in Africa over the last century demand the re-examination of priorities and policies. The introduction of developed medical and other human technologies into the continent has contributed to increases in population and a rapid, unsustainable increase in the utilization of resources. This in turn has led to the destruction of flora and fauna on an unprecedented scale with little real improvement in the human condition. One factor in this has been the increase in livestock in line with human demographic growth, as it is a traditional livelihood of many African peoples. In recent years the growth in livestock populations has slowed owing to a cycle of degradation and disease, affecting especially traditional pastoral systems with a close physical association between people, livestock, and wild animals. Pathogens benefit hugely from the dynamic state created by animal migration, although to some extent the livestock and certainly wildlife show considerable tolerance to this. One of the grave economic consequences of this increase in disease has been collapse of the export trade. In order for Africa to fully benefit and share in world trade, the zoosanitary situation must show improvement. To do this without destroying the natural resource base and traditional pastoral systems, will require a careful, future-oriented land-use policy along ecologically sound criteria. Export livestock will have to be maintained in areas, probably free of ruminant wildlife, with strict veterinary controls. If this can be balanced with sufficient areas retained for traditional pastoralism and wildlife, with perhaps the main income from recreational tourism and local consumption, the benefits will be considerable. The answer may be community-based, low-cost, decentralized health systems for pastoral communities, with less stringent sanitary mandates, a private/parastatal sector servicing, with specialization in wildlife, dairy or export livestock and a central veterinary policy, related to surveillance and monitoring using small well-resourced professional teams to carry out regulatory and statutory duties.

KEYWORDS: pastoral societies; wildlife; Africa; disease transmission

INTRODUCTION

The dramatic changes in the human and animal populations of Africa over the last century demand the re-examination of priorities and policies set for animal health during pre-independence times and still adhered to in many government depart-

Address for correspondence: Dr. Richard Kock, OAU IBAR Pan African Programme for the Control of Epizootic Diseases, P.O. Box 30786, Nairobi, Kenya. Voice: 254-2-318086; fax: 254-2-226565.

richard.kock@OAU-IBAR.org

Ann. N.Y. Acad. Sci. 969: 24–33 (2002). © 2002 New York Academy of Sciences.

ments. The historical background to this started with the rapid introduction of medical and other human technologies into the continent over the last century and disruption of the social and political systems through colonization. This contributed to a burgeoning of population and a rapid, unsustainable increase in the utilization of resources and degradation of land in many areas, with an estimated 73% of the agricultural dry lands on the continent now affected.[1–3] For Africa, where >65% of the population are involved in agriculture (some 70 million dependent on livestock) this is a critical issue. It was fashionable to blame livestock for this cycle of land degradation, but research shows it is a complex issue and livestock-associated degradation is only relevant to wetter ecosystems. Most pastoralists occupy arid lands, or so-called non-equilibrium environments, and the traditional livestock systems of the past had little impact on rangeland resources or the environment.[4] The problem more recently is associated with changes in land use in arid zones, which includes the settlement of pastoralists and excessive use of key resource areas.[5]

The rapid withdrawal of the colonial powers in the 1960's, left behind weak political and socio-economic structures, which could not cope well with the demands of the growing communities. This in turn contributed to the economic ills and the destruction of wild ruminants on an unprecedented scale,[6] with little real improvement in the human condition during the latter years.[7] This is a key difference from the development history of the Northern hemisphere.

LIVESTOCK AND WILDLIFE TRENDS

In Africa there was an increase in livestock in line with human demographic growth, as it is a traditional livelihood of many African peoples and meat is a preferred source of protein,[8] but it was insufficient at ~1–2% per annum to cater for the growing population (see FIG. 1).

The growth in livestock populations has slowed over recent years as available grazing resources have been exceeded and many livestock populations are at best stable or even decreasing. As a result, Africa is now a net importer of livestock and livestock products spending up to three times, what it earns (US$900 million in 1998) from livestock exports.[9] In order for the developing nations of Africa to halt this trend and achieve poverty alleviation and food security, there will need to be increased consumption of indigenous livestock, commercial production, and *de facto* there will need to be much greater attention given to livestock productivity and health, including post-harvest processing and marketing.[8]

The trend in wildlife populations (except in southern Africa) is downwards. The causes are related to human activity and the demand for land and meat. Few accurate figures are available, but for instance in Kenya between 1974 and 1996 wildlife in range lands declined by 33% whilst livestock declined by only 10%.[10] In Uganda the decline over the similar period was 73% of all large mammal biomass including four species extinctions (Lamprey, personal communication).

Since the greatest diversity of grazing ruminants evolved in Africa, it is common sense that it is a good environment for livestock. This idea is supported by the diverse pastoral societies, which evolved over the millennia on the continent. With this ecological background and the increasingly liberal global trade policies towards Africa, some negotiated as long ago as 1986 (Uruguay Round Agricultural Agreement,

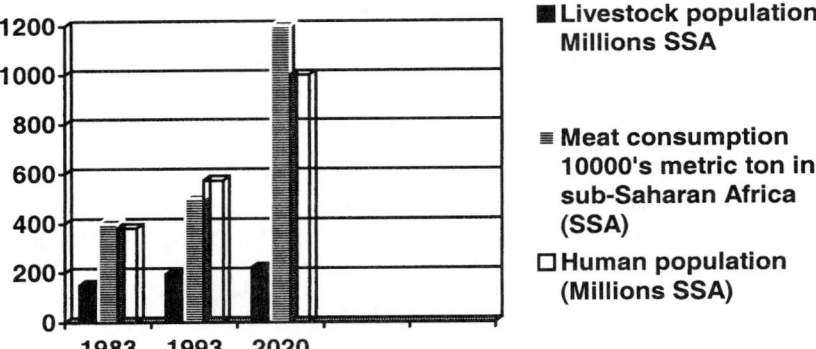

FIGURE 1. Livestock population, meat consumption, and human population in sub-Saharan Africa; data are from Delgado *et al.*[8]

UR), Africa should capitalize on its potential. The major block on this is Africa's failure to fulfill the sanitary measures negotiated at the time.

The impact of livestock economics is also subtle in seemingly remote rural areas, where natural resources are still available. Here the deficit in, and high cost of, meat has been compensated for by the availability of bush meat (Tanzania's wildlife meat "production" was worth US$30 million in 1988[11]) but this is unsustainable. The collapse of large wild mammal populations has already occurred in many African countries or is imminent. The lost economic potential through tourism is huge and the ecological consequences will be dramatic with, for example, the loss of seed dispersal mechanisms and bush encroachment.

DISEASE TRENDS

The changing ecological conditions are also leading to more fertile ground for disease, affecting especially pastoral systems where there is a close physical association between people, livestock and wild animals. Viral and other pathogens benefit hugely from the dynamic state created by animal migration,[12] and the increasing pressure on scarce resources from all human and animal populations with more frequent contact improves the opportunity for disease transmission. The recent incursion of rinderpest virus into Kenyan wildlife populations, associated with cattle in the Somali pastoral ecosystem, is an example of this.[13] It is worth noting here that in Somalia over 50% of the population are pastoralists,[14] and it is therefore not surprising that this should be one of the last reservoirs of a disease that Africans, with assistance from the international community, have been trying to eradicate for over a century.

To some extent the local breeds of livestock and wildlife show tolerance to many pathogens (e.g, blood parasites, foot-and-mouth disease (FMD), African swine fever (ASF)) but unfortunately, the economic consequence of poor zoosanitary conditions has been the collapse of the export trade, especially to the lucrative markets of Europe and the Middle East. The recent cessation in trade from the horn of Africa to Saudi Arabia and the Gulf as a result of the spread of Rift Valley fever are contemporary examples of this problem. For countries like Somalia and Ethiopia the effects on the local economy, which is almost exclusively dependent on livestock, is dire.

THE DECLINE OF VETERINARY INFRASTRUCTURE IN AFRICA

In many African countries the zoosanitary situation is worsening, with a virtual collapse of the state veterinary services established before independence. This is demonstrated by the steady spread of contagious bovine pleuropneumonia (CBPP) through the continent. Despite this situation, governments continue to follow entrenched policies of disease control within national borders, which are clearly not succeeding, based on a high staffing level (salaries consuming up to 90% of the recurrent budget) and without effective operating budgets.[28] This means that personnel are static and unmotivated, carrying out few field investigations and submitting unsubstantiated and unrepresentative reports on disease incidence, which ultimately provide the sanitary trade authority (OIE) with a false impression of the status. There is, in general, a lack of confidence from trade organizations in the ability of many African countries to achieve a sanitary mandate, hence the trade restrictions persist.

To be fair, with the complex cross-border ecosystem dynamics, transhumance, and inability to implement sanitary regulations owing to political and economic constraints, it is not surprising that the present systems are not working.

One specific reason for the decline in services is that public investment in the livestock sector has decreased significantly over recent years in absolute and relative terms. Investment was measured in Cameroon, Ethiopia, Kenya, Mali, Tanzania, and Uganda through examination of gross domestic product (GDP). The input from livestock was >5% of the total GDP compared to the expenditure on livestock production as a proportion of GDP at <3%. If the livestock proportion is broken down, the animal health service delivery component is extremely low at <3% of livestock GDP in all countries and as low as 0.5% in some (see FIG. 2).[27]

This decrease in funding is partly due to the increasing demands on the national exchequer from human health programs, education, security and military spending, urban infrastructure, and rural development, but perhaps also due to a perceived failure of the outdated veterinary policies to bear fruit. This is a mistake given the analyses in some countries such as Kenya, where public investments in animal health and services (PAHE) have been shown to play a statistically significant role in increasing livestock production.[15] With erratic funding however, these gains cannot be sustained.

Politics plays a major role in public investment and another explanation for the decline in funding the livestock sector is that the main lobby group, the backbone of which is the pastoral community, has been increasingly marginalized—socially and politically—in most African countries.[4]

A JUSTIFICATION FOR VETERINARY SERVICES

It is clear that in order for more countries in Africa to achieve food security with an increasing demand for meat and livestock products and fully benefit and share in the world trade in livestock, the zoosanitary situation must show improvement. Unless the demands of the wealthier nations for disease free animals and sanitary "safe" products

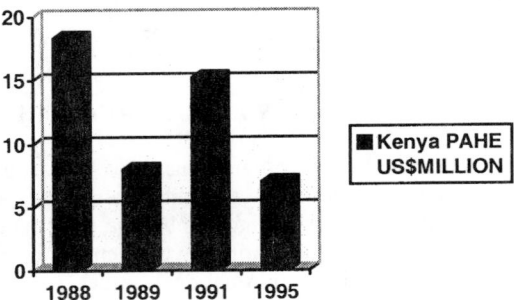

FIGURE 2. Public investments in animal health and services (PAHE) in Kenya; data from Thambi & Maina.[27]

are relaxed, which is unlikely in the short term given the massive investment by the private and public sector in protecting their industries, the situation will deteriorate.

To achieve the sanitary mandate will require an efficient and effective veterinary service in the broadest sense, combining public, private and community based human resources, with realistic goals and appropriate funding.

CONFLICTS—WILDLIFE CONSERVATION AND PASTORALISM

What is relatively new in this socio-agro-political debate amongst Africans is the realization that the wildlife resource is part of the overall equation. African wildlife has been a food and material resource for Africans for millennia, and this continues in many parts, supplementing the diet and providing a safety net at times of drought or conflict, but its commercial potential has only been realized by a few. Wildlife has contributed significantly to African GDP (the sector is worth US$7 billion and is growing at 5% per annum), mainly in East and Southern African countries through consumptive and non-consumptive tourism with up to 30% of the foreign exchange earnings derived from this sector in Kenya.[16] However, much of this activity has been promoted and until recently controlled by Africans of European origin and expatriates with necessary high-level political support (usually with a vested interest).[17] The money has come from donors, foreign investors and some wealthy Africans.

In Kenya, wildlife outside of protected areas (privately and publicly funded) is declining at a rate of 3–4% per annum whilst livestock is only increasing at 0.6% per annum,[18] so it is a net loss of resource. In any case the wildlife is only surviving where it is not competing directly for the land—and this is usually in pastoral systems—but even here with the increase in availability of automatic weapons, the populations have declined precipitously in most areas.

In pastoral systems in eastern Africa, the major disease concerns vary with the climate, habitat, etc. and include CBPP, contagious caprine pleuropneumonia (CCPP), *Rift Valley fever (RVF)*, bluetongue, lumpy skin disease (LSD) malignant catarrhal fever (MCF), *mange, diarrhea (rinderpest where it still exists)*, lameness (e.g., *FMD*), *helminths, orf/pox*, PPR, enterotoxemia, *tick borne disease* (e.g., *East*

Coast fever, ECF), *trypanosomosis*, mastitis, *anthrax*, black quarter, brucellosis, *ringworm*, and *ecto-parasites*.[19–21] Many diseases (italics) involve wildlife epidemiologically, but in reality there are only a few species (e.g., buffalo, *Syncerus caffer,* wildebeest, *Connochaetes taurinus),* which contribute significantly to the important epidemics affecting livestock. Wild pigs in East Africa are important in ASF, but their role is not well documented in the West African region where the recent panzootic problem is one of free-ranging domestic pigs. The diseases of major concern to livestock trade presently are CBPP, CCPP, ASF, FMD, RVF, rinderpest, and peste des petites ruminants (PPR).

THE CHANGING PARADIGM IN DISEASE CONTROL

With improving trade conditions and efficiencies in the transport of animals and animal products (global trade), there is an even greater need for new sanitary mandates to prevent disease transfer than hitherto. The recent outbreak of FMD in the United Kingdom at a cost estimated at >7 billion US$ with a "modern" relatively well-resourced veterinary service is evidence of the need to adapt to changing epidemiological conditions.

To achieve an improved health status without destroying the natural resource base and traditional pastoral systems in doing this, will require a careful future oriented land use policy. Given the socio-economic and political situation in Africa, the only realistic option is zoning of land along ecologically sound criteria. Export livestock will have to be maintained in designated areas, probably free from ruminant wildlife and pastoral livestock, with strict veterinary controls. This to some extent has been the policy of countries, which are exporting products to lucrative markets (Botswana/South Africa/Zimbabwe). If this can be balanced with sufficient areas retained for traditional pastoralism including protected areas for wildlife, the benefits will be considerable. The main income for the pastoral sector coming from improved marketing (for local consumption) of livestock meat and products, as well as from wildlife recreational tourism.

The animal health delivery system to support such a land use should be three tiered.

(1) a community based, low-cost, decentralized system for pastoral and remote communities, with less stringent sanitary mandates for local markets applied, with a focus on improving productivity and reducing epidemic and zoonotic health risks;

(2) a private/parastatal sector servicing specialized entities, e.g., wildlife, dairy and export livestock, laboratories with a strict sanitary mandate; and

(3) a central government veterinary service specializing in policy formulation, epidemio-surveillance and monitoring as well as carrying out disease control, regulatory, and statutory duties with small well-resourced professional teams.

In order to make an impact, policy makers need to be realistic and promote these changes **now** for the future. It may take 50 years to achieve, but if professionals and policy makers continue to delay action, the hopes for poverty alleviation by 2015 in Africa often quoted by the donor community are nothing but a pipedream.

PROMOTING THE CHANGE

These ideas are not new, and many organizations and countries in Africa—Organisation African Unity, Inter African Bureau Animal Resources (OAU IBAR), Pan African Rinderpest Campaign (PARC), Pan African programme for the Control of Epizootics (PACE), Community based Animal Health and Participatory Epidemiology (CAPE)—have been active, but there is still the need to seek dialogue with policy makers, professionals and communities to seek solutions.

In the field of Community-based initiatives there have been some notable successes and the OAU IBAR is promoting this approach throughout the continent.[23] It is lamentable that the developed world has invested so much in the veterinary profession in Africa, through support to veterinary institutions such as Universities and Veterinary departments, without addressing the real need at the community level. Veterinarians have been trained to a high level in sciences that have little application to provide a service that is not required, and not surprisingly the levels of unemployment amongst vets is extremely high.

In the field of privatization there has been progress, but as with community-based initiatives there has been reluctance from the government sector to devolve responsibility and, inevitably, jobs in this way. The reluctance is also understandable in countries where livestock value and pet ownership are minimal. The economics for veterinary practice simply do not add up.

In contrast, the involvement of veterinarians in the wildlife sector has increased, and the realization of their role is increasing amongst Veterinary and Wildlife Management Authorities.

In order to improve and quantify knowledge of wildlife livestock interactions in pastoral lands in relation to disease, there have been attempts to develop models.[24,25] These approaches suffer from being perhaps over-ambitious and are lacking in resources for obtaining sufficient data to make the model accurate for a representative number of ecosystems. One zone that has attracted considerable interest for modelling owing to the relative abundance of data for the area is the Greater Serengeti system. It has the disadvantage of being a somewhat unusual, highly politicized zone, and its relevance as a model for much of the sub-Saharan system is questionable.

Perhaps the main reason for the decline in environmental health in general and veterinary services in particular, is a lack of policy integration and some misunderstanding between different stakeholders.

- *Conservationists and environmentalists* blame people and livestock for the decline in biodiversity and land degradation.
- *Livestock keepers* (pastoralists) blame government for reducing their available resource for survival and for not providing a veterinary service. They blame wildlife for spreading and maintaining disease without often understanding the epidemiology.
- *Veterinary authorities* blame the wildlife for acting as disease reservoirs and the pastoralists for not following disease control regulations, particularly relating to animal movement. They argue that wildlife and people who ignore government laws and regulations are the reason for the poor zoosanitary conditions.
- *Donors and the international communities* blame the governments and seek quick fashionable solutions, through private sector and NGOs, which change all too frequently.

- *Different Government Ministries* often act in conflict at a policy level and frequently change policy direction according to prevailing political conditions.

It is a complex politically charged debate, which needs to be brought to all levels with a clear understanding of the issues, facts, and needs. Perhaps the communication revolution will facilitate improved understanding in this regard.

There is no doubt room for compromise, but this will not be a simple process to achieve. On the issue of land use, which is central to the change, zoning is clearly possible if the people and government have the political will. African Nations as a continental community will need to decide where they wish to go. If there cannot be agreement on a regional basis taking into consideration ecosystems as opposed to national borders, disease control will not be achievable. There are difficult questions to answer:

- How much land for conservation is necessary to sustain the environment and biodiversity?
- How much land is required for agriculture?
- How much land is required to sustain pastoralism?

These issues are debated at high levels and in academic circles: there is rarely dialogue with the local communities. If pastoralism is to survive and develop in a modern socio-economic sense, it will mean that at the very least, some areas of higher agricultural productivity and wildlife use areas will need to be accessed by pastoralists.[26] On top of this, the young pastoralists will not be satisfied with the marginal life of their fathers and mothers. There is evidence for this everywhere in Africa, with migration from the rural areas to cities and trends from pastoral to agro-pastoral systems, but often without the appropriate land being made available; the result has been conflict, degradation of land, increasing urban squalor, and loss of livelihoods. There has to be economic empowerment of communities if this trend is to be slowed down.

In return the pastoral societies will have to contribute more actively to the custodianship of the land (where conservation is a priority) and contribute economically especially for the use of higher potential land. The notion that pastoral people have actively conserved natural resources for the benefit of all is also something of a myth. The balance between these communities and the environment, wildlife, etc. was an evolutionary process, over millennia. It was essentially a passive relationship with each species exploiting resources as the need arose. The dominance that humans achieved in relatively recent times has upset this balance.

The actions of communities will have to change to reduce the negative impact of human dominance over the environment. This change could be expressed though actions of the individual and through the politics and actions of the nation state. Perhaps there are other alternatives, but the present status quo will only lead to extinction of these societies, loss of livelihoods, or their assimilation into more dominant ethnic groups, as has happened to most hunter-gatherer societies in Africa.

CONCLUSION

In countries with a substantial wildlife–livestock interface within pastoral systems, zoosanitary conditions cannot be improved without a better understanding of the epidemiology and closer collaboration between the livestock and wildlife sectors. This is important to reduce conflict of interest, and it is particularly pertinent in the health sector. Perhaps the single most important reason for the decline in environmental health in general and veterinary services in particular is a lack of policy integration and some misunderstanding between different stakeholders (conservationists and environmentalists, livestock keepers, e.g., pastoralists, veterinary authorities, donors, and the international agencies and government ministries).

The animal health delivery system to support the mixed land use so prevalent in sub-Saharan Africa should be three tiered and should include (1) a community-based, low-cost, de-centralized system for pastoral and remote communities, (2) a private/parastatal sector servicing specialized entities, e.g., wildlife, and (3) a central government veterinary service specializing in policy formulation, regulatory and statutory duties with small well-resourced professional teams for epidemio-surveillance and disease control.

With some diseases (e.g., FMD) without radical measures such as fencing and major disturbance to the habitat and environment, there is little or no possibility of eradication of a pathogen, and it is only through endemic stability that "control" is achieved. It should be recognized that there are limits to the ability of the very best health delivery system with infinite resources to achieve sanitary conditions given specific epidemiological conditions; this fact is critical to the policy development and implementation of sanitary mandates in Africa.

REFERENCES

1. FAO. 1997. Report of the World Food Summit, Part 1: 13–17. FAO Publications. Rome.
2. THRUPP, L.A. 1998. Critical Links: Food Security and the Environment in the Greater Horn of Africa. Background Paper—Stakeholders Analysis and Dialogue. World Resources Institute and IUCN East Africa Office, Nairobi Kenya.
3. IUCN. 1986. A long term strategy for environmental rehabilitation. IUCN. Gland, Switzerland.
4. SCOONES. I., Ed. 1994. Living with Uncertainty. Intermediate Technology. London.
5. ROTH, E.A. 1996. Traditional pastoral strategies in a modern world: an example from northern Kenya. Human Org. 55 (No.2): 219–224.
6. IUCN. 1999. African Antelope Database. Rod East, Ed. IUCN/SSC. Gland, Switzerland and Cambridge.
7. Le Monde. 1997. Bilan Economique et social 1996. 22e annee. Paris.
8. DELGADO, C., M. ROSEGRANT, H. STEINFELD, et al. 1999. Livestock 2020: the next food revolution. In 2020 Vision. Brief 61, International Food Policy Research Institute June, 1999.
9. THAMBI, E.N., O.W. MAINA & R. BESSIN. 2001a. Animal and animal products trade in Africa: new development perspectives in international trade for Africa. OAU IBAR. Nairobi, Kenya.
10. ODI. 1999. Can Livestock and Wildlife Co-exist? An Interdisciplinary Approach. D. Bourn & R. Blench, Eds.: 58. ODI. Portland House, Stag Place, London SW1E 5DP.
11. CHARDONNET, P. 1995. Faune Sauvage Africaine La Ressource Oubliee. Vols. 1 & 2. CECA-CE-CEEA. Bruxelles, Belgium.
12. MACPHERSON, C.N.L. 1995. The effect of transhumance on the epidemiology of animal diseases. Prev. Vet. Med. 25(2): 213–224.
13. KOCK, R.A., J.M. WAMBUA, J. MWANZIA, et al. 1999. Rinderpest epidemic in wild ruminants in Kenya 1993–7. Vet. Rec. 145: 275–283.

14. IUCN, Somalia. 1997. I. Cuthbert Preliminary Institutional Stakeholder Analysis: Key Institutions and Programs in the Food Security-Environment Management Nexus Somalia Report–IUCN.
15. THAMBI, E.N., O.W. MAINA & T.F. RANDOLPH. 2001b. An analysis of the impact of public animal health expenditures on the performance of the livestock sub-sector in Kenya. OAU IBAR. Nairobi, Kenya.
16. PDG. 1997. The Costs of Environment Degradation to the Kenyan Economy. Policy Development Group. Nairobi, Kenya.
17. IIED. 1994. Whose Eden? An Overview of Community Approaches to Wildlife Management. International Institute for Environment and Development. London.
18. BARROW, E. 1996. Development and Conservation in Pastoral Areas: A Conflicting Interest or an Unrecognised Partnership. Proceedings of the Kenya Pastoralist Forum Meeting. 1st Topic Meeting Wildlife and Pastoralist's Utilisation and Conservation Rights and Privileges. Ufungamano House, Nairobi, Kenya, Feb. 8, 1996.
19. KARIUKI, D.P. & W. LETITYA. Livestock Production and Health Challenges in Pastoral Areas. Samburu District, Kenya. Kenya Agricultural Research Institute, P.O. Box 57811, Nairobi, Kenya, p. 7.
20. BENGIS R., R.A. KOCK & J. FISCHER. 2002. The wildlife livestock interface in sub-Saharan Africa. *In* Infectious Diseases of Wildlife. Sci. Tech. Rev. OIE **21** (1): 53–62.
21. THOMSON, G.R. 1999. Alternatives for controlling animal diseases resulting from the interaction between livestock and wildlife in Southern Africa. South African J. Sci. **95**: 71–76.
22. KOCK, M.D., G. MULLINS & J. PERKINS. 2002. Veterinary Disease Control in Botswana: Impacts on Wildlife Health, Ecosystems and Rural Livelihoods. Conservation Medicine; Ecological Health in Practice. Oxford University Press. New York. In press.
23. CATLEY A. & T. LEYLAND. 2001. Community participation and the delivery of veterinary services in Africa. Prev. Vet. Med. **49**: 95–113.
24. COUGHENOUR, M.B. 1992. Spatial modelling and landscape characterisation of an African pastoral ecosystem. *In* Ecological Indicators, Vol. 1. D.E. Hyatt & V.J. Macdonald, Eds.: 787–810. Elsevier Applied Science. London/New York.
25. COUGHENOUR, M.B. 1993. The Savanna Model. Future Harvest PMB 238. 2020 Pennsylvannia Ave., N.W., Washingtond, DC 20006-1846.
26. ALRMP. 1997. ALRMP Study of Land Tenure and Resource Management in Kenya. Research and Training Consultants. P.O. Box 66799, Nairobi, Kenya (Commissioned by Office of the President Department of Relief and Rehabilitation).
27. THAMBI, N.E. & W.O. MAINA. 2000. Financing livestock and animal health services in sub-Saharan Africa: the case of Cameroon, Ethiopia, Kenya, Mali, Tanzania and Uganda. Background Paper, Economics Unit OAU-IBAR PACE, P.O. Box 30786 Nairobi, Kenya.
28. HOWE, R., R. BOONE, J. DEMARTINI, *et al.* A spatially integrated disease risk assessment model for wildlife/livestock interaction in Ngorongoro Conservation Area, Tanzania. In press.

Health Monitoring and Conservation of Wildlife in Sweden and Northern Europe

TORSTEN MÖRNER

Department of Wildlife, National Veterinary Institute, SE-751 89 Uppsala, Sweden

ABSTRACT: Monitoring of wildlife diseases started in Scandinavia as sporadic postmortem examinations in the early 20th century. In 1945 a monitoring program for wildlife health was initiated. The program is today an integrated part of the National Environmental Monitoring programs in Sweden. The total material today comprises more than 80 000 recorded investigations. There are similar programs in Denmark, Finland, and Norway, but no comparable program exists in other Northern European countries. The program has led to discoveries of new diseases in many mammals and birds, and demonstration of several environmental pollutants, such as mercury, lead, and cadmium, in wildlife. The success of the program is due to several factors such as: a rich wildlife with economically important game species; location of the program at the National Veterinary Institute with excellent facilities and competent staff, good cooperation with hunter and conservation organizations, stable financial support, a cool climate, and a successful relationship with media. Current work also includes more focused investigations on different specific pathogens and pollutants, as well as investigations in single animal species.

KEYWORDS: environment; health monitoring; pathology; wildlife diseases; game

BACKGROUND

In the early 20th century knowledge of the disease panorama among wildlife in Scandinavia was limited. A few studies were carried out by individual researchers at different veterinary colleges and laboratories, for example the report by Thötta in 1930 about tularemia in Norway.[1] In 1935 Christiansen published a survey of different infectious wildlife diseases in Denmark.[2]

In Sweden a health-monitoring program for wildlife was started in 1945, sponsored by the Swedish Hunters Association, the Swedish Environmental Protection Agency, and the Swedish Government. The program was lead by Dr. Karl Borg at the National Veterinary Institute (NVI), in those years located in Stockholm. The program was based on investigations on dead animals found in the wild and on monitoring of normal material from different animal species. Swedish hunters initiated the monitoring program with funds originating from the annual hunting fee. The program is today an integrated part of the National Environmental Monitoring Programs

Address for correspondence: Dr. Torsten Mörner, Department of Wildlife, National Veterinary Institute, SE-751 89 Uppsala, Sweden. Voice +46 18 67 42 14; fax +46 18 30 91 62.
Torsten.Morner@sva.se

Ann. N.Y. Acad. Sci. 969: 34–38 (2002). © 2002 New York Academy of Sciences.

in Sweden. On an annual basis 1 000–2 000 animals are investigated and the total material today comprises more than 80 000 recorded investigations.

There are several explanations for why the program has become a natural part of the health-monitoring program in Sweden. Among these are: (1) the economic importance of game and hunting in Sweden, (2) the regulation of hunting with the hunting rights linked to the landownership, (3) the awareness of the public that human and wild animal health are linked, (4) the location of the program to the National Veterinary Institute with excellent facilities and the devotion of a competent staff with an interest in wildlife, (5) the importance of diseases possibly transmissible between wildlife and domestic animals, (6) the potential of zoonoses having wildlife reservoirs, (7) the discovery of the impact of environmental pollutants, such as mercury, lead and cadmium, (8) a good cooperation with hunter and conservation organizations, (9) a stable financial support from government funds, (10) a cool climate allowing material of good quality, and (11) a very successful relationship with media with frequent reports supporting the monitoring program.

Similar programs are today in place in Denmark, Finland, and Norway. Close contact and cooperation is established between the different Scandinavian Wildlife programs with exchange of experience, and also cooperative studies. The different groups in Scandinavia meet on an annual basis. No comparable program exists in other Northern European countries.

HEALTH MONITORING PROGRAM

The health-monitoring program is mainly a "passive" collection and investigation of dead wild animals, submitted to the laboratory by landowners, hunters, or the public. All kinds of wildlife, including both game and protected species, are investigated. Annually around 600–800 mammals, including deer, hares, rodents, carnivores, and others; and 600–800 birds of different species are investigated. The examination is free of charge for the submitter and financed mainly by government funds generated from annual hunting fees. The submitter receives an answer about findings and the cause of death (if possible to determine). The results of the investigation and different collected specimens are also included in monitoring programs for certain microorganisms, parasites, or environmental pollutants.

The "passive" collection of dead animals represents a statistical sample of different diseases and causes of death. The program gives only to a limited extent information about changes in the wildlife populations, since the submission of animals to NVI can depend on several factors and does not always reflect increased mortality.

However, in order to study the impact of diseases on wildlife populations, focused studies are performed at regular intervals.

The cool subarctic climate with relatively short summers with maximum temperatures of 25–30°C and long winters with temperatures below freezing guarantees that most material submitted will be in good condition. Examination of well-preserved carcasses is preferred, and rotten material is rejected, with the exception of forensic cases where illegal hunting is suspected. It is also preferable to examine whole body carcasses, instead of specimens sampled by less experienced pathologists in the field.

DISCOVERIES—DISEASES

A large number of "new" diseases have been discovered during the 50 years the program has been running. Viral infections have included Inclusion Body Hepatitis in Eagle owls (*Bubo bubo*),[3] papilloma virus in moose (*Alces alces*),[4] myxomatosis in rabbits (*Oryctolagus cuniculi*),[5] European Brown Hare Syndrome (EBHS) in hares (*Lepus* spp.)[6] and Rabbit Haemorrhagic Disease in rabbits.[7]

Several diseases caused by bacteria have also been studied. Long before the program started, in 1911, Hülphers reported[8] a newly discovered bacterial species in rabbits, today known as *Listeria monocytogenes*. This bacterium has continuously been isolated from Swedish wildlife.[9,10] Infections with *Francisella tularensis* (tularemia) has also frequently been studied in hares and other species,[11,12] as well as infections caused by *Yersinia pseudotuberculosis*,[9,10] *Mycobacterium bovis* and *M. avium*,[13] and others.

Infections with *Sarcoptes scabiei* in red fox (*Vulpes vulpes*), arctic fox (*Alopex lagopus*), lynx (*Lynx lynx*) and marten (*Martes martes*),[14] and with *Elaphostrongylus* spp. in moose and other deer[15] are the most important parasitic diseases studied.

Management actions are normally not taken in Sweden if disease outbreaks occur in wild populations, with some exceptions. Action can be taken to manage wildlife diseases in cases of zoonoses where wildlife act as a reservoir, or where diseases transmissible between wild and domestic animals are found, for example, bovine tuberculosis in deer, or when diseases threaten endangered populations. An example of this is the discovery of sarcoptic mange among arctic foxes in the North of Sweden, when 23 foxes, approximately 10% of the total Swedish population, were caught and treated for mange since the disease had occurred in one small isolated population.[16]

DISCOVERIES—POLLUTANTS

In the early 1950s, the intoxication of wild birds with mercury, originating from seed-dressing, was discovered as a result of pathological studies in combination with analytical chemistry.[17] Since 1950, further environmental toxicological studies have been in progress at NVI, mainly concentrating on cadmium and lead.[9,10] Several studies have also been performed on organic compounds like phenoxy acids.[18]

COOPERATION WITH LANDOWNERS, HUNTERS, CONSERVATION ORGANIZATIONS AND ANIMAL WELFARE GROUPS

According to the Swedish law, the right of hunting belongs to the landowner or the person/persons renting the hunting rights for the land. Because of this, landowners and hunters are always interested in diseases and causes of death in "their" wildlife. This is true for both game species and protected species. Very close cooperation is therefore maintained with the Swedish Hunting Association (SHA) and its game wardens. SHA has approximately 25 field stations and approximately 75 employees, with several of them being involved in the system of reporting and submitting material to NVI. Cooperation with other conservation organizations like the Swedish Society for Nature Conservation and the Swedish Ornithological Society is also an important factor in the monitoring program's success.

MEDIA

One of the most important collaborators for a successful program is the media, including daily papers, weekly magazines, specialist press, radio, and TV. The attitude of the "health program" is always an open one towards the media. All possible information is provided upon request. Several journalists visit NVI and the postmortem room regularly and are given relevant information about wildlife, wildlife health and pollutants. Only with forensic cases, which are handled under security, is access restricted

THE FUTURE

The wildlife health-monitoring program today is a well-recognized program in the Swedish scientific world as well as among the public, hunters, conservationists, and media. Continued support for this important part of the management and conservation of wildlife and nature in Sweden and Northern Europe is expected.

REFERENCES

1. THJÖTTA, T. 1930. Tularemia och dess forekomst i Norge. Nord. Med. Tidskr. **2:** 177–180. (In Norwegian)
2. CHRISTIANSEN, M. 1935. De vigtigste smittsamme Sydomme hos vilt. Medd. Statens Vet. Serumlab. **157,** 92 pp. (In Danish)
3. BORG, K. 1972. A brief report on virus hepatitis in the eagle owl. Research report from the National Veterinary Institute, Stockholm, 6/1972.
4. MORENO-LOPEZ, J. 1981. Characterization of a papilloma virus from the European elk (EEPV). Virology **112:** 589–595.
5. BORG, K. 1963. Dissemination of myxomatosis by birds. Nord. Vet. Med. **15:** 159–166.
6. GAVIER-WIDÉN, D. 1991. Epidemiology and diagnosis of the European brown hare syndrome in Scandinavian countries: a review. Rev. Sci. Tech. Off. Int. Epizooties **10:** 453–457.
7. GAVIER-WIDÉN, D. 1993. Viral hepatitis of rabbits and hares in Scandinavia. Zoo & Wild Animal Medicine. W.B. Saunders Co. Philadelphia, USA, pp. 322–325.
8. HÜLPHERS, G. 1911. Liver necrosis in rabbit caused by a heretofore not described microorganism. Svensk Vet.Tidskr. **16:** 265–273. (In Swedish)
9. BORG, K. 1975. Viltsjukdomar. LTs förlag, 191 pp. (In Swedish)
10. MÖRNER, T. 1991. Liv och död bland vilda djur. Sellin & Partner. Stockholm, 169 pp. (In Swedish)
11. MÖRNER, T. 1986. The occurrence of tularemia in Sweden. *In* Proceedings from der 28 Internationalen Symposiums uber die Erkrankungen der Zootiere. Rostock, DDR, pp. 327–331.
12. MÖRNER, T. 1992, A review of the ecology of tularaemia, Rev. Sci. Tech. Off. Int. Epizooties **11**(4): 1123–1130.
13. MÖRNER, P.A. 1990. Mycobacterial infections in Swedish Wildlife. [abstract] VIth International Conference on Wildlife Diseases, Berlin, GDR, p. 48.
14. BORNSTEIN, S. 2001. *Sarcoptes scabiei* and sarcoptic mange. Parasitic diseases of wild mammals. Iowa State University Press, Iowa, USA, pp. 107–121.

15. STEEN, M. 1991. Elaphostrongylosis. Ph.D thesis, Swedish University of Agricultural Sciences, Uppsala, Sweden.
16. MÖRNER, T. 1988. Successful treatment of Wild Arctic Foxes (*Alopex lagopus*) infested with *Sarcoptes scabiei* var. *vulpes* [abstract]. 37th WDA Annual Conference, Athens, Georgia, USA, p. 29.
17. BORG, K. 1966. Mercury poisoning in Swedish Wildlife. J. Appl. Ecol. **3:** 171.
18. ERNE, K. 1966. Studies on the animal metabolism of phenoxy acetic herbicides. Acta Vet. Scand. **7:** 264–271.

Relating National Veterinary Services to the Country's Livestock Industry

Case Studies from Four Countries—Great Britain, Botswana, Perú, and Vietnam

ROGER S. WINDSOR

The SB Co, Middlefield House, by Dumfries, DG1 3SF, Scotland

ABSTRACT: At the end of WW II, the British Government of the time decided that it was essential for Britain to become self-sufficient in food. In consequence there was a large investment in services to agriculture and in particular many new veterinary investigation centers were opened to help farmers produce more animal products. The upsurge in world trade led the Government of Mrs. Thatcher to decide that livestock was just another commodity and so there has been a massive scaling down of money available to assist the livestock farmer. For Botswana the livestock industry is vital to the well-being of the people and successive Governments have continued to invest in veterinary services. As a consequence, Botswana has one of the best and most efficient Veterinary Services in Africa. By contrast, the livestock industry in Perú has an insignificant effect on the gross national product. The fiber exports from camelids are a small international market, while the dairy industry is unable to provide sufficient milk for the nation. Partly as a result of this, the Peruvian Government invests very little in the livestock industry or the veterinary services that support it. Vietnam is in a transitional stage: there is a large but as yet unorganized livestock industry with a mass of smallholder farmers. The Government has made a large investment in people in the Department of Animal Health but without a concomitant investment in equipment and training. If the industry is to develop, it will require much more investment from the government. These countries will be discussed in more detail and an attempt will be made to show how by relating the services to the livestock industry, governments can improve services and at the same time cut the costs.

KEYWORDS: veterinary services; government investment; livestock

INTRODUCTION

There are considerable calls on the financial resources of governments of countries: hospitals, schools, roads, defense are obviously of major importance, and as the demand for these grow so the amount of money for other projects is reduced. The past 50 years has seen massive increases in the populations of some countries, and

Address for correspondence: Dr. Roger S. Windsor, The SB Co., Middlefield House, by Dumfries, DG1 3SF, Scotland.
thesbco@aol.com

Ann. N.Y. Acad. Sci. 969: 39–47 (2002). © 2002 New York Academy of Sciences.

TABLE 1. The importance of livestock to the economies of Botswana, Great Britain, Perú, and Vietnam

Country	Size (km^2)	Human population (millions)	Livestock populations	Value of agriculture as % of GDP
Botswana	600,370	1.57	Cattle from 3 to 6 million[a]	4.0%
			Sheep < 1 million	
			Pigs NS	
			Poultry < 1 million	
Great Britain	244,000	59.5	Cattle 15 million	1.7%
			Sheep 40 million	
			Pigs 5 million	
			Poultry > 100 million	
Perú	1,285,216	22.8	Cattle < 1million	13%
			Sheep[b] 1–2 million	
			Pigs < 1 million	
			Poultry 20million	
Vietnam[7]	331,041	78.8	Cattle[c] 7.0 million	26%
			Sheep 500,000	
			Pigs 18.3 million	
			Poultry[d] 168.6 million	

The goat population is included in the figure for sheep.
[a]Cattle population decreases in time of drought.
[b]Sheep population includes 250,000 alpacas and llamas.
[c]Cattle population includes buffalo.
[d]Poultry population includes ducks.
Unless stated this information has been obtained from web-sites dedicated to the different countries.

there have not been concomitant increases in the resources of these countries. As budgets are stretched, governments seek to reduce spending in any way that is politically possible. If the governments of Perú or Vietnam sought to reduce the spending on agricultural services it is not likely that there would be massive public unrest, whereas should the Botswana Government seek to reduce spending on livestock services there would be serious political repercussions. The object of this paper is to demonstrate the importance of livestock to the economy and to relate the involvement of the state to this importance. An attempt is made to illustrate this involvement using as examples the livestock industries of Botswana, Great Britain, Perú, and Vietnam. TABLE 1 shows details of the countries with areas, populations both human and livestock, and the importance of agriculture to the economy.

CASE STUDIES
Great Britain

The outbreak of cattle plague (rinderpest) that was imported into Britain in June 1865, resulted in the setting up of the Veterinary Department of the Privy Council Office: the State Veterinary Service (SVS) has existed in one form or another ever since.[1] After the eradication of cattle plague, attention was turned to other diseases: sheep pox (eradicated 1866), contagious bovine pleuropneumonia (1896), sheep scab (1952, but later reintroduced), classical swine fever (1969, reintroduced 2000 and eradicated in the same year), Newcastle Disease (eradicated 1966 but subsequent reintroductions), glanders (1928), rabies (1902, several subsequent reintroductions), and foot and mouth disease (FMD) (not finally eradicated until 1962, but three subsequent reintroductions, the last, this year). Eradication of the major livestock diseases enabled the British to realize unprecedented gains in productivity.[1]

After WW II, during which there were serious problems in feeding the people because the enemy sank the food supply ships, the government decided that Britain would never again be dependent upon the major foodstuffs being imported and that Britain would become self-sufficient in cereals, root crops, sugar, and animal products (meat, milk and eggs). To achieve this there was a massive investment in agricultural advisory services, veterinary research and investigation laboratories, and veterinary field services.[1]

The emergence of the global market, the marked increase in world free trade, and most of all the election of Mrs. Margaret Thatcher as Prime Minister in Britain brought this to an end. As imports of foodstuffs of animal origin—beef from Argentina and Botswana; pork products, milk, butter, and cheese from various countries in the EU; lamb from New Zealand; and eggs from as far away as China—have flooded the British market, so the relative importance of agriculture in Britain has declined. Today the gross national income from farming is less than the profits of any two of the larger supermarket chains combined. As farming has declined, so rural industries (recreation, including hotels, rural museums, boating, walking, golf courses) have boomed. Today farming produces revenue of £1.2 billion, which is only 10% of that of other rural industries. The current outbreak of FMD has devastated not only the farming communities of many areas of Britain, but by closing these areas to tourism it has also caused massive hardship for the whole rural community. Concomitant with the down-sizing of farming has been an equivalent diminution of services offered by government to farming. The old National Agricultural Advisory Service has been almost completely disbanded, with large sections of it privatized into the hands of the advisers themselves. The Central Veterinary Laboratory at Weybridge has been hived off and made into an Agency, and many state organizations have had to become self-financing. The Veterinary Investigation Service has reduced the number of laboratories from 29 to 13 and there is now a charge for almost every service. The reorganization of the Veterinary Field Service in 1995 slashed the number of senior posts and amalgamated county-based offices into regional based offices;[2] this, of course, was the reason why the State Veterinary Service (SVS) was, at the start, unable to cope with the current outbreak of FMD.

"The number of vets employed full time in the SVS has halved over the past 20 years. ... the number of veterinary surgeons employed by the SVS in 1979 (full time equivalents) was 597. By 1997 the number had fallen to 289 ... . By 2001 there were

286 permanent staff. Of these 286, 220 were field veterinary officers." [2] The savings have been enormous. until now! Where the savings were in millions, the government is now paying out billions of pounds in compensation to farmers and to the people involved in the eradication campaign.

If a country wishes to have high production and sophisticated livestock then it must be prepared to pay the price of disease security. There must be regulatory systems in place to prevent the entrance of exotic disease. There must also be a service that is trained and equipped to respond rapidly to any emergency.

Botswana

Most of Botswana is semi-arid savannah with low rainfall and a fragile vegetation, suitable only for extensive ranching of cattle (1 animal per 20 hectares). Although the Limpopo and Molopo rivers form the boundaries on the east and southeast of the country, respectively, the only river to flow within the country is the Okavango, which breaks up into an inland delta and the water seeps into the Kalahari sands. There is, therefore, no ready source of water for irrigation and hence no arable farming. The population of cattle in Botswana varies enormously depending upon the rainfall, and in times of good rain the cattle numbers can expand up to 7 million. However, in periods of drought animals are slaughtered and the number can fall as low as 3.5 million. In times of drought it can be difficult for Botswana to reach its quota of meat for export to Europe.

The major revenue earner for the country is the mining of diamonds, with some coal and copper mining also bringing in foreign exchange. Although the contribution of the livestock sector to the GNP is not great, almost 80% of the human population has an association of some sort with livestock, and in particular with cattle. While the export of diamonds benefits the state, the export of beef benefits the people. The former President of Botswana, Sir Seretse Khama, stated that "the people cannot eat diamonds" (Falconer, 1980, personal communication). The people therefore have a keen interest in the success of their export sales. Were the exports of beef to cease, the value of cattle would be drastically reduced. There is therefore a great political incentive to keep FMD under control: this requires a well-staffed and efficient veterinary service.

Botswana has an excellent Veterinary Service: the Districts are now all manned by veterinary surgeons who are responsible for the work of trained Livestock Officers and Veterinary Assistants—in this way the Field Services has a presence in almost every village in the country. Despite the size of the country the numbers employed in the Veterinary Department are small—there are less than 40 veterinary surgeons in the country—but because of the investment in training of lay people, who then work under the guidance of veterinary surgeons, the veterinary cover is excellent. In the early 1980s Botswana invested more than $4 million in the construction of a National Veterinary Laboratory, and in 1995 this magnificent building was extended by the addition of new laboratories to examine for residues in meat. The laboratory is well equipped with modern machinery and staffed by laboratory-trained veterinary surgeons and technical/scientific staff. The laboratory serves the Field staff and also the Abattoir staff. The three modern abattoirs of Lobatse, Maun and Francistown are staffed by veterinary surgeons trained in meat inspection and food hygiene and trained meat inspectors working under their direction. All services to farmers, with the exception of drugs, are provided free of charge, although the District Veterinary Officers are allowed to charge for the out-of-hours clinical services that they give. However, the farmers are charged indirectly for their services, as every animal slaughtered in the export abattoirs has to pay a slaughter fee (formerly $25) and this money is used to finance the Veterinary Department. Disease control is important to Government, politicians, and livestock owners. As long as the country continues to export meat and meat products to Western markets, money will be made available for adequate disease control.

That the country is conscious of its disease-free status is evidenced by the outbreak of contagious bovine pleuro-penumonia (CBPP) in 1995. After the disease had been imported from Namibia it spread unchecked for some months in northwest Botswana. By the time that the Veterinary Department diagnosed the disease, it had spread extensively. In order to eradicate the disease 320,000 cattle were slaughtered.[3] With the cost of compensation for slaughtered animals, the cost of control measures, and the socio-economic costs of looking after people who had lost their livelihoods it has been conservatively estimated that the country spent over $200 million (Amanfu 2000, personal communication). This is strong evidence that when the livestock industry is of economic importance a country will heavily invest in its veterinary services.

Perú

The geography of Perú is not conducive to agriculture: the coastal strip along the Pacific Ocean which comprises 5% of the land mass is a complete desert, but it is where 80% of the population (total 23 million) live. The eastern part of the country, comprising 81% of the area, is Amazonian jungle in which live 5% of the population. Between these two lie the Andes (14%), with peaks of almost 7000m and here live 15% of the people. The desert coastal strip is farmed where the rivers come down to the sea and there is water for irrigation. This is used for arable agriculture including, sugar and cotton, and more recently cash crops such as tomatoes, onions, garlic, melons, and asparagus which are grown for the export markets. In Arequipa and Cajamarca there are thriving dairy industries. However, the major agricultural crop is cocaine, which is grown on the eastern side of the Andes in an area known as the *seja de selva* (eyebrow of the jungle). Livestock other than dairy cattle is only of importance in the Andes, where they keep camelids, cattle, and sheep. A consequence of this is that veterinary services are not of major importance to the country. It was not until after WW II that the first Peruvian veterinary school was founded.

As with many Latin American countries, Perú has a very large and complicated bureaucratic system. The veterinary staff are all centrally employed by the Ministry of Agriculture and there is a central direction in Lima with a Departmental Service in one unified organization. However, chains of command are long and the senior personnel change with regularity. Each time the Minister changes, the Director of Agriculture and all twenty-four of the Departmental Directors of Agriculture (RDA) change, as do the Regional Directors of Livestock, and the Regional Directors of Animal Health (RDAH). It should be pointed out that it is by no means certain that even the RDAH is a veterinary surgeon: because the veterinary profession was late on the scene, most senior posts on the Ministry of Agriculture are held by agriculturalists. In the six years 1986–92, no veterinary surgeon held the post of Director of Agriculture and only one veterinary surgeon held the post of RDA—in the Department of Loreto, a huge department in the Amazon with almost no livestock!

From this it can be seen that the livestock industry in Perú is not of national importance and consequently, veterinary surgeons are not held in high esteem. They are often employed directly on a farm being paid a pittance and working under the farm manager. The major epidemic diseases such as FMD and rabies are mostly kept under control by the veterinary staff of the Ministry of Agriculture, and in the dairy Departments of Arequipa and Cajamarca, following pressure from the Farmers' Cooperatives, there have been attempts to control tuberculosis and brucellosis (Lozada, L., 1986, personal communication).

British Aid projects in Cajamarca (1970–83) and Arequipa (1986–95) had demonstrated to farmers the value of a good laboratory diagnostic service, and in Arequipa the benefits of a clinical service that operated all day every day. The Ministry of Agriculture had participated in developing both laboratories but had no money, and less will, to establish similar laboratories in other Departments of the country. However, the projects stimulated a demand in other Departments for clinical and laboratory services. At present there is no likelihood of these demands being fulfilled. In conclusion it can be said that livestock is unimportant to the Peruvian economy; although the campesinos (small holder farmers) in the Andes depend upon their livestock for survival, they are too small a group to have any power, and so veterinary services are low on the list of government priorities. Because the veterinary profession is also small and without power, there is little likelihood of the Government being forced to change its priorities.

Vietnam

The last 50 years have not been kind to Vietnam: the country has been heavily engaged in three major wars which killed many of its people, destroyed its industries and its cities, and laid to waste much of the countryside, with the concomitant effects on agriculture and livestock. For almost half a century Vietnam has had a communist government, and traditionally communist governments invest heavily in the countryside and agriculture; the Vietnamese Government is no exception. At present there are several national, six regional, and 60 provincial veterinary laboratories.[4] These laboratories are all over-staffed and under-equipped, and because they charge for their services they are under-used. There are approximately 25,000 employees in the provincial veterinary field services.[5] The National Government employs approximately 270 veterinary staff[6] and runs the National and Regional Laboratories, but each Province is autonomous and is run by its own Peoples' Committee. They employ the veterinary and ancillary staff in the Provincial laboratories and the field staff at Provincial, District and Commune levels. Most of the provincial staff are employed at the lower levels of the scale, namely the Community Animal Health Workers (CAHW) who are frequently paid no salaries, but generate incomes from private veterinary practice and participation in disease control campaigns that are paid for by the farmers themselves. Some of the CAHW team leaders receive small incentive allowances from the provincial authorities. Those who do not receive a salary continue to work because this enables them to take part in disease control campaigns that are paid for by the farmers themselves and so they are able to obtain an income. As a general rule their overall level of income from veterinary work reflects the livestock industries in their area; thus CAHWs in the Delta and around the main cities may do very well, while those in the poorer more remote areas generate very small incomes from veterinary work and have other means of income, usually farming.[5]

The whole government bureaucracy—in all fields, not just in veterinary medicine—is grossly overstaffed, and so the majority of the budget goes to paying the staff (usually very low salaries). This in turn results in the staff looking for other work to enable them to survive. This vicious circle means that the services are poor, and so less work comes in, which, because the institutions charge for their services, results in lower income for the service and so it continues. Money is then not available to purchase reagents or drugs and so the staff are less able to perform their work. There is little incentive to work and so the young people become demoralized or they leave the service. Since there are few opportunities outside the government services, only the best can find work with private companies and so the best leave. Future management of services will, therefore, not be in the hands of the most able. There are glittering exceptions to this picture, where some particularly bright members of staff have found ways to improve the income of their centers. This is particularly true of offices or laboratories near the ports where meat inspection and food hygiene examinations are required for the export of meat and meat products.[3]

The vast majority of livestock production is in the hands of small holder farmers. Of the total of 11.97 million farm households in the country, 9.53 million (79.6%) were engaged in livestock production of one sort or another.[7] Of families keeping ruminants (1.84 million), 61% kept only one buffalo and 52.75% kept only one bovine (these are kept mainly for draught power). Of the 7.4 million households who keep pigs, 82.6% keep only one or two animals.[7] It is impossible to provide such people with economic veterinary services and the people do not have the money to pay for such services. It could be said that the CAHW are providing the community-based services ("barefoot vets") seen in Africa.

Vietnam has long, sparsely populated borders with Cambodia, Laos, and China and it is therefore impossible to prevent the ingress (and indeed the egress) of animals carrying such infections as FMD or classical swine fever viruses. It is therefore imperative that any attempt to control such infections be carried out on a regional basis. Vietnam could have a very productive livestock industry with the potential to export pigs, pigmeat, and poultry to its rich neighbours: for this to happen it would be necessary to control the major epidemic diseases and there would need to be a drastic rationalization of animal keeping. The country has many calls on its national budget, with schools and hospitals being at the top of the list. The staple national diet is rice, and so the main priority of the government is to keep rice production at a level which will feed the people and allow for exports. There is little left over in the agricultural budget to pay for veterinary services. However a major overhaul of these services would improve their efficiency, delivery, and value for money. The project "Strengthening Veterinary Services in Vietnam," which is financed by the European Union, is attempting this Herculean task.

DISCUSSION

It could be argued that there is no need for any country to have a veterinary department and that animal disease should be the concern of the farmers themselves.

The money saved could be used for new hospitals, schools, or roads. This may happen by default in some African countries, e.g., in Tanzania, the Department of Animal Health has withdrawn many services as it has seen its funds reduced. The counter argument is that it is essential to have an organization to control the major epidemic diseases and particularly those that have zoonotic importance such as rabies, tuberculosis, and brucellosis, or there will be a serious risk to human health. Leaving it to the individual can put animals at risk. If a farmer refuses to take action to control a disease, it may be that not only he, but all the farmers in the neighborhood may suffer. The sacrifices made by the farmers in the Western Province of Zambia have kept the remainder of that country free from CBPP. In effect Western Province has been in quarantine for more than 50 years; their animals are vaccinated on an annual basis and they are unable to sell them outside the area: the prices paid are consequently much lower. These people would be far better off without a veterinary department, but what about the rest of the country?

Of the four countries discussed, the only one in which livestock is of major political importance is Botswana, and it is the only one in which the Department of Veterinary Services has a major voice. In Britain when the Prime Minister wished to call an election and was concerned that FMD would prevent such an election, he turned to the Chief Scientist and the Professor of Epidemiology at Imperial College, University of London (neither of whom had had any veterinary training), and they recommended killing all animals on contiguous farms and for an area of 3 km around every diseased farm, in the certainty that such a massive slaughter would stop the disease in its tracks: it almost did. The Prime Minister was able to hold his election, but 2 million healthy animals were slaughtered in the process. The policy has cost the country in excess of £2 billion to control the outbreak, and it is said that the rural community has lost a further £10 billion. When Botswana had a similar disastrous outbreak of disease, the 1995/6 outbreak of CBPP, they did not call in chemists and mathematicians, but they listened to their veterinary surgeons, and brought the disease under control with the minimum loss of animal life. Perú and Vietnam do not have slaughter policies for animal diseases, but try to contain them by vaccination. In both countries the farmers have to pay for vaccinations and so there is a variable take-up, which results in diseases continuing to grumble on. This is of little importance to Perú because they are unconcerned about exporting livestock or meat. Vietnam on the other hand will have to take active steps to control FMD and classical swine fever if it wishes to expand its trade in pigs and pig products with countries in southeast Asia and beyond.

It is barely possible for Britain to pay the costs of the current outbreak of FMD. The social fabric of the country has been damaged, not by the disease, but by the extraordinary way in which the outbreak was brought under control. Farming will change, the financing of farming will change, more attention will be given to countryside maintenance and less to the production of food. Britain will import more of its food (if that is possible) and the British countryside will become a sort of Disneyworld. There will then be no need of a state veterinary service. What remains of it will police animal welfare, make sure that dogs and other pets coming into the country have had the correct vaccinations and possess the right certificates. With the death of farming in Britain will come the death of the large animal veterinary profession. We will not have to worry about bovine tuberculosis because the cows will be few and far between. Only when the badgers start to die in large numbers will the public realize that there is no longer a State Veterinary Service.

Botswana, on the other hand will be required to export more meat to Britain to make up for the loss, and so there will be continuing pressure on its politicians to ensure that their veterinary service is well staffed, well trained and well equipped. The large animal veterinary profession has a great future in Botswana. While the effects of the British projects are still felt in Perú, there will continue to be a demand for veterinary services, but these will wither with the passage of time and the Peruvian veterinary services will wither with them. There is still hope for a veterinary service in Vietnam. Their livestock industry will continue to expand and consolidate, and with larger units will come more demand for improved veterinary services. Because there is a tremendous potential for exports, there may develop a political demand for increased government veterinary intervention which, in turn, will allow the trade to expand. There is hope for the future of the veterinary profession in Vietnam.

There is no hope at all for the veterinary profession if it continues to allow its students to be taught primarily by molecular biologists and mathematical modelers, by cell biologists and pure scientists, with almost no veterinary input. Until the veterinary profession takes its own future in hand, there is no future.

REFERENCES

1. ANONYMOUS. 1965. Animal Health—A Centenary. J.W.R. Pearce, L.P. Pugh, and Sir John Ritchie, Eds. Her Majesty's Stationary Office, London.
2. QUIN, J. 2001. SVS Staffing Levels, quoted in The Veterinary Record **148:** 643.
3. AMANFU, W., S. SEDIADIE, K.V. MASUPU, et al. 2000. Comparison between c-ELISA and CFT in detecting antibodies to *Mycoplasma mycoides* biotype SC in cattle affected by CBPP in Botswana. Ann. N.Y. Acad. Sci. **916:** 364–369.
4. WINDSOR, R.S. 2000. Mission Report on Diagnostic Laboratory Services in Viet Nam, SVSV, PMU. Cuc Thu Y, Phuong Mai Ward, Dong Da, Hanoi, Vietnam.
5. HUNTER, A.G. 2000. Report on the training plan for animal health in Vietnam. SVSV, PMU. Cuc Thu Y, Phuong Mai Ward, Dong Da, Hanoi, Vietnam.
6. HUNTER, A.G. & N.D. TAM. 1999. Report on the assessment of training needs in animal health and husbandry at regional centers and sub-departments of animal health in Vietnam. SVSV, PMU. Cuc Thu Y, Phuong Mai Ward, Dong Da, Hanoi, Vietnam.
7. LAN, L.T.K 1999. SVSV, Desk-Study on Major Livestock Production Systems in Vietnam. PMU. Cuc Thu Y, Phuong Mai Ward, Dong Da, Hanoi, Vietnam.

Public Health Considerations in Human Consumption of Wild Game

ALWYNELLE S. AHL,[a] DAVID NGANWA,[b] AND SAUL WILSON[b]

[a]USDA Fellow,Center for the Integrated Study of Food, Animal and Plant Systems at Tuskegee University, Tuskegee, Alabama 36083, USA

[b]College of Veterinary Medicine, Nursing and Allied Health, Tuskegee University, Tuskegee, Alabama 36083, USA

ABSTRACT: The role of a few microorganisms, like *Brucella* and *Mycobacterium* and certain parasites of food animals, in causing human disease has been recognized for a hundred years. By the 1990s, other microorganisms derived from food animals were recognized as contributing to human illness. Handling and/or consumption of wild game may result in human exposure to novel microorganisms; these unrecognized or unknown agents or diseases in wild species may cross into humans and cause "new" diseases with which we are not familiar.

KEYWORDS: emerging diseases; food safety; wildgame consumption; public health

FOOD SAFETY AND HUMAN HEALTH

As a species, our mucous membranes are constantly bombarded by bacteria, viruses and other microbial agents. Our digestive tracts are exposed to numerous bacteria with every bite we eat. Most of the time we don't get sick,[1] but when we do the results can be personally devastating. Ongoing work in foodborne diseases has increased understanding of the array of hazards and diseases and the likelihood of their occurrence.[2–4] Most of these studies have emphasized concern for domestically produced food; however, some research papers focus on game. Farmed game present much the same hazards as those presented by meat from domestic animals,[4] and these hazards are related to husbandry practices as well as contamination of food and water. Wild harvested game may present similar hazards, but the likelihood of harboring agents unlike those of domestically raised relatives is increased. This may present unrecognized hazards to consumers.

Wild game or bushmeat was the original meat protein source for the human species and continues to contribute significant amounts of protein to human populations in poorer countries or poorer areas of the more developed countries. Also, hunting and game consumption continues to be a popular activity in many societies. The ex-

Address for correspondence: Dr. Alwynelle S. Ahl, USDA Fellow, Center for the Integrated Study of Food, Animal and Plant Systems at Tuskegee University, Tuskegee, Alabama 36083. asahl@tusk.edu

Ann. N.Y. Acad. Sci. 969: 48–50 (2002). © 2002 New York Academy of Sciences.

port of wild game, whether farmed or wild-harvested, provides income for local individuals while satisfying desires for unique cuisines from other locales. Consumer concerns in developed countries for safety of domestic meat related to bovine spongiform encephalopathy (BSE) has resulted in depopulation of many herds in Europe as well as fear of consuming that which remains. Thus, red meat supplies in Europe are decreased and the many concerns have led to increased interest in and consumption of "naturally produced" meat such as game.

HAZARDS

Hazards to human health may be caused by parasites, viruses, or bacterial agents. Environmental contaminants, such as chemicals, toxins, or drugs used to treat sick animals, may find their way into the game and be transmitted to humans. Hazards caused by microorganisms can be avoided by careful handling of the carcass and thorough cooking of the meat before eating. Wild game is likely less affected by chemicals or toxins unless they have access to domestic foods, which may harbor mycotoxins (seasonal) or other toxins found in domestic animals. However, since a single human is unlikely to be exposed to a lot of game from a single source, the risk to any one person is likely negligible.

Viruses may pose special problems about which we know too little. One hypothesis about the origin of AIDS is that it came originally from handling and consumption of bushmeat. Ebola virus has an endemic focus in the wild and may be transmitted to human through contact with or consumption of such wild hosts. More frightening is the secondary transmission of diseases such as AIDS and Ebola directly from human to human contact and not necessarily through further contact with wildlife. In general, thorough cooking of meat is sufficient to kill viruses and bacteria, thus preventing transmission to the consumer. However, risk of illness or disease to the persons who handle game or prepare the uncooked meat may remain.

New diseases such as variant Creutzfeldt-Jacob Disease (vCJD) have developed from consuming domestic meat contaminated with BSE. Precisely how BSE arose in cattle is yet unresolved.[5] Nonetheless, humans have learned through hard experience that novel agents can appear associated with food and cause illness and death in consumers, especially the young, elderly or immunosuppressed individuals. In the USA, chronic wasting disease (CWD) of deer and elk, a prion disease related to BSE and scrapie, appears to be passed among animals through contact with infected nasal and salivary secretions.[6] A major public health problem could be created should this disease cross into cattle and then with the same transmission pattern, cross into humans. Though CWD is known only in the USA and Canada at present, the lack of world-wide surveillance and monitoring of cervids indicates one cannot rule out its occurrence elsewhere. The possibilities related here should be monitored since the prion agent is not affected by thorough cooking or other known disinfection agents.

Colonizing the gastrointestinal tract of humans is a vast array of symbiotic and commensal bacteria that have profoundly important effects on many host activities, including immune function, nutrient processing, and others.[6] Bacteria from game, novel to the consumer, can potentially present unknown hazards and effects. In addition, movement of an agent from one species to another may change the nature of the agent and cause it to behave in entirely different ways in the new host. In fact, our tendency to keep infants and children shielded from bacteria appears to have an influence on development of our intestinal tract and flora. Exposure to new agents as adults can have unwanted consequences, both acute and chronic. These facts argue strongly for careful handling of game and thorough cooking of such meat for consumers.

SUMMARY

The world-wide emphasis on food safety has focused primarily on the safety of domestically produced food, considering agents such as *Escherichia coli* O157:H7, *Listeria monocytogenes, Campylobacter, Salmonella enteritidis*, and other *Salmonella* species. However, it is prudent to provide hunters and game harvesters with information on safe handling of game carcasses. Public health authorities should remain vigilant in seeking new foodborne diseases. Researchers need to better understand the role of commensal bacteria in the development and functioning of the human hosts.[7] Finally, though not preventative for all hazards associated with game, careful carcass handling and thorough cooking of the meat before consumption can go a long way toward ensuring human health and safety relating to this alternate protein source.

REFERENCES

1. LEVIN, B.R. & R. ANTIA. 2001. Why we don't get sick: the within-host population dynamics of bacterial infections. Science **292** (5519): 1112–1115.
2. ST. LOUIS, M.E., D.L. MORSE, M.E. POTTER, *et al.* 1988. The emergence of Grade A eggs as a major source of *Salmonella enteritidis* infections. J. Am. Med. Assoc. **259** (14): 2103–2107.
3. CENTERS FOR DISEASE CONTROL AND PREVENTION. 1992-93. Update: multistate outbreak of *Escherichia coli* O157:H7 infections from hamburgers—Western United States. MMWR **42:** 257–263.
4. AHL, A.S. & P. SUTMOLLER, Eds. 1997. Contamination of animal products: prevention and risks for public health. Rev. Sci. Tech. Off. Int. Epizoot. **16** (2): 307–715.
5. DESEO, J. 2001. Out of the barn: can the mad cow be contained? Inside Laboratory Management, May/June.
6. ENSERINK, M. 2001. America's own prion disease. Science **292:**1641.
7. HOOPER, L.V. & J.I. GORDON. 2001. Commensal host-bacterial relationships in the gut. Science **292** (5519):1115–1118.

Emerging Morbillivirus Infections of Marine Mammals

Development of Two Diagnostic Approaches

JEREMIAH T. SALIKI, EMILY J. COOPER, AND JONATHAN P. GUSTAVSON

Oklahoma Animal Disease Diagnostic Laboratory, College of Veterinary Medicine, Oklahoma State University, Stillwater, Oklahoma 74078, USA

ABSTRACT: In the last 13 years, four viruses belonging in the *Morbillivirus* genus of the Paramyxoviridae family have emerged as significant causes of disease and mortality in marine mammals. The viruses involved are canine distemper virus (CDV) in seals and polar bears, dolphin morbillivirus (DMV) and porpoise morbillivirus (PMV) in cetaceans, and phocine distemper virus (PDV) in pinnipeds. The two cetacean morbilliviruses (DMV and PMV) are now considered to be the same viral species, named cetacean morbillivirus (CMV). All three morbillivirus species (CDV, CMV, and PDV) are genetically and antigenically related and cross-react in various serological tests. The diagnosis of morbilliviral infections in marine mammal specimens poses two challenges. First, various marine mammal species can be infected by more than one closely related but distinct morbilliviruses, making definitive virus identification unattainable by classical virology methods. Second, standard immunological reagents such as anti-species conjugates are unavailable for most marine mammal species, rendering definitive serological diagnosis difficult by classical serological techniques. The objectives of this study were to develop two diagnostic approaches that alleviate these difficulties, providing simple, rapid, and cost-effective diagnostic methods. For nucleic acid detection, reverse transcription-polymerase chain reaction (RT-PCR) and restriction endonuclease digestions were used to differentiate the three viruses. For antibody detection, a monoclonal antibody-based competitive enzyme-linked immunosorbent assay (c-ELISA) was used on sera from several species, thus avoiding the need for multiple anti-species enzyme conjugates.

KEYWORDS: *Morbillivirus*; canine distemper virus; dolphin morbillivirus; porpoise morbillivirus; phocine distemper virus; RT-PCR; c-ELISA

INTRODUCTION

Four viruses belonging in the *Morbillivirus* genus of the Paramyxoviridae family have emerged during the past 13 years as significant causes of disease and mortality in marine mammals. The viruses involved are canine distemper virus (CDV) in

Address for correspondence: Dr. Jeremiah T. Saliki, Oklahoma Animal Disease Diagnostic Laboratory, Farm Road and Ridge Road, Oklahoma State University, Stillwater, OK 74078. Voice: 405-744-6623; fax: 405-744-8612.
jsaliki@okstate.edu

Ann. N.Y. Acad. Sci. 969: 51–59 (2002). © 2002 New York Academy of Sciences.

seals[1] and polar bears,[2,3] dolphin morbillivirus (DMV) and porpoise morbillivirus (PMV) in cetaceans,[4–7] and phocine distemper virus (PDV) in pinnipeds.[8,9] Several mass-mortality events have been attributed to these viruses. First, in 1987 to 1988, about half of the population of bottlenose dolphins (*Tursiops truncatus*) along the Atlantic coast of the United States died during the first recognized marine morbilliviral epizootic.[6] Second, in 1987 CDV killed thousands of Siberian seals (*Phoca sibirica*) in Lake Baikal, Russia.[1,10] Third, in 1988 a PDV epizootic killed approximately 17,000 harbor seals (*Phoca vitulina*) in the North sea.[9,11] Finally, between 1990 and 1991 a DMV epizootic killed thousands of striped dolphins (*Stenella coeruleoalba*) in the western Mediterranean.[7,12,13]

The morbilliviruses are closely related antigenically and genetically. The two cetacean morbilliviruses (DMV and PMV) are so closely related that they are now considered to be the same viral species, named cetacean morbillivirus (CMV).[14] The definitive diagnosis of morbillivirus in a host's tissues or secretions relies on isolation of the virus, detection of viral antigens by immunohistochemical staining, or detection of viral RNA. Nevertheless, the close relationship among members of the group renders species differentiation difficult. The geographical distribution and host range of morbilliviruses in general and marine morbilliviruses in particular keeps increasing. Recently detected new hosts or new environments for morbilliviruses include CDV in African wild cats[15] and in Alaskan and Russian polar bears[2,13] and an apparently new member of the morbillivirus group in a long-finned pilot whale (*Globicephalus melas*) on the U.S. Atlantic coast.[16] The expanding host and geographical ranges of these viruses underscore the need for specifically identifying each virus in the diagnostic laboratory. It is particularly important to determine which virus is involved when morbillivirus infection is initially detected in a new location or new host.

The morbilliviruses are difficult to culture in the laboratory, and only a few laboratories worldwide routinely attempt morbillivirus isolation from diagnostic specimens. Serological diagnosis is possible using the virus neutralization test (VNT). Wide use of the VNT is hampered, however, by lack of cell culture facilities, lack of the appropriate live virus stocks, high cost, and a long incubation period of 4–6 days. Previous papers have described either individual RT-PCR tests for various morbilliviruses[17,18] or a consensus RT-PCR for the group.[19,20] This study pursued two goals: (a) to develop a rapid and cost-effective PCR-based test scheme to detect and differentiate the three marine morbilliviruses (CDV, CMV, and PDV) in cell cultures and animal tissues and (b) to develop a monoclonal antibody-based C-ELISA for morbillivirus serological diagnosis.

MATERIALS AND METHODS

PCR Primer Selection

This study focuses on differentiating among CDV, CMV, and PDV. To avoid having to perform three separate PCR tests, a single consensus RT-PCR was performed, followed by restriction fragment length polymorphism (RLFP) analysis of the PCR product to differentiate the viruses. Previously described[19,20] universal primers (antisense: 5′-ATT GGG TTG CAC CAC TTG TC–3′; sense: 5′–ATT AAA AAG GG(G/C) ACA GGA GAG AGA TCA GCC–3′) were used to amplify an 80-bp product in the phosphoprotein (P) gene. These primers had been shown to amplify RNA from formalin-fixed, paraffin-embedded tissues.[19,20] Because RNA obtained from formalin-fixed tissues is significantly fragmented,[21] it was necessary to use primers that amplified as small a product as possible. Primers were purchased from a custom DNA supplier.

RNA Isolation and Reverse Transcription PCR

Total RNA was isolated from virus isolates (Rockborn strain of CDV, PDV strain 1-2-6A, and the Belfast strains of DMV and PMV), using a commercially available kit and from formalin-fixed, paraffin-embedded (FFPE) tissues using previously described methods[22] with the following modifications: 5 µL of polyacryl carrier was added to coprecipitate the RNA before precipitation with 1 mL cold 100% ethanol. The precipitate was pelleted, washed with 75% ethanol, dried, and resuspended in 30 µL RNase-free water. The FFPE tissues were obtained from three sources (Dr. S. Kennedy, Department of Agriculture and Rural Development, Belfast, Northern Ireland; Dr. P.Y. Daoust, Atlantic Veterinary College, University of Prince Edward Island, Charlottetown, Prince Edward Island, Canada; Dr. P. Duignan, Massey University, New Zealand) and had been previously tested for morbillivirus antigens and/or nucleic acid by immunohistochemical staining or RT-PCR. Following RNA isolation, 2 µL of total RNA was added to a mixture containing final concentrations of 0.5 mM $MgCl_2$, 1 × PCR buffer (10 mM Tris, 50 mM KCl, and 0.1% Triton® X-100), 0.5 mM of each dNTP, 1 U/µL RNase inhibiter, 2.5 U/µL reverse transcriptase, 0.7 µM antisense primer, and RNase-free water for a 20-µL total reaction volume per sample. Samples were then thermal cycled in 0.2 ml thin-walled PCR tubes for 1 cycle at 37°C for 1 hour, 99°C for 5 minutes, and 4°C to hold. For PCR, 80 mL of PCR mixture containing 1.5 mM $MgCl_2$, 1 × PCR buffer (10 mM Tris, 50 mM KCl, and 0.1% Triton® X-100), 0.28 µM sense primer, and 0.03 U/µL Taq DNA polymerase was added to the RT product. Amplification was carried out in 40 cycles at 94°C for 30 seconds, 55°C for 30 seconds, and 72°C for 30 seconds followed by a final extension at 72°C for 7 minutes and 4°C to hold.

Restriction Digest and Electrophoresis

P gene sequences for CDV (Genebank M32418), PDV (Genebank X75960), and DMV (Genebank Z47759) were aligned; and unique restriction endonucleases were selected to differentiate between the viruses (FIG. 1). TaqI, MspA1I, and BseLI specifically cut CDV, PDV, and CMV products yielding fragments of sizes 59/21, 50/30, and 35/45 bp, respectively. Ten microliters of amplicon was digested according to the manufacturer's instructions. Following amplification and digestion, 10 mL of uncut PCR product and 10 mL of each of the three digestions were electrophoresed on a high-percentage gel (either 5% agarose-TBE or a precast 15% polyacrylamide-TBE). A 10-bp DNA ladder was used as a reference marker.

Serum Samples

A total of 736 marine mammal serum samples belonging to four different orders or families were used in this study. These included 113 *Canidae*, 36 *Mustelidae*, 118 *Cetacea*, 405 *Pinnipedia*, and 64 samples from undetermined species. The mor-

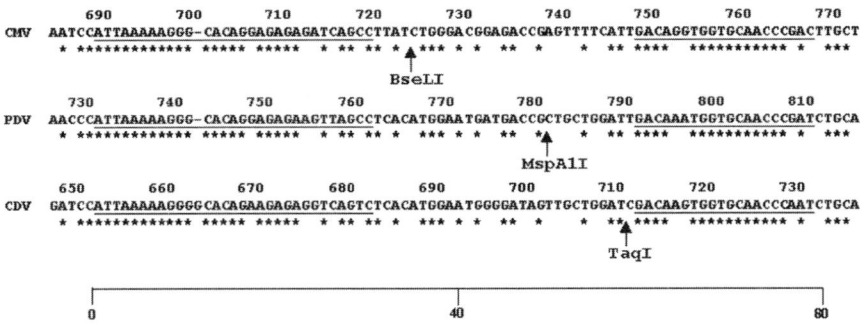

FIGURE 1. Nucleotide sequence of the P gene region of *Morbillivirus* RNA showing unique restriction enzyme sites. Numbers correspond to individual sequences with Genebank accession numbers: Z47758 (DMV), X75960 (PDV), and M32418 (CDV).

billivirus antibody status of each sample was determined using the virus neutralization test (VNT), with the four viruses as indicators. Following the VNT, all samples were frozen at −70°C until they were tested by c-ELISA.

Competitive ELISA

The c-ELISA was developed using a monoclonal antibody (mAb) generated against CDV and shown to be reactive with CDV and PDV. The mAb was also able to compete with positive sera for binding to morbillivirus antigen in an ELISA.[23] The c-ELISA was performed as described.[23] Briefly, serum was diluted 1:10 in PBS containing 0.05% Tween 20 (PBST) and reacted with antigen-coated plates for 30 minutes. The mAb diluted in PBST was then added, and the plates incubated for 1 hour. After washing, the plates were reacted with peroxidase-conjugated anti-mouse IgG for one hour and washed again. A substrate–chromogen mixture consisting of 0.01% hydrogen peroxide and 0.1 mg/ml of 3,3′,5,5′-tetramethylbenzidine (TMB) (Sigma Chemical Co., St. Louis, MO) in 0.05 M citrate/phosphate buffer (pH 5.0) was added, and the plates incubated for 25 minutes. Color reaction was stopped by adding 2 M sulfuric acid. Optical density (OD) readings were taken at a wavelength of 450 nm, using a computer-interfaced ELISA plate reader.

The c-ELISA depends on the ability of serum antibody to compete with a monoclonal antibody for binding to antigen. Competition is detected as a reduction in the OD reading of serum–mAb wells when compared to control wells with mAb alone. Because the OD signal is determined solely by the amount of mAb that binds, quenching of the signal indicates competition and, by extension, presence of specific antibody in the serum. The OD values were used to calculate the percent inhibition induced by each serum, using the formula:

$$\text{Percent inhibition} = [1 - (OD_{Ser}/OD_{mAb})] \times 100$$

Where OD_{Ser} = mean OD of wells with serum and mAb and OD_{mAb} = mean OD of wells with mAb alone.

TABLE 1. Estimates of c-ELISA performance relative to VNT

VNT antibody specificity	Animal group	Sensitivity	Specificity	Kappa
CDV, PDV, and CDV/PDV	Canidae	100.0	91.4	0.94
	Pinnipedia	90.0	99.0	0.78
	Canidae/Pinnipedia	98.8	98.4	0.95
DMV, PMV, DMV/PMV	Cetacea	69.2	95.2	0.62

Statistical Analyses of c-ELISA Results

All serum samples were tested by c-ELISA and the standard VNT. Results of both tests were expressed as positive or negative for each sample to allow for a qualitative comparison. Using the VNT as the gold standard, sensitivity and specificity and exact binomial confidence intervals for these estimated parameters of the c-ELISA were calculated.[24] Agreement between VNT and c-ELISA beyond chance was estimated by calculating the agreement quotient (kappa).[25]

For statistical evaluations of the c-ELISA, sera were excluded that had positive but undetermined antibody specificity for VNT ($n = 8$). Sera were also excluded that had unknown family or species identification ($n = 64$). Other deletions included 36 sera from sea otters (*Mustelidae*), which had no VNT or c-ELISA positive results, and three sera that had unusual VNT-positive results, which were not considered to be representative of marine mammals (two sera that were positive to both DMV and PDV and one serum sample from a whale that was positive for PDV). After these exclusions were made, 625 serum samples from 109 *Canidae*, 117 *Cetacea*, and 399 *Pinnipedia* were used to evaluate c-ELISA performance (TABLE 1).

RESULTS

The RT-PCR methods used in this paper proved to be sensitive and specific in detecting and differentiating morbilliviruses in formalin-fixed, paraffin-embedded (FFPE) tissues and virus isolates (FIGS. 2 and 3). Results from the FFPE specimens tested by RT-PCR and RFLP were in complete agreement with immunohistochemistry and/or RT-PCR results obtained previously.

The c-ELISA permitted the testing of 736 serum samples from several marine mammal species in one test. The criterion for designation of a homologous virus in the VNT was set such that a serum sample had to yield at least a twofold higher titer against a single virus before that virus would be determined to have induced the antibody in the serum. On the basis of this criterion, of the 105 sera that had a positive VNT antibody titer, the homologous virus could be determined in 54% (57/105). Of the remainder, 31% (33/105) were CDV/PDV, 6% (6/105) were DMV/PMV, 1% (1/105) were DMV/PDV, and 8% (8/105) were of undetermined antibody status. In recognition of this apparent failing of the "gold standard" to be more definitive, all data analyses on positive samples were performed using the two pairs CDV/PDV and DMV/PMV rather than the individual viruses. The relative sensitivity and specificity values ranged from 69.2 to 100% and from 91.4 to 99%, respectively, while the kappa

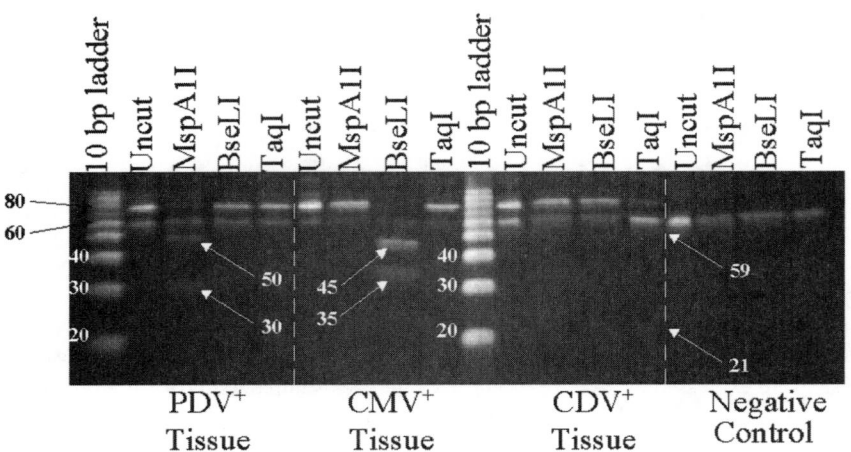

FIGURE 2. Restriction enzyme digest of RT-PCR amplified *Morbillivirus* RNA from formalin-fixed, paraffin-embedded tissue specimens.

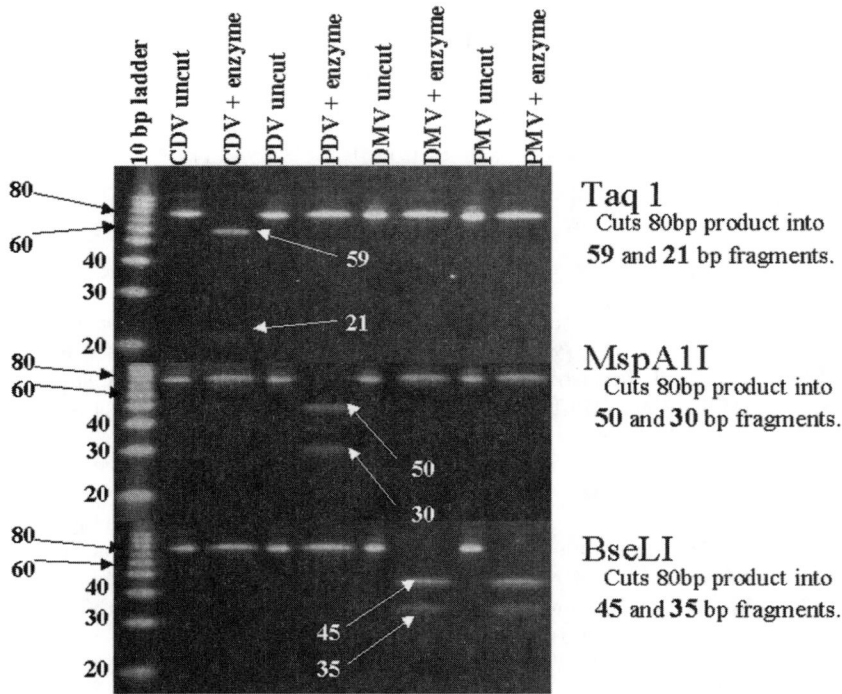

FIGURE 3. Restriction enzyme digest of RT-PCR amplified *Morbillivirus* RNA from virus isolates.

values ranged from 0.62 to 0.95 (kappa values ≥0.5 are considered good). These results provided evidence that the c-ELISA was a valid test.

Evaluation of the c-ELISA according to animal groups produced expected results. The greatest sensitivity (100%) occurred in sera from the Canidae family. Samples from Pinnipedia provided the greatest specificity (99%). These two families involved the combination of CDV/PDV virus pairs from VNT. The sensitivity and specificity for these two families combined both exceeded 98%. The results stated above for the DMV/PVM virus pairs were entirely from Cetacea. The sensitivity was significantly lower for sera from this family (69.2%) based on evaluation of 95% confidence intervals compared to corresponding intervals for samples from Canidae or Pinnipedia. The specificity (95.2%) was intermediate between the corresponding specificity for Canidae (91.4%) and Pinnipedia (99.0%). All of the 95% confidence intervals for specificity overlapped among the different animal group or virus pair comparisons, which indicated no significant difference among these specificity estimates.

DISCUSSION

Analysis of the U.S. Atlantic coast dolphin epizootic in 1987–1988 revealed that approximately one-third of the specimens showing histologic evidence of viral infection tested negative using immunohistochemical techniques because of postmortem autolysis.[6] However, 35 of the 36 dolphins tested were positive for morbilliviral RNA by RT-PCR.[26] The RT-PCR protocol used in this study was specifically designed for use on diagnostic specimens containing degraded RNA either from formalin fixation or postmortem tissue decomposition. The addition of restriction endonuclease digestion allows diagnosticians to rapidly identify the specific morbillivirus found in the sample. This information will be useful in studying the epidemiology of these viruses in new and existing hosts and geographical locations. However, the main difficulty with studying the epidemiology of viruses of marine species is obtaining representative samples from the population. To date, the majority of the diagnostic samples obtained are from animals that have died in the wild or shortly after stranding. The RT-PCR test system developed in this study would allow for rapid, cost-effective screening of live animals using samples such as peripheral blood mononuclear cells. The test scheme might also be useful in identifying new morbilliviruses in the marine mammal population.

It was surprising in this study to observe that the CDV/PDV-specific mAb competed against both CDV/PDV-specific sera and DMV/PMV-specific sera for binding to solid-phase CDV antigen. A possible explanation for this cross-reactivity is that steric hindrance caused by cross-reactive serum antibody binding to epitopes close to the specific epitope recognized by the mAb prevented it from binding. Although this outcome was not expected at the beginning, it was useful, because a single mAb-based c-ELISA could be used to detect antibody against the four morbilliviruses.

Morbillivirus infections currently occur in marine mammals in the Pacific and Atlantic oceans and the Mediterranean, Caspian, and North Seas.[16] Serology is a major epidemiological tool used to detect the occurrence of morbillivirus infections in marine mammal populations in which clinical disease has not been observed. For example, serological evidence indicates that morbillivirus infections occur in polar bears, although clinical morbillivirus disease has not yet been described.[2,3] The availability of a simple, fast, reliable, and cost-effective test would provide a tool that can be readily used by various laboratories for diagnostic and epidemiological purposes. The c-ELISA described in this study fits that role.

ACKNOWLEDGMENTS

This work was supported in part by a grant from the Morris Animal Foundation (98Z0-29). We thank Drs. S. Kennedy, P.Y. Daoust, and P.J. Duignan for providing formalin-fixed, paraffin-embedded tissue samples and the histopathology, serology, and virology laboratories at the Oklahoma Animal Disease Diagnostic Laboratory for their assistance with this project.

REFERENCES

1. GRACHEV, M.A., V.P. KUMAREV, L.V. MAMAEV, et al. 1989. Distemper virus in Baikal seals. Nature 338: 209.
2. FOLLMANN, E.H., G.W. GARNER, J.F. EVERMANN, et al. 1996. Serological evidence of morbillivirus infection in polar bears (Ursus maritimus) from Alaska and Russia. Vet. Rec. 138: 615–618.
3. GARNER, G.W., J.F. EVERMANN, J.T. SALIKI, et al. 2000. Morbillivirus ecology in polar bears (Ursus maritimus). Polar Biol. 23: 474–478.
4. KENNEDY, S., J.A. SMYTH, P.F. CUSH, et al. 1992. Morbillivirus infection in two common porpoises (Phocoena phocoena) from the coasts of England and Scotland. Vet. Rec. 131: 286–290.
5. LIPSCOMB, T.P., S. KENNEDY, D. MOFFETT, et al. 1996. Morbilliviral epizootic in bottlenose dolphins of the Gulf of Mexico. J. Vet. Diagn. Invest. 8: 283–290.
6. LIPSCOMB, T.P., F.Y. SCHULMAN, D. MOFFETT, et al. 1994. Morbilliviral disease in Atlantic bottlenose dolphins (Tursiops truncatus) from the 1987–88 epizootic. J. Wildl. Dis. 30: 567–571.
7. VISSER, I.K.G., M.F. VAN BRESSEM, R.L. DE SWART, et al. 1993. Characterization of morbilliviruses isolated from dolphins and porpoises in Europe. J. Gen. Virol. 74: 631–641.
8. DUIGNAN, P.J., J.T. SALIKI, D.J. ST. AUBIN, et al. 1994. Neutralizing antibodies to phocine distemper virus in Atlantic walruses (Odobenus rosmarus rosmarus) from Arctic Canada. J. Wildl. Dis. 30: 90–94.
9. OSTERHAUS, A.D. & E.J. VEDDER. 1988. Identification of a virus causing recent seal deaths. Nature 20: 335.
10. VISSER, I.K.G., V.P. KUMAREV, C. ORVELL, et al. 1990. Comparison of two morbilliviruses isolated from seals during outbreaks of distemper in North West Europe and Siberia. Arch. Virol. 111: 149–164.
11. OSTERHAUS, A.D., E.J. GROEN, H.E.M. SPIJKERS, et al. 1990. Mass mortality in seals caused by a newly discovered morbillivirus. Vet. Microbiol. 23: 343–350.
12. DOMINGO, M.L., L. FERRER, M.A. PUMAROLA, et al. 1990. Morbillivirus in dolphins. Nature 336: 21.
13. DOMINGO, M.L., M. VILAFRANCA, J. VISA, et al. 1995. Evidence of chronic morbillivirus infection in the Mediterranean striped dolphin (Stenella coeruleoalba). Vet. Microbiol. 44: 229–239.
14. BARRETT, T., I.K. VISSER, L. MAMAEV, et al. 1993. Dolphin and porpoise morbilliviruses are genetically distinct from phocine distemper virus. Virology 193: 1010–1012.
15. HARDER, T.C., M. KENTER, M.J. APPEL, et al. 1995. Phylogenetic evidence of canine distemper virus in Serengeti's lions. Vaccine 13: 521–523.
16. TAUBENBERGER, J.K., M.M. TSAI, T.J. ATKIN, et al. 2000. Molecular genetic evidence of a novel morbillivirus in a long-finned pilot whale (Globicephalus melas). Emerg. Infect. Dis. 6: 42–45.

17. BLIXENKRONE-MOLLER, M., G. BOLT, E. GOTTSCHALCK, *et al.* 1994. Comparative sequence analysis of the gene encoding the nucleocapsid protein of dolphin morbillivirus reveals its distant evolutionary relationship to measles virus and ruminant morbilliviruses. J. Gen. Virol. **75:** 2829–2834.

18. FRISK, A.L., M. KONIG, A. MORITZ, *et al.* 1999. Detection of canine distemper virus nucleoprotein RNA by reverse transcription-PCR using serum, whole blood, and cerebrospinal fluid from dogs with distemper. J. Clin. Microbiol. **37:** 3634–3643.

19. KRAFFT, A., J.H. LICHY, T.P. LIPSCOMB, *et al.* 1995. Postmortem diagnosis of morbillivirus infection in bottlenose dolphins (*Tursiops truncatus*) in the Atlantic and Gulf of Mexico epizootics by polymerase chain reaction-based assay. J. Wildl. Dis. **31:** 410–415.

20. REIDARSON, T.H., J. MCBAIN, C. HOUSE, *et al.* 1998. Morbillivirus infection in stranded common dolphins from the Pacific ocean. J. Wildl. Dis. **34:** 771–776.

21. FINKE, J., R. FRITZEN, P. TERNES, *et al.* 1993. An improved strategy and a useful housekeeping gene for RNA analysis from formalin-fixed, paraffin-embedded tissues by PCR. Biotechniques **14:** 448–453.

22. MASUDA, N., T. OHNISHI, S. KAWAMOTO, *et al.* 1999. Analysis of chemical modification of RNA from formalin-fixed samples and optimization of molecular biology applications for such samples. Nucleic Acids Res. **27:** 4436–4443.

23. SALIKI, J.T. & T.W. LEHENBAUER. 2001. Monoclonal antibody-based competitive enzyme-linked immunosorbent assay for detection of morbillivirus antibody in marine mammal sera. J. Clin. Microbiol. **35:** 1877–1881.

24. GREINER, M. & I.A. GARDNER. 2000. Epidemiologic issues in the validation of veterinary diagnostic tests. Prev. Vet. Med. **45:** 3–22.

25. MARTIN, S.W., A.H. MEEK & P. WILLEBERG. 1988. Veterinary Epidemiology. Iowa State University Press. Ames, IA. pp. 73–75.

26. SCHULMAN, F.Y., T.P. LIPSCOMB, D. MOFFETT, *et al.* 1997. Histologic, immunohistochemical, and polymerase chain reaction studies of bottlenose dolphins from the 1987–1988 United States Atlantic Coast epizootic. Vet. Pathol. **34:** 288–295.

PCR and Molecular Detection for Differentiating *Vibrio* Species

O.A.E. SPARAGANO,[a,b] P.A.W. ROBERTSON,[a] I. PURDOM,[a] J. McINNES,[a] Y. LI,[c] D.-H. YU,[c] Z.-J. DU,[c] H.-S. XU,[c] AND B. AUSTIN[a]

[a]*Centre for Marine Biodiversity and Biotechnology (CMBB), Department of Biological Sciences, Heriot-Watt University, Riccarton, Edinburgh EH14 4AS, Scotland, UK*

[b]*School of Agriculture, Food and Rural Development, University of Newcastle upon Tyne, England*

[c]*Department of Marine Biology, Ocean University of Qingdao, 5 Yushan Road, Qingdao 266003, Shandong, China*

ABSTRACT: Vibriosis is an economically important disease of fish, marine invertebrates (particularly penaeid shrimps), and large marine mammals and is responsible for high mortality rates in aquaculture worldwide. Some *Vibrio* species are also responsible for zoonoses, whereas others are relatively non-pathogenic. Using 16S- and 23S-based PCR reactions, we obtained species-specific patterns and a 470-bp band, respectively. DNA sequences obtained on the 23S rRNA gene allowed us to identify species-specific probes for *Vibrio parahaemolyticus, V. alginolyticus, V. anguillarum* and for a cluster of taxonomically related species: *V. carchariae/harveyi/campbelii.* A phylogenetic tree based on the 23S sequences confirmed previous results obtained by Western blotting.

KEYWORDS: vibriosis; 16S PCR reactions; 23S PCR reactions; *Vibrio* species; aquaculture

INTRODUCTION

Vibriosis is responsible for important economic losses in aquaculture.[1] In terms of public health, *Vibrio* species can be responsible for diseases in marine animals[2,3] and in humans,[4] especially when contaminated seafood products are consumed.

Not all *Vibrio* species are pathogenic, however, and within the same species we can see a broad range of pathogenicity. Some *Vibrio* species, found in healthy marine animals, are considered opportunistic and can lead to health problems for the carrier under conditions of stress.[5]

Therefore, it is important to implement techniques that are able to target taxonomic groups at the subspecies level in order to investigate environmental risks. This

Address for correspondence: Dr. O.A.E. Sparagano, School of Agriculture, Food and Rural Development, University of Newcastle upon Tyne, Newcastle upon Tyne, NE1 7RU, UK. Fax: (00.44)191-222-7811.

olivier.sparagano@ncl.ac.uk

Ann. N.Y. Acad. Sci. 969: 60–65 (2002). © 2002 New York Academy of Sciences.

TABLE 1. Bacterial cultures used in this study

Sample/reference code	Species	Origin
A (SF1)	*Vibrio carchariae*	PRC, cultured fish
B (SF3)	*V. carchariae*	PRC, cultures fish
C (D1040)	*V. harveyi*	PRC, cultured fish
D (D1048)	*V. harveyi*	PRC, cultured fish
E (D1232)	*V. harveyi*	PRC, seawater
F (V72)	*V. anguillarum*	Norway, cod (type strain)
G (V283)	*V. alginolyticus*	Spoiled horse mackerel (type strain)
H (V284)	*V. alginolyticus*	Type strain LMG 4409 (Belgium)
I (V285)	*V. campbellii*	Sea water (type strain)
J (V286)	*V. carchariae*	Brown shark (type strain)
K (V295)	*V. harveyi*	Dead amphipod (type strain)
L (V304)	*V. parahaemolyticus*	Patient with food poisoning (type strain)

paper presents different molecular techniques used by the authors and others to specifically identify *Vibrio* species and their pathogenicity.

MATERIALS AND METHODS

Sample Preparation and DNA Extraction

The 12 *Vibrio* isolates used in this study are presented in TABLE 1. The cultures were grown on tryptone soya agar (Oxoid, Basingstoke, U.K.) supplemented with 1% (wt/vol) sodium chloride at 18°C for 2–3 days. DNA was extracted from axenic cultures using a Qiagen Dneasy™ Tissue Kit as outlined in the manufacturer's protocol (QIAGEN Ltd, West Sussex, UK).

PCR Methods

16S-based PCR: 16S1 (5′-AGAGTTTGATCCTGGCTCAG-3′) and 16S4 (5′-TTGTACACACCGCCCGTC-3′) primers amplifying a 1543-bp fragment of the 16S rRNA gene were used as previously described by Gurtler and Stanisich.[6]

23S-based PCR: 23S5 (5′-ACGGTGGATGCCCTGGCA-3′) and 23S10 (5′-CCTTTCCCTCACGGTACTG-3′) primers amplifying a 474-bp fragment of the 23S rRNA gene were used as previously described by Gurtler and Stanisich.[6]

PCR reaction mixes for both PCR reactions included a *Taq* antibody to enable a hot-start reaction and UDG and dUTP as described before by Gubbels *et al.*[7] Annealing temperature were 51°C and 57°C for 16S and 23S rRNA PCR reactions, respectively.

A

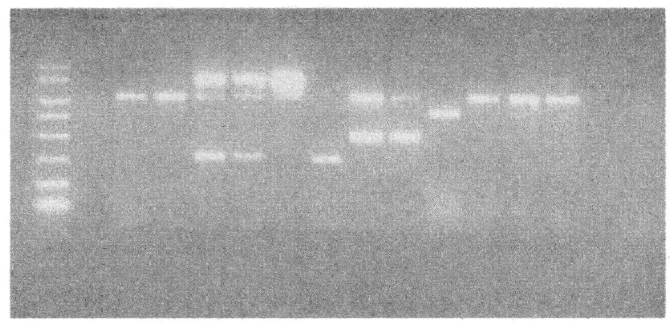

B

FIGURE 1. A: PCR results with 16S1 and 16S4 primers (Marker bands: 50, 150, 300, 500, 750, 1000, 1500, and 2000 bp). **B:** PCR results with 23S5 and 23S10 primers (Marker bands: 50, 150, 300, 500, 750, 1000, 1500, and 2000 bp).

RESULTS

FIGURES 1A and 1B show PCR results for 16S and 23S rRNA PCR, respectively. FIGURE 1A shows that more than one band was amplified by the PCR reaction, giving band patterns for all 12 *Vibrio* isolates. The patterns observed for the three *V. carchariae* isolates matched those for *V. harveyi* and *V. parahaemolyticus*. Isolates from the same species, such as *V. harveyi* (PRC) and *V. alginolyticus* showed the same patterns. FIGURE 1B shows the same 474-bp fragment for all 12 *Vibrio* isolates, which were subsequently sequenced.

The sequencing results are presented in FIGURE 2. Although the majority of the sequences are similar among the 12 isolates, we were able to find three variable zones (between 100 and 120, 140 and 170, and 300 and 315 bp). A phylogenetic tree based on the sequences obtained in FIGURE 2 is presented in FIGURE 3. Isolates from

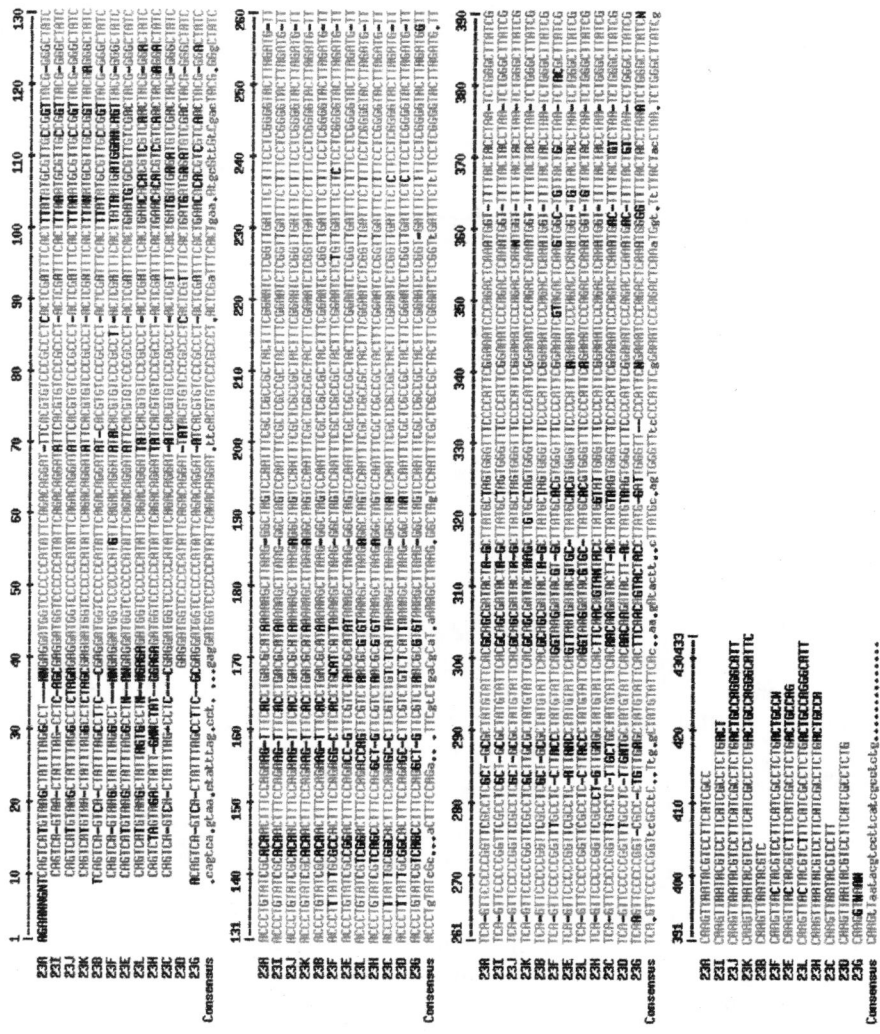

FIGURE 2. DNA sequences and alignment obtained with 23S5 and 23S10 primers.

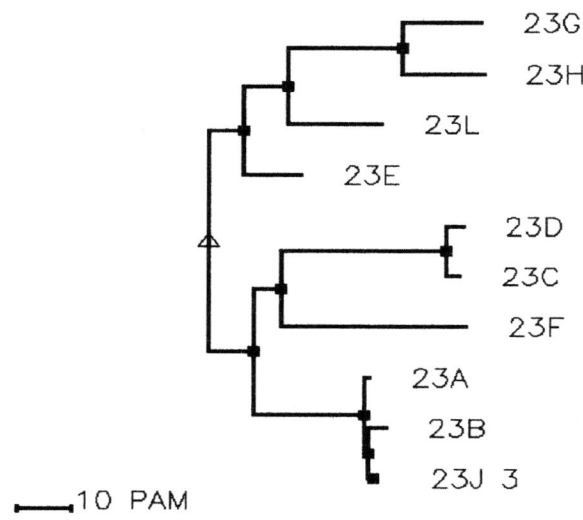

FIGURE 3. Phylogenetic tree based on the 23S rRNA sequencing.

the same species are usually closely linked on the phylogenetic tree. In particular, *V. carchariae* isolates are very closely related genetically to *V. campbellii* and *V. harveyi* (Scotland), in confirmation of earlier studies using ELISA and Western blot techniques.[8] Furthermore, *V. alginolyticus* (23G, 23H) and *V. parahaemolyticus* (23L) and *V. harveyi* (23C, 23D) and *V. anguillarum* (23F) seem to represent independent clusters.

CONCLUSION

Molecular techniques can be very powerful and, as shown here, can discriminate between closely related *Vibrio* species. It helps to genetically relate strains or isolates in order to evaluate the occurrence of mixed infections and the interactions between pathogens. As molecular tools are usually more sensitive than traditional techniques, they can also give information regarding population dynamics. Our objective is to further develop this technology for the *Vibrio* species and related species such as *Listonella* and *Photobacterium*. We are also developing integrated techniques able to identify several pathogen species in one test to give a better epidemiological picture and reduce costs and time constraints. Multiple species identification techniques already exist for the detection of other environmental pathogens; for example, the reverse line blot hybridization (RLB) has been developed successfully for parasites and bacteria.[7,9,10]

This new approach will be developed in our laboratory with reference strains and environmental isolates, then will be validated directly in field experiments.

ACKNOWLEDGMENTS

The authors would like to thank the Scottish Higher Education Fund for Scotland (SHEFC) for financing this research (Grant Number 106).

REFERENCES

1. AUSTIN, B. & D.A. AUSTIN. 1999. Bacterial fish pathogens disease of farmed and wild fish. 3rd (revised) edit. Springer-Praxis. Godalming.
2. MUROGA, K. 1995. Viral and bacterial diseases in larval and juvenile marine fish and shellfish—a review. Fish Pathol. **30:** 71–85.
3. VANDERBERGHE, J., Y. LI, L. VERDONCK, *et al.* 1998. Vibrios associated with *Penaeus chinensis* (Crustacea: Decapoda) larvae in Chinese shrimp hatcheries. Aquaculture **169:** 121–132.
4. KAIN, K.C., R.L. BARTELUK, M.T. KELLY, *et al.* 1991. Etiology of childhood diarrhea in Beijing, China. J. Clin. Microbiol. **29:** 90–95.
5. NASH, G., C. NITHIMATHACHOKE, C. TUNGMANDI, *et al.* 1992. Vibriosis and its control in pond-reared *Penaeus monodon* in Thailand. *In* Diseases in Asian Aquaculture I. Fish Health Section. M. Shariff, R.P. Subasinghe & J.R. Arthur, Eds.: 143–155. Asian Fisheries Society. Manila, Philippines.
6. GURTLER, V. & V.A. STANISICH. 1996. New approaches to typing and identification of bacteria using the 16S-23S rDNA spacer region. Microbiology **142:** 3–16.
7. GUBBELS, J.M., A.P. DE VOS, M. VAN DER WEIDE, *et al.* 1999. Simultaneous detection of bovine *Theileria* and *Babesia* species using reverse line blot hybridization. J. Clin. Microbiol. **37:** 1782–1789
8. ROBERTSON, P.A.W., H-S. XU & B. AUSTIN. 1998. An enzyme-linked immunosorbent assay (ELISA) for the detection of *Vibrio harveyi* in penaeid shrimp and water. J. Microbiol. Methods **34:** 31–39.
9. SPARAGANO, O., M.J. GUBBELS, A.P. DE VOS & F. JONGEJAN. 1999. Multiple and specific identification of Piroplasmidae in hosts and vectors using an integrated molecular technique. Epidémiol. Santé Animale **35:** 81–85.
10. SCHOULS, L.M., I. VAN DE POL, S.G.T. RIJPKEMA & C.S. SCHOT. 1999. Detection and identification of *Ehrlichia*, *Borrelia burgdorferi* sensu lato, and *Bartonella* species in Dutch *Ixodes ricinus* ticks. J. Clin. Microbiol. **37:** 2215–2222.

Early Diagnosis of Johne's Disease in the American Bison by Monoclonal Antibodies Directed against Antigen 85

JEFF G. LEID,[a] DAVID HUNTER,[b] AND C.A. SPEER[c]

[a]Center for Biofilm Engineering and Center for Bison and Wildlife Health, Montana State University, Bozeman, Montana 59717, USA

[b]Turner Enterprises, Inc., 1123 Research Drive, Bozeman, Montana 59718, USA

[c]College of Agricultural Sciences and Natural Resources and Agricultural Experiment Station, The University of Tennessee, Knoxville, Tennessee 37901-1071, USA

ABSTRACT: Several monoclonal antibodies derived from hybridomas from mice that had been immunized with recombinant *Mycobacterium bovis* antigen 85 (Ag85) were tested for reactivity against antigen 85 (Ag85) from *M. bovis* and against sera from 100 bison inoculated with *M. paratuberculosis* and from 100 control bison from a disease-free herd. Monoclonal antibodies mAb85.1, mAb85.44.1, mAb85.44.9, and mAb85.96 reacted against three or four 30–33-kDa bands of the Ag85 complex of *M. bovis*. Importantly, these mAbs also reacted with bands of similar molecular weight in the sera of bison inoculated with *M. paratuberculosis*. Additionally, when sera from 198 bison in four herds were reacted against mAb85.1 and mAb85.96, 26 bison reacted positively for the presence of Ag85 by either mAb or by both. These preliminary results indicate that monoclonal antibodies may eventually lead to a reliable diagnostic test for the early detection of *M. paratuberculosis* infections in ruminants as well as to a means for identifying contaminated dairy products.

KEYWORDS: Johne's disease; *Mycobacterium paratuberculosis*; *Mycobacterium bovis*; monoclonal antibodies; antigen 85

INTRODUCTION

Johne's disease, caused by *Mycobacterium paratuberculosis*, affects numerous ruminants, including the American bison (*Bison bison*), in which it is manifested as a chronic wasting disease exhibiting clinical signs only in older animals. In bison, the disease usually appears in animals 6–10 years old.[1–3] Although diagnostic assays are available for *M. paratuberculosis*, they are time-consuming, labor intensive, and usually incapable of detecting infections in young animals.[4] Antibodies against *M. paratuberculosis* are generally not present in young animals, nor do young infected

Address for correspondence: Dr. C.A. Speer, College of Agricultural Sciences and Natural Resources and Agricultural Experiment Station, The University of Tennessee, Knoxville, TN 37901-1071. Voice: 1-865-974-7303; fax: 1-865-974-9329.

caspeer@utk.edu

Ann. N.Y. Acad. Sci. 969: 66–72 (2002). © 2002 New York Academy of Sciences.

animals consistently shed the bacterium in their feces.[5] Antigen 85 (Ag85) is a highly conserved complex of proteins that is secreted by *Mycobacterium*-infected macrophages.[6] The Ag85 protein complex consists of fibronectin-binding proteins that are secreted early during infection by various species of *Mycobacterium*, including *M. tuberculosis*, *M. bovis,* and *M. paratuberculosis.*[7] Additionally, Ag85 has been shown to be important in cell wall biosynthesis in *M. tuberculosis.*[8] Thus, diagnostic assays that are based on the detection of Ag85 might provide a means of early detection of *Mycobacterium* infections.

Recently, antigen 85 has been the focus of much work in a variety of settings. A current study has shown that recombinant bacillus Calmette-Guérin (BCG) vaccines expressing the *Mycobacterium tuberculosis* 30-kDa major secretory protein induce greater protective immunity against tuberculosis than conventional BCG vaccines.[9] Additionally, a DNA vaccine encoding Ag85A from *M. bovis* demonstrated protection against Buruli ulcer.[10] Antigen 85C has also been crystallized, and the data from that study have suggested potential drug and vaccine targets that may aid in the fight against mycobacterial infections.[11]

Diagnostic assays are also now beginning to use antibodies and combinatorial strategies to detect antigen 85 from *M. tuberculosis* in humans and orangutans, and it is likely that this approach will also work well with bison.[12,13] The mAbs that we have produced in this study may be the first step toward such an aim. Additionally, the fact that these mAbs were generated against *M. bovis* Ag85 and reacted with Ag85 in the sera of bison inoculated with *M. paratuberculosis* suggests that global screening of herds may be accomplished to test for mycobacterial infections, a tool that would help guide management decisions.

MATERIALS AND METHODS

Animals

Balb/c mice were housed in the Animal Resource Center at Montana State University. American bison were housed on various private ranches in western Montana.

Immunizations

Female Balb/c mice aged 6–8 weeks were immunized i.p. with purified *M. bovis* antigen 85-MBP fusion protein generously provided by Dr. Gerhardt Schurig at Virginia Tech School of Veterinary Medicine. For the first immunization, 50 μg of the antigen was mixed with TiterMax™ (Sigma Chemical Co., St. Louis, MO) according to the manufacturer's instructions. Additional immunizations of 50 μg in PBS (Sigma) were carried out every three weeks until antibody titers were sufficiently high: greater than 1:1000 dilution by Western blot analysis. A final boost was administered i.p., and the spleen cells harvested four days later for production of monoclonal antibodies.

Generation of Monoclonal Antibodies

A fusion was performed on spleen cells to produce mAbs as described.[14] Briefly, spleen cells were harvested by tissue emaciation in a tissue grinder. The cells were counted in the presence of Trypan blue (Sigma) at a 1:1 ratio, and viable cells noted. SP2/0 myeloma cells were previously grown to confluence in T-175 flasks (Fisher Scientific Co., Pittsburgh, PA), counted as above, and viable cells noted. Spleen and SP2/0 cells were fused at a ratio of 2:1 in 50% PEG (Sigma) over two minutes, centrifuged, and added to a 1× and ½× flask containing peritoneal feeder cells and HAT. The cells from each flask were plated onto 48-well plates at a final volume of 500 μL and incubated without disturbance for 5–7 days at 37°C and 10% CO_2. The wells were then visually checked for the presence of clones.

Testing of Clones

Supernatant fluid (~100 μL) from wells with clones was aspirated, and antibody reactivity tested by Western blot. Briefly, purified antigen 85, generously provided by Dr. Gerhardt Schurig, was suspended in 1× running buffer, loaded onto a precast 8% polyacrylamide gel (BioRad, Hercules, CA), and electrophoresed. The proteins were transferred to nitrocellulose (Sigma), blocked for 45 min with equine serum (Sigma), and rinsed with TBST. The nitrocellulose was placed in a miniblot apparatus (BioRad), sealed, and 80 μL of the supernatant fluid added to each lane and incubated for 1 hr at room temperature. After incubation, the blot was washed with 200 ml of TBST, and 80 μL of second-stage goat anti-mouse IgG and IgM alkaline phosphatase (1:250) was added to each lane. The blot was then incubated again for 45 min at room temperature. It was washed again with 200 mL of TBST and developed by the addition of 133 μL of Nitroblue (Sigma) and 67 μL of 5-bromo-4-chloro-3-indolyl phosphate (Sigma) in 20 mL of AP buffer. Positive clones were identified by their reactivity with the specific antigen 85 bands seen from ~30–35 kDa.

Subcloning of Positive Clones

Once positive clones were identified, they were transferred to 24- or 6-well plates, depending on their confluency, and immediately subcloned. Viable cells were counted as above, and peritoneal feeder cells collected. Dilutions were made from a 1×10^4 stock solution of hybridoma cells and plated into flat-bottomed 96-well plates as follows: One plate was plated at a density of 50 cells/mL, two plates were plated at 5 cells/mL, and a final two plates were plated at 2.5 cells/mL. The plates were then incubated at 37°C and 10% CO_2 for 3–4 days, at which point the wells were visually screened for single, clonal colonies. Once identified, supernatant fluid from these colonies was collected and tested for reactivity as above. Positive clones were then grown to confluency in 5-liter roller bottles; and mAbs isolated, purified, and characterized again for their ability to recognize specific antigen 85 bands by Western analysis.

Screening of Inoculated American Bison Serum

American bison sera were collected from bison calves inoculated with 1×10^8 *Mycobacterium paratuberculosis* organisms and from bison known to be free of Johne's disease. The sera were electrophoresed as above and probed for the presence of antigen 85 by Western analysis with the mAbs generated as described above. The presence of antigen 85 in the sera was noted by specific reactivity of the antigen 85 protein (~30–35 kDa) with the anti-antigen 85 mAbs.

American Bison Herd Screening

Bison sera samples were obtained from peripheral blood, electrophoresed, transferred to nitrocellulose, and probed for Ag85 reactivity by mAbs Ag85.1 and Ag85.96. The presence of antigen 85 was noted by reactivity with either of these mAbs, and the results reported in table format. A total of 198 samples from four separate herds was tested.

RESULTS AND DISCUSSION

Several mAbs were generated against recombinant *M. bovis* Ag85 that specifically recognize Ag85 (consists of three or four bands at 30–33 kDa) in Western blots of the purified antigen and in the serum of bison experimentally inoculated with *M. paratuberculosis* (FIGS. 1–3). Eighty 2- to 4-month-old bison were inoculated five times with *M. paratuberculosis*: 40 of them received high doses of 10^8 bacteria, and 40 received low doses of 10^6. Additionally, 20 yearling bison were inoculated with the high dose. One hundred bison from a disease-free herd were used as controls. At 180 days after the last inoculation, sera obtained from these bison and purified Ag85 as a control were tested in Western blots with Ag85-specific mAbs, principally mAb85.1, mAb85.44.1, mAb85.44.9, and mAb85.96. All mAbs reacted with recombinant Ag85 (FIGS. 1–3), and mAb85.1 and mAb85.96 (the only ones tested) reacted with Ag85 complexes in the sera from animals inoculated with *M. paratuberculosis*; no reactions occurred with sera from control animals (FIG. 3).

In an additional study, mAb85.1 and mAb85.96 were used in Western blots to test for the presence of Ag85 in the sera of 198 bison selected from four large herds. One hundred and one, 71, 20, and 6 bison were tested from the four herds, of which 5,

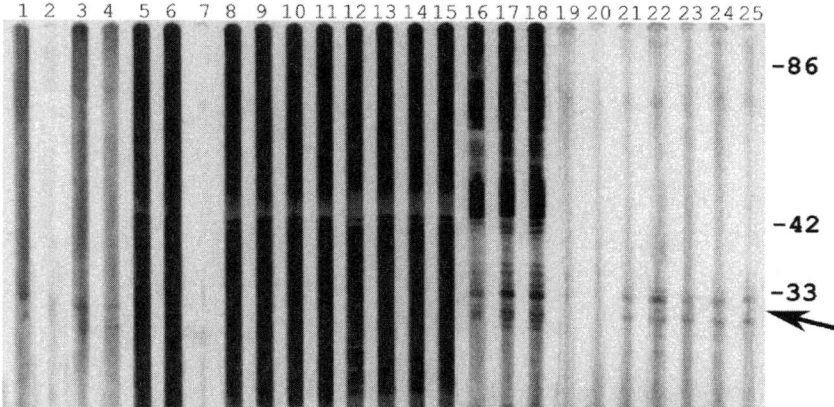

FIGURE 1. Western blot of subclones of two hybridomas generated against purified Ag85 from *Mycobacterium bovis*. *Lanes 1–4* show reactivity of supernatant fluid obtained from four wells containing subclones of mAb85.1; *lanes 5–9* show reactivity of supernatants of five wells containing subclones of mAb85.96. *Arrow* indicates location of Ag85, which consists of three or four primary bands ranging from 30 to 33 kDa. Approximate molecular weights are shown at the right side of the figure.

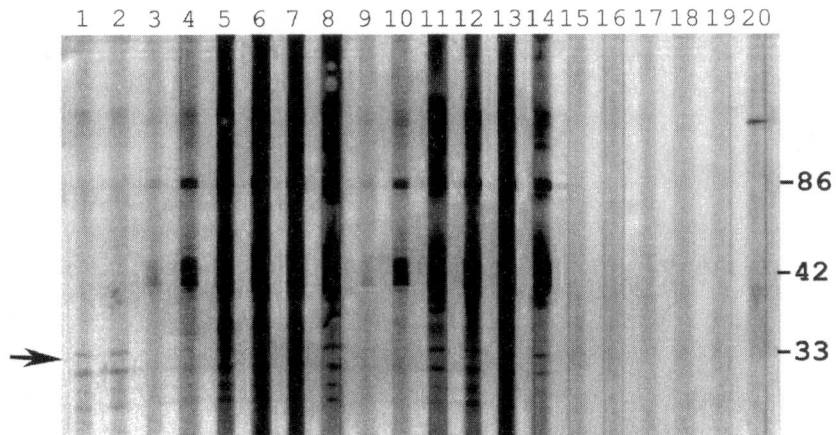

FIGURE 2. Western blot of purified mAbs reacting against purified *M. bovis* antigen 85. *Lanes 1* and *2* were reacted with 50 and 100 µg/mL of mAb85.96; *lanes 3–8* contain 10, 50, 100, 250, 500, and 1000 µg/mL of mAb85.44.9; lane 9 is supernatant fluid from unpurified mAb85.44.9; *lanes 10–13* contain 50, 100, 500, and 1000 µg/mL of mAb85.44.1; *lane 14* is supernatant fluid from unpurified mAb85.44.1; *lanes 15–19* contain 50, 100, 500, and 1000 µg/mL of mAb85.1. *Lane 20* is supernatant fluid from unpurified mAb85.1. *Arrow* shows location of Ag85 bands. Molecular weight markers are shown on the right.

15, 6, and 0, respectively, reacted positively for the presence of Ag85 with mAb85.1 or 85.96 or both (TABLE 1).

Antibody-based tests to detect Ag85 early during mycobacterial infections need to be developed that specifically differentiate between various species of *Mycobacterium*. These preliminary results indicate that monoclonal antibodies against Ag85 from *M. bovis* and *M. paratuberculosis* might be used to provide a general screen of public and private bison herds across the United States. Any positive animals may then be given extra attention both by further visual diagnosis and other diagnostic assays available. The combinatorial approach may eventually lead to a more reliable diagnostic assay that could be used to detect early infections with *M. paratubercu-*

TABLE 1. Screening of American bison herds for reactivity with serum Ag85 by mAb85.1 and mAb85.96

Animals tested	No. positive	mAb85-1	mAb85-96	Both
FZ herd–71	15	6	2	7
AY herd–20	6	0	2	4
VZ herd–101	5	5	0	0
#'s herd–6	0	0	0	0

NOTE: total samples tested = 198; total samples positive = 26. American bison sera samples were tested for reactivity with Ag85-specific mAbs by Western blot analysis. Samples were categorized as either positive by mAb mAb85.1 reactivity, mAb mAb85.96 reactivity, or by reactivity with both mAbs.

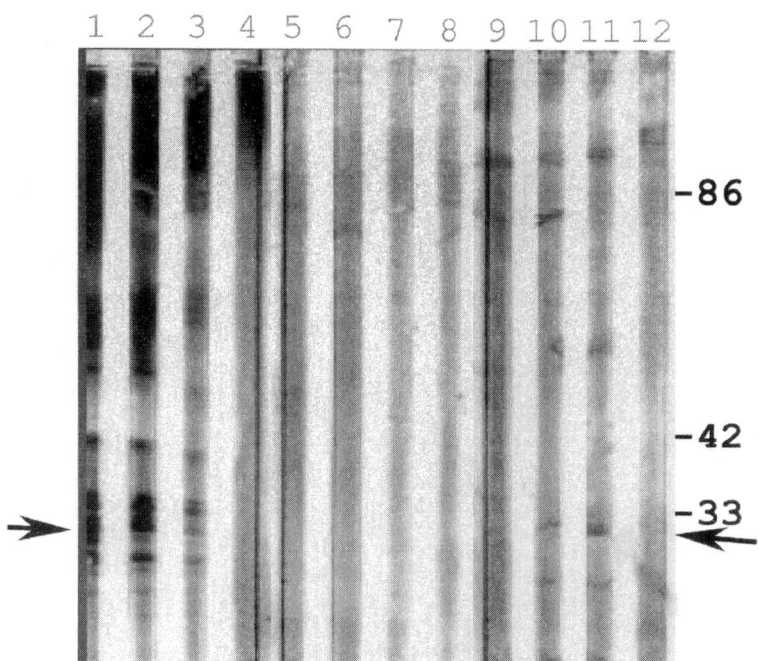

FIGURE 3. Western blot analysis of mAb85.96 and mAb85.1 reacted against purified Ag85 from *M. bovis* and sera from control bison and bison inoculated with *M. paratuberculosis. Lanes 1–4* show reaction of 500, 100, 50, and 1 µg/mL of purified mAb85.96 with Ag85; *lanes 5* and *6* show nonreactivity of 10 and 100 µg/mL of mAb85.96, respectively, with serum from noninoculated bison; *lanes 7* and *8* show nonreactivity of 10 and 100 µg/mL of mAb85.1, respectively, with serum from noninoculated bison; *lanes 9–12* show positive reactions of serum from *M. paratuberculosis*-infected bison with mAb85.96 (lanes 9 and 10 contain 10 and 100 µg/mL serum, respectively) and mAb85.1 (lanes 11 and 12 contain 100 and 10 µg/mL serum, respectively). *Arrows* show location of Ag85 bands; molecular weight markers are on the right side.

losis in the American bison as well as other ruminants. Such tests might also be used to detect *Mycobacterium* in dairy products including milk and cheese, which are suspected sources of *M. paratuberculosis* infections in humans associated with Crohn's disease.[15,16]

REFERENCES

1. HARRIS, N.B. & RG. BARLETTA. 2001. *Mycobacterium avium* subsp. *paratuberculosis* in veterinary medicine. Clin. Microbiol. Rev. **14:** 489–512.
2. KENNEDY, D.J. & G. BENEDICTUS. 2001. Control of *Mycobacterium avium* subsp. *paratuberculosis* infection in agricultural species. Rev. Sci. Tech. **20:** 151–179.
3. MANNING, E.J. & M.T. COLLINS. 2001. *Mycobacterium avium* subsp. *paratuberculosis*: pathogen, pathogenesis and diagnosis. Rev. Sci. Tech. **20:** 133–150.

4. LINNABARY, R.D., G.L. MEERDINK, M.T. COLLINS, *et al.* 2001. Johne's disease in cattle. Counc. Agric. Sci. Technol. Rep. **17:** 1–10.
5. STABEL, J.R. 2000. Transitions in immune responses to *Mycobacterium paratuberculosis.* Vet. Microbiol. **77:** 465–473.
6. WIKER, H.G. & M. HARBOE. 1992. The antigen 85 complex: a major secretion product of *Mycobacterium tuberculosis.* Microbiol. Rev. **56:** 648–661.
7. ABOU-ZEID, C., T.L. RATLIFF, H.G. WIKER, *et al.* 1998. Characterization of fibronectin-binding antigens released by *Mycobacterium tuberculosis* and *Mycobacterium bovis* BCG. Infect. Immun. **56:** 3046–3051.
8. BELISLE, J.T., V.D. VISSA, T. SIEVERT, *et al.* 1997. Role of the major antigen of *Mycobacterium tuberculosis* in cell wall biosynthesis. Science **276:** 1420–1422.
9. HORWITZ, M.A., G. HARTH, B.J. DILLON & S. MASLESA-GALIC'. 2000. Recombinant bacillus Calmette-Guérin (BCG) vaccines expressing the *Mycobacterium tuberculosis* 30-kDa major secretory protein induce greater protective immunity against tuberculosis than conventional BCG vaccines in a highly susceptible animal model. Proc. Natl. Acad. Sci. USA **97:** 13853–13858.
10. TANGHE, A., J. CONTENT, J.P. VAN VOOREN, *et al.* 2001. Protective efficacy of a DNA vaccine encoding antigen 85A from *Mycobacterium bovis* BCG against Buruli ulcer. Infect. Immun. **69:** 5403–5411.
11. RONNING, D.R., T. KLABUNDE, G.S. BESRA, *et al.* 2000. Crystal structure of the secreted form of antigen 85C reveals potential targets for mycobacterial drugs and vaccines. Nat. Struct. Biol. **7:** 141–146.
12. LANDOWSKI, C.P., H.P. GODFREY, S.I. BENTLY-HIBBERT, *et al.* 2001. Combinatorial use of antibodies to secreted mycobacterial proteins in a host immune system-independent test for tuberculosis. J. Clin. Microbiol. **39:** 2418–2424.
13. KILBOURN, A.M., H.P. GODFREY, R.A. COOK, *et al.* 2001. Serum antigen 85 levels in adjunct testing for active mycobacterial infections in orangutans. J. Wildl. Dis. **37:** 65–71.
14. JUTILA, M.A., G. WATTS, B. WALCHECK & G.S. KANSAS. 1992. Characterization of a functionally important and evolutionarily well-conserved epitope mapped to the short consensus repeats of E-selectin and L-selectin. J. Exp. Med. **175:** 1565–1573.
15. CHIODINI, R.J. 1989. Crohn's disease and the mycobacterioses: a review and comparison of two disease entities. Clin. Microbiol. Rev. **2:** 90–117.
16. STABEL, J.R. 2000. Johne's disease and milk: do consumers need to worry? J. Dairy Sci. **83:** 1659–1663.

Pan-Mediterranean Comparison for the Molecular Detection of *Theileria annulata*

OLIVIER A.E. SPARAGANO,[a,b] GRAZIA CARELLI,[c] LUIGI CECI,[c]
VARDA SHKAP,[d] THEA MOLAD,[d] FABRIZIO VITALE,[e]
GUIDO R. LORIA,[e] STEFANO REALE,[e] SANTO CARACAPPA,[e]
ALI BOUATTOUR,[f] SONIA ALMERIA,[g] JOAQUIM CASTELLA,[g]
EDUARDO CORCHERO,[h] AND MIGUEL HABELA[h]

[a]*School of Agriculture, Food and Rural Development, University of Newcastle, Newcastle upon Tyne NE1 7RU, U.K.*

[b]*Department of Biological Sciences, Heriot-Watt University, Edinburgh EH14 4AS, U.K.*

[c]*Dipartimento di Sanità e Benessere Animale, Facoltà Veterinaria di Bari, Bari, Italy*

[d]*Kimron Veterinary Institute, Beit Dagan, Israel*

[e]*Istituto Zooprofillatico Sperimentale della Sicilia "A. Mirri," Palermo, Italy*

[f]*Institut Pasteur de Tunis, Tunis, Tunisia*

[g]*Facultad Veterinaria de Barcelona, Barcelona, Spain*

[h]*Facultad Veterinaria de Caceres, Caceres, Spain*

ABSTRACT: Seven laboratories decided to compare their molecular diagnostic techniques to identify Mediterranean theileriosis caused by *Theileria annulata*. Each laboratory used either PCR or PCR and reverse line blot hybridization (RLB) to identify *T. annulata*. Five laboratories sent their own samples to laboratory 4 to be recoded and passed on to at least two other laboratories. A total of 120 blood samples were analyzed during this study, generating 540 results. Laboratory 1 sent only *T. annulata*–infected samples (positive control batch), and all the laboratories testing this batch found 100% infection. Laboratory 2 sent only negative samples from a Mediterranean area where *T. annulata* was unknown, and two laboratories out of three found a few positive samples in these negative samples. For the remaining samples, detection performance was variable. Agreement between laboratories ranged from 21.4 to 91.3%. The overall mismatch between laboratories was around 30% by whatever technique used. This paper describes the methodological parameters that could explain the variation of results.

KEYWORDS: *Theileria annulata*; molecular diagnostic techniques; Ixodid ticks; cattle; Mediterranean coast fever; tropical theileriosis

Address for correspondence: Dr. O.A.E. Sparagano, School of Agriculture, Food and Rural Development, University of Newcastle, Newcastle upon Tyne, NE1 7RU, UK. Fax: 00 (44).191.222.7811.
olivier.sparagano@ncl.ac.uk

Ann. N.Y. Acad. Sci. 969: 73–77 (2002). © 2002 New York Academy of Sciences.

TABLE 1. Methods used in this study

Laboratory	Sample processed	Method	Amplified fragment (bp)	Targeted gene	Probe concentration (picomoles)	Reference
1	119	PCR	727	TAMS	N/A	Shiels et al.[5]
2	120	RLB	450	18S	100–200	Gubbels et al.[8]
3	119	PCR	721	TAMS	N/A	D'Oliveira et al.[4]
4	96	RLB	450	18S	50–100	Gubbels et al.[9]
5	24	PCR	721	TAMS	N/A	D'Oliveira et al.[4]
6	24	RLB	450	18S	50–100	Gubbels et al.[8]
7	38	PCR	900	TAMS	N/A	Katzer et al.[9]

INTRODUCTION

Theileria annulata[1] is a tick-borne protozoan that causes an infection in cattle also known as Mediterranean coast fever in the Mediterranean countries or tropical theileriosis. This pathogen is mainly transmitted by Ixodid ticks of the genus *Hyalomma* and poses a risk of exposure for hundreds of millions of cattle in North Africa, southern Europe, and Asia.[2] Imported exotic breeds of cattle are more susceptible to this infection, and mortality rates ranging between 40 and 60% have been reported.[3] Because of a lack of specificity and/or sensitivity of traditional techniques such as tick salivary gland staining, blood smear, or serological assays for detection of the pathogen or exposure to infection, numerous molecular techniques have been developed to improve the ability to detect *T. annulata* infections. Polymerase chain reaction (PCR) targeting the *Tams1* gene[4,5] or the 18S rRNA6 were the first tests developed to identify *T. annulata* in cattle or ticks, followed by the development of nested PCR7 or reverse line blot hybridization tests.[8] Nevertheless, no comparison has been done to evaluate the validity and usefulness of each test. Seven laboratories decided to compare their results by exchanging coded DNA samples and comparing results with their own test.

MATERIALS AND METHODS

Sample Preparation

EDTA-vacutainer tubes were used by five laboratories (1, 2, 3, 5, and 6) to collect blood samples from 24 cattle in their own countries. Laboratory 1 collected the positive samples (from 24 animals vaccinated with a *T. annulata* cell culture vaccine); Laboratory 2 collected negative samples; and Laboratories 3, 5, and 6 collected field samples. DNA was extracted from all samples following a common protocol based on phenol-chloroform and were sent to Laboratory 4 for recoding. Each participating laboratory decided to work on a different number of samples (see TABLE 1). Because of logistical difficulties, Laboratories 5 and 6 each tested the samples they collected in their own country.

TABLE 2. Number of contradictory results for each laboratory (including field samples and true negative samples)

Laboratory	Contradictory results	Error (%)	Positive/negative samples
1	3/119	2.50	3+
2	1/120	0.83	1+
3	8/119	6.72	5+, 3−
4	3/96	3.12	3+
5	1/24	4.17	1+
6	2/24	8.34	1+, 1−
7	5/38	13.16	5−

Molecular Techniques

As shown in TABLE 1, three laboratories used a combination PCR/RLB targeting a 450-bp fragment on the 18S rRNA gene of *T. annulata*, and four laboratories used PCR targeting of different fragment sizes on the TAMS gene of *T. annulata*.

RESULTS

Testing of Control Sample Batches

Laboratories 1, 2, 3, and 4 processed the 24 positive control samples and found all of them positive for *T. annulata*. Laboratories 1, 2, and 3 processed the 24 negative control samples, and their results agreed for 20 of them. Laboratories 1 and 3 found 3 and 1 samples positive, respectively, among the negative control samples.

Field Samples

Of the 72 field samples, the results of 25 (34.7%) were the same for all the laboratories that processed them (12 being positive and 13 being negative for all participating laboratories). The majority of the laboratories (all except one) working on the field samples agreed on a further 18 (25.0%) samples. Laboratories 1, 2, 3, 4, 5, 6, and 7 failed to agree with all the other laboratories for 0, 1, 6, 3, 1, 2, and 5 results within this second group, respectively. For the 29 (40.3%) remaining samples, there was no clear majority in agreement of results.

The correlation between the test results of the seven laboratories is presented in TABLE 2. The agreement in the results between any two laboratories ranged from 21.4% (between laboratories 6 and 7) to 91.3% (between laboratories 1 and 5). Average match of results between laboratories ranged from 44.78% (for laboratory 7) to 77.7% for laboratory 5.

In terms of techniques used, for the RLB-based test results, a match 69.9% was detected among the laboratories that used this technique for testing the samples, whereas PCR-based tests alone gave an average match of results of 65.0%. On average PCR-based tests detected 45.53% positive samples, whereas RLB-based tests detected 63% positive samples.

TABLE 3. Percentage of matching results among laboratories

Laboratory	1	2	3	4	5	6	7	Average	Average (without Laboratory 7)
1	100	77.5	66.2	73.2	**91.3**	50.0	76.3	72.4	71.6
2	77.5	100	60.6	76.4	83.3	58.3	44.7	66.8	71.2
3	66.2	60.6	100	67.6	65.2	79.2	52.6	65.2	67.8
4	73.2	76.4	67.6	100	70.8	75.0	28.9	65.3	72.6
5	**91.3**	83.3	65.2	70.8	100	N/A	N/A	77.7	77.7
6	50.5	58.3	79.2	75.0	N/A	100	**21.4**	56.8	65.6
7	76.3	44.7	52.6	28.9	N/A	**21.4**	100	44.78	N/A

NOTE: N/A: Not applicable. Extreme examples are given in bold.

CONCLUSION

The overall average agreement among laboratories was about 70% (reaching 83% and 100% for negative samples and positive samples [vaccinated animals], respectively), showing that the major disagreements of results arose with field samples from endemic regions. To minimize the variation among methods, we collected blood and extracted DNA following the same technique. This was more constraining for some laboratories than others, however. Furthermore, three laboratories (laboratories 1, 3, and 5) followed the same PCR method published by d'Oliveira et al.,[4] and three other laboratories (laboratories 2, 4, and 6) followed the protocol published by Gubbels et al.[8] Although every effort was made to keep the variation in sample handling and processing to a minimum, there were still some technical constraints that affected the way the PCR and PCR/RLB were performed. Some parameters were uncontrollable and included (1) each laboratory in each country bought their reagents from different manufacturers; (2) transportation of samples between countries could affect the quality of the DNAs exchanged between colleagues (one custom service held the samples for laboratory 7 for several weeks under unknown storage conditions); (3) interpretation of borderline results may affect the overall agreement between the tests; and (4) PCR, electrophoresis, blotting, and color development steps were performed by each laboratory using variable probe or primer concentrations, power sources, or exposure time. For instance laboratories 2 and 4, following the same RLB protocols but with different probe concentrations on the membrane and using two different developer/fixer sources, achieved a 76.4% match between their results.

This study showed a few differences between laboratories and also pinpointed some individual problems that each laboratory should consider for future work. For instance, TABLE 2 shows that laboratories 1 to 6 usually disagree with the other partners by finding additional positive samples, whereas laboratory 7 got five false-negative results.

In this study there was no problem with samples collected from positive animals, but we raised some concerns about the validity of the tests for carrier animals and negative herds because some partners had contradictory results. This could be of economic relevance when these tests are used for importation clearance or during routine tests.

In conclusion, there is an obvious need for standardization and uniformity, as well as for understanding the limits of each diagnostic test, which laboratories should take into consideration.

REFERENCES

1. DSCHUNKOWSKY, E. & J. LUHS. 1904. Die Piroplamosen der Rinder. Rinder. Zentralbl. Bakteriol. Parasitenkd. Infektionskr. **35:** 486–492.
2. ROBINSON, P.M. 1982. *Theileria annulata* and its transmission—a review. Trop. Anim. Hlth. Prod. **14:** 3–12.
3. BROWN, C.G.D. 1990. Control of tropical theileriosis (*Theileria annulata* infection) of cattle. Parassitologia **32:** 23–31.
4. D'OLIVEIRA, C., M. VAN DER WEIDE, M.A. HABELA, *et al.* 1995. Detection of *Theileria annulata* in blood samples of carrier cattle by PCR. J. Clin. Microbiol. **33:** 2665–2669.
5. SHIELS, B., C. D'OLIVEIRA, S. MCKELLAR, *et al.* 1995. Selection of diversity at putative glycosylation sites in the immunodominant merozoite/piroplasm surface antigen of *Theileria* parasites. J. Mol. Biochem. Parasitol. **72:** 149–162.
6. DE KOK, J.B., C. D'OLIVEIRA & F. JONGEJAN. 1993. Detection of the protozoan parasite *Theileria annulata* in *Hyalomma* ticks by the polymerase chain reaction. Exp. Appl. Acarol. **17:** 839–846.
7. MARTIN-SANCHEZ, J., J. VISERAS, F.J. ANDROHER & P. GARCIA-FERNANDEZ. 1999. Nested polymerase chain reaction for detection of *Theileria annulata* and comparison with conventional diagnostic techniques: its use in epidemiology studies. Parasitol. Res. **85:** 243–245.
8. GUBBELS, J.M., A.P. DE VOS, M.. VAN DER WEIDE, *et al.* 1999. Simultaneous detection of bovine *Theileria* and *Babesia* species using reverse line blot hybridization. J. Clin. Microbiol. **37:** 1782–1789.
9. KATZER, F., S. MCKELLAR, L. BEN-MILED, *et al.* 1998. Selection for antigenic diversity of Tams 1, the major merozoite antigen of *Theileria annulata*. Ann. N.Y. Acad. Sci. **849:** 96–108.

Reverse Line Blot Hybridization Used to Identify Hemoprotozoa in Minorcan Cattle

SONIA ALMERIA,[a] JOAQUIM CASTELLÀ,[a] DAVID FERRER,[a] JUAN FRANCISCO GUTIÉRREZ,[a] AGUSTIN ESTRADA-PEÑA,[b] AND OLIVIER SPARAGANO[c]

[a]Parasitology, Department of Animal Health, Veterinary School, Autonomous University of Barcelona, 08193 Bellaterra, Barcelona, Spain

[b]Parasitology, Veterinary School Zaragoza, Zaragoza, Spain

[c]School of Agriculture, Food and Rural Development, University of Newcastle, Newcastle upon Tyne, United Kingdom

ABSTRACT: Piroplasmosis, a tick-borne protozoal disease, is an important disease affecting domestic and wild animals. We performed PCR-based reverse line blot hybridization (RLB) assays on blood samples obtained from 133 cattle exposed to ticks in field conditions in Minorca (Balearic Islands, Spain) in three different seasons. The oligonucleotides used were those for *Theileria annulata*, *T. buffeli*, *T. taurotragi*, *T. velifera*, *Babesia bigemina*, *B. bovis*, *B. divergens*, and *B. major*. The RLB technique allowed the simultaneous identification of *T. annulata*, *T. buffeli*, *B. bigemina*, and *B. bovis* as the piroplasms present in cattle in Minorca. Of the 133 animals, only 4 were not infected by any of the studied parasites. The results indicated endemic piroplasm infection in cattle in Minorca; especially important was the presence of *T. annulata*. The RLB was highly sensitive and allowed the simultaneous detection and identification of the *Theileria* and *Babesia* species in carrier cattle, which cannot be achieved by classical identification methods.

KEYWORDS: piroplasmosis; hemoprotozoa; Minorcan cattle; reverse line blot hybridization; *Theileria*; *Babesia*

Piroplasmosis is a tick-borne protozoal disease affecting domestic and wild animals. The causative agents, *Theileria* and *Babesia*, are distributed worldwide and are a serious constraint for animal health and production.[1] Some species (*B. divergens*, *B. microti*) are also involved in zoonoses.[2]

Classical laboratory diagnosis of piroplasmosis is based on the light microscopy detection of the protozoan parasites in thin smears of blood and in the presence of macroschizonts of *Theileria annulata* in Giemsa-stained lymph node biopsies and, unlike *T. parva*, in blood smears.[3] Light microscopy detection of piroplasms has low

Address for correspondence: Dr. Sonia Almeria, Parasitology, Department of Animal Health, Veterinary School, Autonomous University of Barcelona, 08193 Bellaterra, Barcelona, Spain. Voice: 34935812847; fax: 34935812006.
Sonia.Almeria@uab.es

Ann. N.Y. Acad. Sci. 969: 78–82 (2002). © 2002 New York Academy of Sciences.

sensitivity and does not allow the differentiation of the species causing the infection, which differ in their pathogenicity. Serological tests such as the indirect immunofluorescence antibody test (IFAT), commonly used to screen for the presence of benign theileriosis, also have disadvantages, such as cross reactivity with antibodies directed against other species, which limits their specificity.[4]

In recent years, highly sensitive and specific PCR techniques have been developed to detect and identify separate species of several *Theileria* and *Babesia*.[5] Nevertheless, these PCR techniques do not allow the simultaneous detection of *Theileria* and *Babesia* species that could be present in an animal. The most recently developed test to detect and differentiate all known *Babesia* and *Theileria* species of importance in cattle is a PCR-based reverse line blot hybridization assay (RLB). The essence of RLB is to hybridize PCR products to specific probes immobilized on a membrane in order to identify differences in the amplified sequence. The assay allows the simultaneous detection of pathogens against multiple probes. For the detection of piroplasms, the conserved domain of *Theileria* and *Babesia* in the 18 small subunit (SSU) ribosomal RNA (rRNA) is used to amplify the hypervariable V4 region by PCR. Within this region, species-specific oligonucleotides are used.[5] In this study, RLB was performed to detect and identify all *Theileria* and *Babesia* species infecting cattle in the Mediterranean island of Minorca (Balearic Islands, Spain).

MATERIALS AND METHODS

Animals and Samples

The details of the experimental samples have been described elsewhere.[6] Briefly, 133 adult cattle exposed to tick infection in field conditions were sampled depending on farm size over one year. Different numbers of animals were sampled over three time periods: 45 animals in March, 40 in June, and 48 in October. Blood samples were collected in EDTA.

DNA Extraction and PCR-RLB Amplification

DNA was obtained from 200 μL of blood after proteinase K incubation and phenol-chloroform-isoamyl alcohol extraction before being used as a template for PCR. The pair of primers used was RLB1 (5′-biotin-CTAAGAATTTCACCTCTGACAGT) and RLB2 (5′-GACACAGGGAGGTAGTGACAAG), which hybridized with regions conserved for *Theileria* and *Babesia*. The reactions were performed as described by Gubbels *et al.*[5] using an automated DNA thermal cycler (Perkin Elmer, California). Four microliters of DNA was added to 50 μL total reaction. To minimize nonspecific amplification, a touchdown PCR program, as described by Schouls *et al.*,[7] was used. To monitor for the occurrence of false-positive PCR results, negative controls were included during extraction of DNA from blood samples. In addition, each time that the PCR was performed, negative and positive control samples were included. Positive control samples used included *T. annulata* (kindly provided by Dr. Habela, Faculty of Veterinary Medicine, Cáceres, Spain), *B. bovis* (kindly provided by Dr. Jongejan, Utrecht, The Netherlands), and *B. bigemina* (from a clinical case diagnosed in our laboratory). Amplification products were analyzed by electrophoresis in a 1.2% agarose gel. The reverse line blotting technique has been described elsewhere.[5,7] Briefly, denatured DNA products were hybridized onto an activated Biodyne C membrane (Pall, Gelman Sciences, Michigan) onto which species-specific oligonucleotides were covalently linked. The oligonucleotides used were those for *Theileria annulata* (CCTCTGGGGTCTGTGCA), *T. buffeli* (GGCTTATTTCGGWTTGATTTT, where W indicates A or T), *T. taurotragi*, (TCTTGGCACGTGGCTTTT), *T. velifera* (CCTATTCTCCTTTACGAGT), *Babesia bigemina* (CGTTTTTTCCCTTTTGTTGG), *B. bovis* (CAGGTTTCGCCTGTAAT-TGAG), *B. divergens* (GTTAATATTGACTAATGTCGAG), and *B. major* (TCCGACTTTGGTTGGTGT), including a catch-all *Theileria* and *Babesia* species control oligonucleotide (TAATGGTTAATAGGARCRGTTG, where R indicates A or G). Every oligonucleotide probe presented an amino-linked group at 5′. The hybridization took place in a miniblotter (Immunetics, Cambridge, MA). After hybridization, the membrane was incubated with peroxidase-labeled streptavidin (Boehringer Mannheim, Mannheim, Germany), incubated with ECL detection fluid (Amersham–Pharmacia, Germany), and the reaction visualized after exposure to an ECL hyperfilm (Amersham–Pharmacia, Germany).

RESULTS AND DISCUSSION

The PCR reaction amplified a 460- to 520-base pair (bp) fragment of the 18 SSU rRNA spanning the V4 region depending on the presence of the species of piroplasms (FIG. 1A). Regardless of whether the PCR yielded a visible fragment on agarose gels, all samples were analyzed by reverse line blot hybridization (RLB). FIGURE 1B shows RLB results of some PCR products analyzed in the assay.

The RLB technique allowed the simultaneous identification of *T. annulata*, *T. buffeli*, *B. bigemina*, and *B. bovis*, as the piroplasms present in cattle in Minorca. *T.*

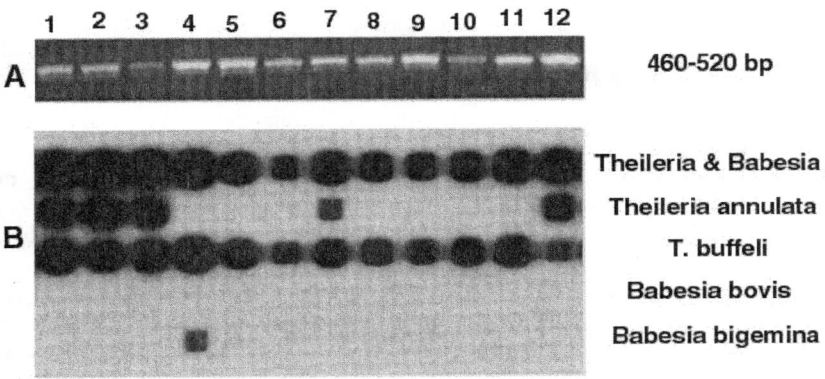

FIGURE 1. (**A**) Amplified PCR fragments of the rRNA gene regions of all *Theileria* and *Babesia* species. (**B**) Reverse line blotting (RLB) products positive for the specific oligonucleotides for *Theileria annulata*, *T. buffeli*, and *Babesia bigemina*, including a catch-all *Theileria* and *Babesia* species control oligonucleotide. In this figure no positive samples for *Babesia bovis* were found.

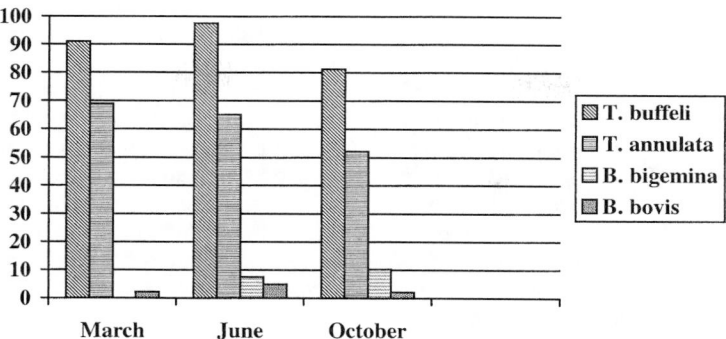

FIGURE 2. Dynamics of the prevalence of infection by the *Babesia* and *Theileria* species found in Minorca in this study.

taurotragi, *T. velifera*, *Babesia major*, and *Babesia divergens* were not detected in the study.

Of the 133 animals, only four were not infected by any of the studied piroplasms. Prevalence of infection of *Theileria* species was very high: 128 out of 133 animals (96.2% of the studied animals) were found to be infected. Of those, 119 (89.5%) were infected by *T. buffeli* and 82 (61.6%) by the pathogenic *T. annulata*. Prevalence infection by *Babesia* species was lower. Twelve animals (9.0%) were infected by *Babesia* species, of those, eight were infected by *B. bigemina* (6.0%) and four by *B. bovis* (3%).

The RLB allowed the detection of the species that simultaneously infected the animals. Seventy-three animals (54.9%) were simultaneously infected by both *T. annulata* and *T. buffeli*; whereas 46 (34.6%) were only infected by *T. buffeli*, and nine (6.8%) were only infected by *T. annulata*. Five animals were not infected by any *Theileria* species. The animals infected by *B. bigemina* were simultaneously infected by at least one species of *Theileria*, while only one animal infected by *B. bovis* was not infected by any other *Babesia* or *Theileria* species. The presence of both *Babesia* species was not found simultaneously in any animal.

There were no statistically significant differences in the prevalence of infection by *T. annulata* or *T. buffeli* among the studied periods. Although, the prevalence of *B. bigemina* showed an increase toward the end of the studied period, differences were not statistically significant among periods ($P < 0.1$). *B. bovis* was observed in a few animals throughout the study (FIG. 2).

In this study, piroplasm infection in cattle in Minorca was analyzed by RLB. The RLB assay allowed the discrimination of *T. annulata* from nonpathogenic *Theileria* species and the simultaneous detection and identification of *Theileria* and *Babesia* species when they occurred in the same animal. The species found infecting cattle in Minorca by this technique were *T. buffeli*, *T. annulata*, *B. bigemina*, and *B. bovis*. Prevalence of nonpathogenic *Theileria* species (*T. buffeli*) was very high, but especially important was the high prevalence of *T. annulata*, the cause of Mediterranean theileriosis. Prevalence of these species was similar throughout the study, indicating an endemic situation as described in a previous study in which separate PCR analyses were performed for the same animals.[6] The RLB showed statistically significant higher sensitivity in the detection of *T. annulata* compared to the PCR analysis performed in the previous study[6] (55 animals vs. 82 by PCR and RLB, respectively). Although RLB detected a higher number of animals infected by *Theileria* spp., species differences were not statistically significant compared to those found by PCR. Prevalence of infection by *Babesia* species in the present study was lower compared to *Theileria*, being *Babesia bigemina* the main *Babesia* species found. The animals infected by *B. bigemina* detected by RLB coincided with those previously found infected when analyzed by specific PCR.[6] Although the presence of *B. bovis* was lower compared to the other species, it was especially interesting because it was described for first time in this area in Spain.[8] RLB detected a higher number of animals infected by *B. bovis* compared to those detected by PCR,[6] although differences were not statistically significant. In conclusion, RLB showed high sensitivity and specificity in the detection of piroplasms of cattle and seems the optimal approach for the detection and discrimination of these important parasites.

REFERENCES

1. JONGEJAN, F. & G. UILENBERG. 1994. Ticks and control methods. Rev. Sci. Tech. Off. Int. Epizoot. **13:** 1201–1226.
2. KJEMTRUP, A.M & P.A. CONRAD. 2000. Human babesiosis: an emerging tick-borne disease. Int. J. Parasitol. **30:** 1323–1338.
3. UILENBERG, G. 1981. Theilerial species of domestic livestock. *In* Advances in the Control of Theileriosis. A.D. Irvin, M.P. Cunningham & A.S. Young, Eds.: 4–37. Martinus Nijhoff Publishers. The Hague. Belgium.
4. PAPADOPOULOS, B., N.M. PERIÉ & G. UILENBERG. 1996. Piroplasms of domestic animals in the Macedonia region of Greece. 1. Serological cross-reactions. Vet. Parasitol. **63:** 41–56.
5. GUBBELS, M.J. *et al.* 1999. Simultaneous detection of bovine *Theileria* and *Babesia* species using a reverse line blot hybridization. J. Clin. Microbiol. **37:** 1782–1789.
6. ALMERIA, S. *et al.* 2001. Bovine piroplasms in Minorca (Balearic Islands, Spain): a comparison of PCR-based and light microscopy detection. Vet. Parasitol. **99:** 249–259.
7. SCHOULS, L.M., *et al.* 1999. Detection and identification of *Ehrlichia, Borrelia burgdorferi* sensu lato, and *Bartonella* species in Dutch *Ixodes ricinus* ticks. J. Clin. Microbiol. **37:** 2215–2222.
8. ALMERIA, S. *et al.* 2001. First report of *Babesia bovis* in Spain. Vet. Rec. **149:** 716–717.

Construction and Evaluation of a Recombinant Foot-and-Mouth Disease Virus

Implications for Inactivated Vaccine Production

HESTER G. VAN RENSBURG[a] AND PETER W. MASON[b]

[a]Onderstepoort Veterinary Institute, Exotic Diseases Division, Onderstepoort, 0110, South Africa

[b]Plum Island Animal Disease Center, USDA, ARS, Greenport, New York 11944, USA

ABSTRACT: The South African Territories (SAT) types of foot-and-mouth disease virus (FMDV) show marked genomic and antigenic variation throughout sub-Saharan Africa. This variation is geographically linked and requires the use of custom-made vaccines. Adaptation of field isolates as vaccine strains is cumbersome, time consuming, and expensive. As an alternative to the adaptation process, the construction of recombinant FMD viruses followed by the production of conventional, inactivated vaccines utilizing these viruses is proposed. The advantage of such a strategy would be the ability to manipulate the antigenicity of these viruses by substituting the antigenic coding regions (i.e., structural proteins) of a full-length cDNA clone of a suitable strain. A chimeric cDNA clone between types A and SAT 2 was constructed by inserting the external capsid-coding region of the vaccine strain ZIM/7/83/2 into the genetic backbone of the A12 cDNA clone. Preliminary evaluation of the recombinant FMD virus revealed a slower growth rate for the recombinant than the parental ZIM/7/83/2, although similar antigen yields could be obtained. The chimera was found to be thermally less stable than the parental strain, suggesting it to be an inferior strain for inactivated vaccine production.

KEYWORDS: South African Territories (SAT); custom-made vaccines; chimeric viruses

INTRODUCTION

Foot-and-mouth disease (FMD) is a highly contagious acute viral disease, affecting all cloven-hoofed animals, including cattle, sheep, goats, and pigs, and a number of wildlife species such as antelope and African buffalo.[1] Control of the disease includes control of animal movement and vaccination. Conventional FMD vaccines can readily be produced from chemically inactivated tissue culture-propagated virus. However, effective vaccination in sub-Saharan Africa requires the use of custom-made vaccines for specific geographic localities due to the genetic and antigenic

Address for correspondence: Hester G. Van Rensburg, Ph.D., Onderstepoort Veterinary Institute, Exotic Diseases Division, Private Bag X05, Onderstepoort, 0110, South Africa. Voice: +27 12 529 9584/93; fax: +27 12 529 9543.

trudi@saturn.ovi.ac.za

Ann. N.Y. Acad. Sci. 969: 83–87 (2002). © 2002 New York Academy of Sciences.

variability of South African Territories (SAT) types of foot-and-mouth disease viruses (FMDVs). Antigenic and genetic characterization of field isolates indicates the independent evolution of these viruses in different geographic regions and argues for the use of custom-made vaccines.[2–4]

Such vaccines require the screening of numerous field strains, usually from buffalo, to identify isolates with properties suitable for large-scale growth in baby hamster kidney (BHK) cells. Adaptation of field isolates to BHK cells has been a tedious process. In addition, if adaptable to BHK cells, the resulting viruses do not reliably produce sufficient amounts of stable vaccine antigen. The screening process is therefore cumbersome, labor intensive, and expensive. Owing to these problems, we have begun a preliminary investigation of the usefulness of recombinant DNA technology in the derivation of synthetic, chimeric viruses that could be used for the production of custom-made, inactivated vaccines for FMD. In this study, a chimeric virus was constructed by substituting the external capsid protein-coding region of a type SAT 2 isolate for the corresponding region on the genome of a type A_{12} virus. The viable chimeric virus was cultivated in BHK cells and evaluated in terms of growth properties and thermal stability.

METHODS AND MATERIAL

RNA was extracted from the SAT 2 strain (ZIM/7/83/2), using the phenol-based Trizol reagent (Life Technologies). Oligonucleotides, targeting the external capsid protein-coding region of this isolate and containing $SspI$ and $XmaI$ restriction enzyme sites, were used to amplify the 2.2-kb region (AdvanTaq™ DNA Polymerase, Clontech) from cDNA derived from the extracted RNA (MMLV RT, Life Technologies). This region was ligated into the $SspI$ and $XmaI$ sites of the A_{12} cDNA clone, pA12MAWT (derived from pRMC35[5] by removal of VP2, VP3, and VP1 coding regions). Following identification of a plasmid (#14) encoding a cDNA corresponding to the full-length chimeric genome, an RNA transcript of the genome was produced using the MEGAscript™ T7 kit (Ambion). This RNA was used to transfect BHK cells by means of Lipofectin™ reagent (Life Technologies). Viable virus was recovered and passaged in BHK cells, as described previously.[5] Comparative growth kinetics were performed for both parental ZIM/7/83/2 and chimeric virus SAT2/A12 in BHK cells using a high multiplicity of infection rates. Samples were taken at specific time intervals, and viral titers (expressed as $TCID_{50}$/50 µL (tissue culture infectious doses)[2] and 146S content (a measurement of intact viral particles in the preparation that is indicative of immunogenicity) were determined. Thermal stability for the two viruses was also determined at 4° and 37°C by measuring the 146S content.

RESULTS AND DISCUSSION

Following the successful construction of a chimeric cDNA clone between types A and SAT 2 (SAT2/A12) (FIG. 1A), viable virus was recovered from BHK cells transfected with synthetic RNA derived from this clone.[5] Comparative growth rates for parental ZIM/7/83/2 and chimeric virus SAT2/A12 revealed a slower antigen

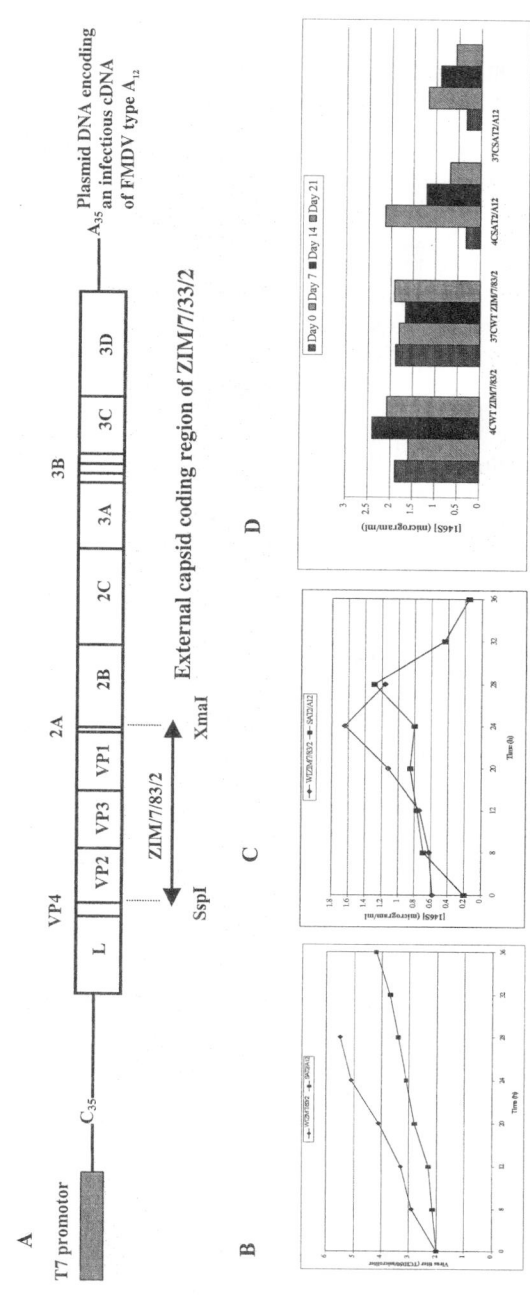

FIGURE 1. (A) Schematic representation of the construction of the chimeric virus #SAT2/A12, containing the external capsid coding region of the SAT2 strain, ZIM/7/83/2, in the genetic background of type A_{12}. (B) Virus growth (viral titers expressed as TCID$_{50}$ measured with time^2) as determined for ZIM/7/83/2 (28h) and #SAT2/A12 (36h). (C) Antigen production (146S content) as determined for ZIM/7/83/2 (28h) and #SAT2/A12 (36h). (D) Thermal stability as determined for parental ZIM/7/83/2 and #SAT2/A12 chimeric virus at 4°C as well as 37°C, was carried out over a 21 day period.

production rate for the chimeric virus (FIG. 1B). The highest 146S yield for ZIM/7/83/2 (1.64 μg/mL) was obtained after 28 hours, whereas the highest yield for SAT2/A12 (1.29 μg/mL) (FIG. 1C) was obtained after only 36 hours. Growth properties similar to those of parental ZIM/7/83/2 were previously reported for A_{12} virus, reaching high titers within 24 hours.[5] Although not performed under the same laboratory conditions, the recombinant SAT2/A12 virus should therefore display similar growth properties. The extended growth rate of 8 hours observed for the chimera could thus be indicative of suboptimal processing of the SAT 2 P1 region by the A_{12} 3C proteinase.

Evident in FIGURE 1D is the stability of ZIM/7/83/2 at both 4° and 37°C. However, after a low initial 146S yield for SAT2/A12, a four- to eightfold increase was obtained at 4°C and 37°C after 7 days. This unexpected appearance of 146S material with time could be explained in terms of the aggregation of the viral particles. Once the aggregates start to dissociate, the yield in 146S might increase. Higher 146S yields for the chimeric virus were obtained after 7 days, but they decreased over the next 2 weeks, suggesting the SAT2/A12 chimera to be less stable than the parental ZIM/7/83/2. The stability of the A_{12} virus derived from the A_{12} cDNA clone, however, has not been determined under these conditions. It is therefore unclear whether the SAT2/A12 chimeric virus displays thermal stability similar to that of the A_{12} virus. In addition, it is important to note that thermal stability testing was carried out on the cell harvest and not on BEA/formaldehyde-inactivated virus. The chemical inactivation process might also influence capsid stability. Therefore, the results presented here may not accurately reflect the relevant capsid stability of the viruses investigated.

Preliminary experiments indicated the chimeric virus to be a slower antigen producer, although comparative antigen yields could be obtained. The chimera was also found to be less stable than the parental virus, indicating that it was an inferior vaccine candidate. The reason for the observed thermal instability is however unclear, because the viruses share the same capsid-coding regions. Based on these preliminary results, the type A_{12} genome may not be the most appropriate genetic background for insertion of the capsid-encoding regions of the SAT 2 viruses. Therefore, alternative chimeric virus construction strategies warrant investigation.

ACKNOWLEDGMENTS

We would like to thank Tina Henry, Jan Esterhuysen, and Billy Phologane for technical assistance, Erika Kirkbride for 146S determinations, and the IAEA for financial support.

REFERENCES

1. THOMSON, G.R. 1994. Foot-and-mouth disease. *In* Infectious Diseases of Livestock with Special Reference to Southern Africa. J.A.W. Coetzer, G.R. Thomson & R.C. Tustin, Eds. :825. Oxford University Press. Cape Town.
2. ESTERHUYSEN, J.J. 1994. The antigenic variation of foot-and-mouth disease viruses and its significance in the epidemiology of the disease in Southern Africa. M.Sc. Thesis, University of Pretoria, South Africa.

3. VOSLOO, W. *et al.* 1995. Genome variation in the SAT types of foot-and-mouth disease viruses prevalent in buffalo (*Syncerus caffer*) in the Kruger National Park and other regions of southern Africa, 1986-1993. Epidemiol. Infect. **114:** 203–218.
4. BASTOS, A.D.S. *et al.* 2001. Genetic heterogeneity of SAT-1 type foot-and-mouth disease viruses in southern Africa. Arch. Virol. **146:** 1537–1551.
5. RIEDER, E. *et al.* 1993. Genetically engineered foot-and-mouth disease viruses with poly(C) tracts of two nucleotides are virulent in mice. J. Virol. **67:** 5139–5145.

Goat Immune Response to Capripox Vaccine Expressing the Hemagglutinin Protein of Peste des Petits Ruminants

A. DIALLO,[a] C. MINET,[a] G. BERHE,[a] C. LE GOFF,[a] D.N. BLACK,[b] M. FLEMING,[b] T. BARRETT,[b] C. GRILLET,[a] AND G. LIBEAU[a]

[a]Cirad, Programme Santé Animale, Campus International de Baillarguet, 34398 Montpellier Cedex 05, France

[b]Institute of Animal Health, Pirbright Laboratory, Pirbright, Surrey, GU 24 ONF, UK

ABSTRACT: Sheep-pox and capripox are contagious diseases of domestic small ruminants for which the causal agent is a poxvirus classified into the *Capripoxvirus* genus. Viruses of this group have a host range specific to sheep, goats, cattle, and possibly buffalo. Thus, they are clearly indicated as vectors for the development of recombinant vaccines for peste des petits ruminants (PPR). Here we report the immune response of goats inoculated with a recombinant capripox-PPR hemagglutinin.

KEYWORDS: capripox vaccine; hemagglutinin protein; immune response; peste des petits ruminants

INTRODUCTION

Sheep-pox and capripox are contagious diseases of domestic small ruminants. They are characterized by fever, lacrimation, and serous nasal discharge, swelling of the eyelids, congestion of mucous membranes, and respiratory distress. These clinical signs are followed by the development of the characteristic skin lesions: macules that evolve into papules, then vesicles or nodules in some cases. The causal agent is a poxvirus classified in the *Capripoxvirus* genus. Viruses of this group have a host range specific to sheep, goats, cattle, and possibly buffalo. Thus, they are strongly indicated for the development of recombinant vaccines for domestic ruminants[2,3] in areas where they are endemic, including Africa, the Middle East, and Asia. In these areas, the most important contagious small ruminant disease is peste des petits ruminants (PPR), a viral disease characterized by erosive stomatitis, catarrhal inflammation of the ocular and nasal mucous membranes, diarrhea, and death in 50–80% of acute cases. The causal agent is a *Morbillivirus* that has two structural proteins inducing a protective immune response, the fusion protein (F) and the viral attachment protein termed the hemagglutinin (H). PPR shares with capripox nearly the same

Address for correspondence: Dr. G. Libeau, Cirad, Programme Santé Animale, TA 30/G, Campus International de Baillarguet, 34398 Montpellier Cedex 05, France. Voice: 33-467-593850; fax: 33-467-593798.

genevieve.libeau@cirad.fr

Ann. N.Y. Acad. Sci. 969: 88–91 (2002). © 2002 New York Academy of Sciences.

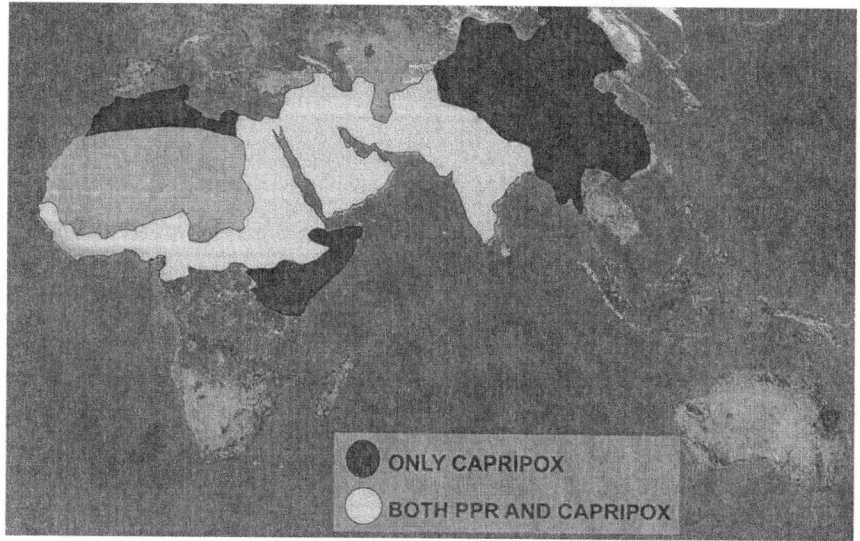

FIGURE 1. Geographical distribution of peste des petit ruminants (PPR) and capripox.

geographic distribution (FIG. 1). The H gene of the PPR virus was inserted into the genome of the attenuated capripox KS-1.[1] The generated recombinant capripox-PPR hemagglutinin can protect goats against the virulent PPR virus. In another study, we demonstrated the dual vaccine property of an attenuated capripox virus expressing the PPR F protein.[4]

MATERIALS AND METHODS

The *Escherichia coli* xanthine-guanine phosphoribosyltransferase gene (*Eco gpt*) was used as a dominant selectable marker for the isolation of the recombinant. Its corresponding DNA and the H PPR cDNA, both under the control of a synthetic promoter, were inserted into the thymidine kinase (TK) gene of the attenuated capripox KS1 genome (FIG. 2), as reported by Romero *et al.*[2,3]

RESULTS AND DISCUSSION

Lamb testis cells (LT) that were infected with one selected recombinant (rec-ca-HPPR) reacted positively from immunofluorescent staining with monoclonal anti-HPPR and FITC-conjugate anti-mouse. This result indicated that the recombinant virus expressed the PPR H protein. Its protective immune response was tested in goats by subcutaneous inoculation. The following doses of the recombinant were tested: 10^5, 10^3, 10, and 0.1 $TCID_{50}$/animal. After a PPR challenge 3 weeks post-

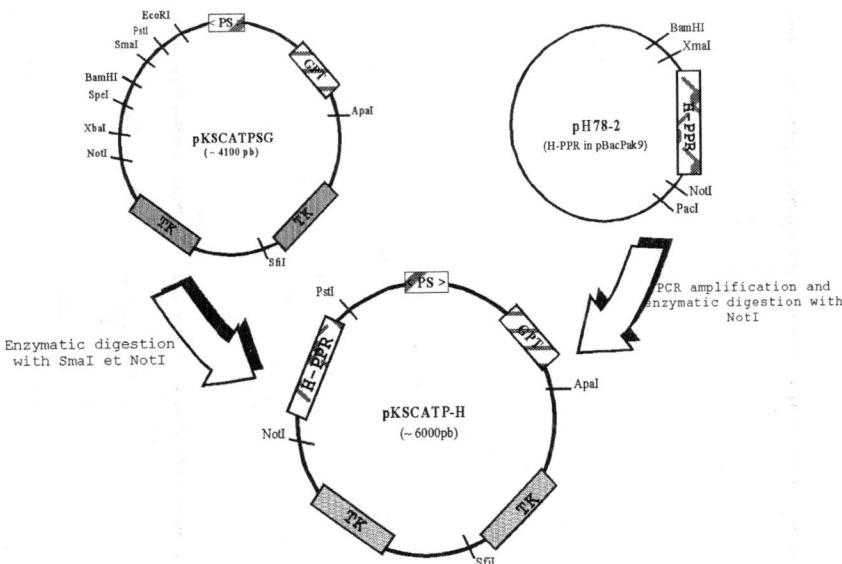

FIGURE 2. Insertion of the H-PPR into the TK gene of the capripox KS1 vaccine strain.

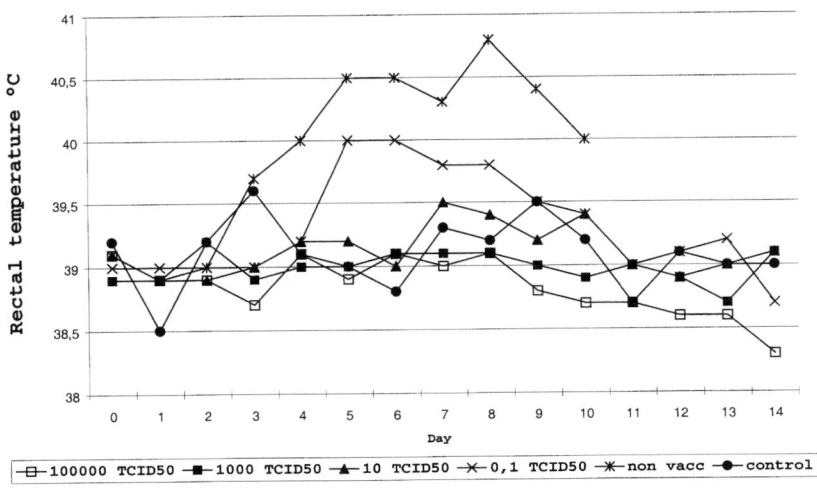

FIGURE 3. Minimum effective vaccine dose. Rectal temperature after PPR challenge.

vaccination, only control animals and those vaccinated with the 0.1 $TCID_{50}$ became sick and died (FIG. 3). These animals showed a dramatic decrease in the number of white blood cells, whereas animals resistant to the challenge did not show a significant change in this biological parameter and also developed PPR neutralizing antibodies (not shown). These results indicate that the recombinant virus re-ca-HPPR, at a dose of at least 10 $TCID_{50}$, can protect goats against virulent PPR virus. This dose is 100 times greater than the capripox-F PPR recombinant[4] that provides a protective immune response at a dose of 0.1 $TCID_{50}$.

REFERENCES

1. KITCHING, R.P., J.M. HAMMOND & W.P. TAYLOR. 1987. A single vaccine for the control of capripox infection in sheep and goats. Res. Vet. Sci. **42:** 53–60.
2. ROMERO, C.H. *et al.* 1993. Single capripox recombinant vaccine for the protection of cattle against rinderpest and lumpy skin disease. Vaccine **11:** 737–742.
3. ROMERO, C.H. *et al.* 1994. A recombinant capripoxvirus expressing the haemagglutinin protein gene of rinderpest virus: protection of cattle against rinderpest and lumpy skin disease viruses. Virology **204:** 425–429.
4. BERHE, G. *et al.* Development of dual recombinant vaccine to protect small ruminants against peste des petits ruminants and capripox infections. Submitted for publication.

Molecular Immunogenetics in Susceptibility to Bovine Dermatophilosis

A Candidate Gene Approach and a Concrete Field Application

JEAN-CHARLES MAILLARD,[a] ISABELLE CHANTAL,[a] DAVID BERTHIER,[a] SOPHIE THEVENON,[a] ISSA SIDIBE,[b] AND HANTA RAZAFINDRAIBE[c]

[a]CIRAD-EMVT, Animal Health Program, Montpellier, France

[b]CIRDES, Bobo-Dioulasso, Burkina Faso

[c]FOFIFA-DRZV, Antananarivo, Madagascar

ABSTRACT: To identify molecular genetic markers of resistance or susceptibility to dermatophilosis in cattle, we used a functional candidate gene approach to analyze the DNA polymorphisms of targeted genes encoding molecules implicated in known mechanisms of both nonspecific and specific immune responses existing in the pathogen/host interface mechanisms. The most significant results were obtained within the Major Histocompatibility Complex (MHC) where the *BoLA-DRB3* and *DQB* genes encode molecules involved in the antigen presentation to T cell receptors. A unique *BoLA* class II haplotype, made up of one *DRB3* exon 2 allele and one *DQB* allele, highly correlates with the susceptibility character ($P < 0.001$). This haplotype marker of susceptibility was also found and validated in other bovine populations. A eugenic marker-assisted selection was developed in the field by eliminating only the animals having this haplotype. The disease prevalence was thereby reduced from 0.76 to 0.02 over 5 years. A crossbreeding plan is in progress to study the genetic transmission of the genotypic and phenotypic characters of susceptibility to dermatophilosis. In conclusion, we discuss several hypotheses at the molecular and cellular levels to better define the exact role of the MHC molecules in disease control and to answer the question: How is MHC diversity selectively maintained by natural selection imposed by pathogens?

KEYWORDS: major histocompatibility complex; dermatophilosis

INTRODUCTION

Bovine dermatophilosis is a severe skin infection inducing a loss in productivity and a 15% mortality rate. This disease is due to the *Dermatophilus congolensis* actinomyces associated with the tick *Amblyomma variegatum*.[1] Currently, no vaccine is expected, and chemoresistance phenomena decrease the means of control (acari-

Address for correspondence: Dr. J.C. Maillard, CIRAD-EMVT, TA30/G, 34398 Montpellier Cedex 5 France. Voice: 33-467-593-835; fax: 33-467-593-798.

maillard@cirad.fr

Ann. N.Y. Acad. Sci. 969: 92–96 (2002). © 2002 New York Academy of Sciences.

cides and antibiotics). Breeders observed that the disease seemed to have a genetic determinism. Using a functional candidate gene approach applied in two extreme groups of zebu Brahman cattle in Martinique (FWI), we studied the DNA polymorphisms of several targeted genes encoding molecules implicated in known mechanisms of both nonspecific and specific immune responses existing in the pathogen/host interface mechanisms.

MATERIALS AND METHODS

Our study has been mainly developed in the zebu Brahman cattle populations of Martinique. Using an 8-year-long ecopathological survey of 568 animals, reared in several herds with the same environmental conditions, we classified 123 unrelated animals of both sexes, into two extreme groups. The 61 most resistant individuals were never infected, whereas the 62 most susceptible individuals showed severe clinical signs and died. The DNA polymorphisms of several genes in the following genetic systems were studied using several biomolecular techniques. The MHC *BoLA* class I specificities was typed by microlymphocytotoxicity. The exon 2 of both class II *BoLA-DRB3* and *DQB* genes were investigated by PCR-RFLP and cloning-sequencing. The lysozyme exons 1 and 2, the lymphotoxine (TNFβ) exon 3, the TNFα exon 4, the Nramp1 exons 9 and 10 and the T cell receptor CD3δ gene polymorphisms were all analyzed by cloning-sequencing. The genomic DNA samples were obtained from buffy coat preparations. The sequences analysis was realized using the DNAsis software.

RESULTS

Identification of New Alleles

In this zebu Brahman population, we have identified 22 new *BoLA-DRB3* alleles, including 7 new PCR-RFLP patterns never previously described and 11 new *BoLA-DQB* alleles.[2–4]

Genetic Markers of Susceptibility

A *BoLA* class II haplotype is the most significant marker ($P < 0.0001$) we found strongly associated with the highest susceptibility to this disease (96%). This haplotype is made up by the two linked alleles of the exon 2 of *DRB3*09* and *DQB*1804* genes.

Field Validations

Field validations have been developed in several other cattle populations either of the same breed or of different breeds in the world, to confirm the strong association between this *DRB3/DQB BoLA* haplotype and susceptibility to dermatophilosis. See results in TABLE 1.

TABLE 1. Comparison of the susceptibility BoLA haplotype *DRB3*09/DQB*1804* phenotypic frequencies (Φ Fq) between different cattle populations

	Susceptible		Resistant	
Cattle populations	Ratio	Φ Fq	Ratio	Φ Fq
Brahman (Martinique)	21/62	0.34	2/61	0.03
Brahman (Madagascar)	2/9	0.22	1/67	0.01
Gudali zebus (Cameroon)	11/36	0.31	1/14	0.07
Zebus (Burkina Faso)	7/20	0.35	2/20	0.10
Baoule (Burkina Faso)	26/119	0.22	3/147	0.02
Creole (Guadeloupe)	3/10	0.30	0/14	0.00

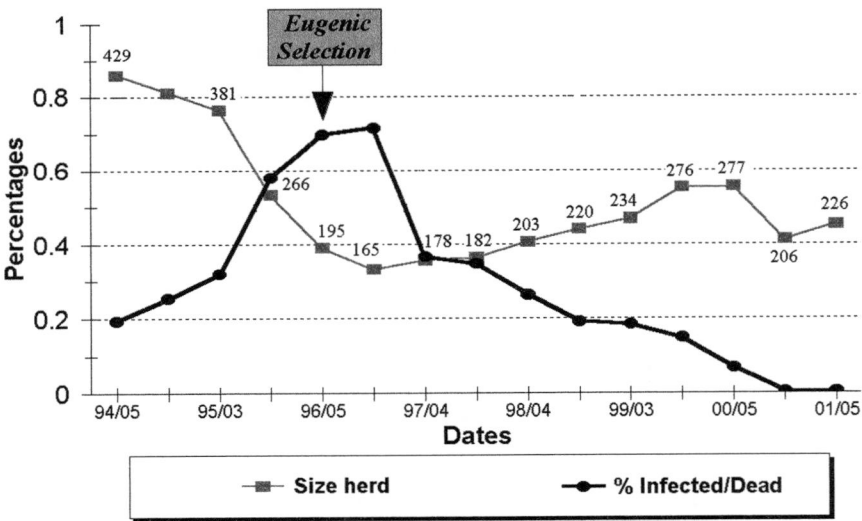

FIGURE 1. Evolution of the clinical status of dermatophilosis after a marker-assisted selection (MAS) based on a eugenic elimination of individuals having the susceptibility *BoLA* haplotype.

Marker-Assisted Selection (MAS)

A practical MAS was developed for 5 years, in several herds, in the field in Martinique Island. Indeed, a eugenic selection based on the elimination of *only* individuals having the *BoLA* haplotype prediction marker of susceptibility has given excellent results with a very significant decrease of the disease prevalence from 76% in 1996 to less than 2% in 2001. See results in FIGURE 1.

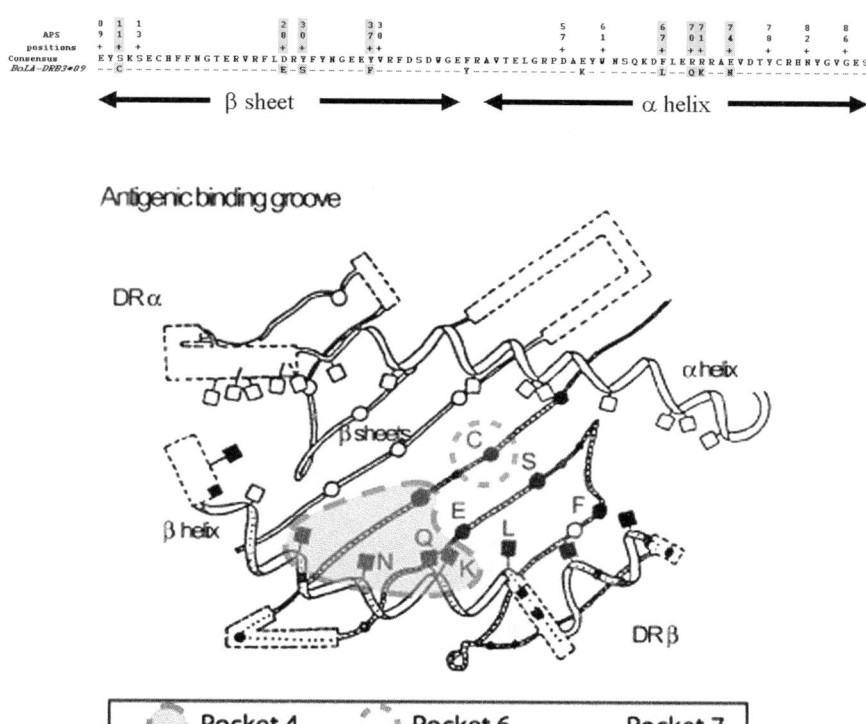

FIGURE 2. a: Amino acid residues constituting the CESFLQKN susceptibility marker in the exon 2 of the *BoLA-DRB3*09* allele. **b:** Spatial localization of the CESFLQKN amino acid involved in the different pockets of the antigen binding groove.

DISCUSSION AND CONCLUSION

This work shows a new example of disease-MHC haplotype correlation, confirming the numerous other associations previously described in several animal and human models.

The antigen presentation site (APS) is a groove made up of several β sheets at the bottom with 2 α helices above. This APS region is encoded by exon 2 of the *DRB3* or *DQB* genes and contains 16 particular polymorphic residue positions implicated in the antigen binding. The susceptibility *BoLA-DRB3*09* allele shows a particular 'C-E-S-F-L-QK-N' amino acid sequence in the APS positions 11-28-30-37-67-70/71-74, which is a motif marker of susceptibility (see FIG. 2a).

The 3-dimensional model we made gave the following probable explanation: the amino acid residues of the particular CESFLQKN marker sequence provoke spatial modifications in the bulk of several binding groove pockets (see FIG. 2b) inducing poor or different specific peptide linkages. Thus, these peptides are possibly exposed to proteases and are poorly—or not at all—recognized by the T cell receptor. Finally, the efficacy of the immune response is specifically and/or quantitatively modified. Such results have been described in other human and animal disease models.[5] This successful example of eugenic field selection assisted by a marker of susceptibility is very applicable to developing countries. Indeed, this model of selection based on markers of a highly polymorphic genetic system like the MHC allows the elimination of only the individuals having the predictive susceptibility marker while conserving the global genetic diversity in the population, with all the other "positive" characteristics. At the population level, the highly allelic polymorphism of the MHC molecules strongly involved in the specific immune response allows control of the biological mechanisms used by the pathogens to escape the host immunity. The "heterozygote advantage" and the "frequency dependence" theories[6] validate this concrete approach. On the quantitative genetic aspect, a cross-breeding plan is currently in progress to study the simultaneous transmission of the identified genotypic markers and the phenotypic clinical characters. Finally, only about 30% of the susceptible animals possess this marker, indicating that it is not a major gene and that other genes are probably also involved in susceptibility in a multigenic and multifactorial context.

REFERENCES

1. AMBROSE, N.C. *et al.* 1999. Immune responses to *Dermatophilus congolensis* infections. Parasitol. Today **15** (7): 295–300.
2. MAILLARD, J.C. *et al.* 1999. Characterization of 18 new *BoLA-DRB3* alleles in zebu Brahman cattle. Animal Genet. **30**: 200–203.
3. MAILLARD, J.C. *et al.* 2001. Sequencing of four new *BoLA-DRB3* and six new *BoLA-DQB* alleles. Animal Genet. **32**: 44–46.
4. *BoLA* Nomenclature Web Site: http://www2.ri.bbsrc.ac.uk/bola/
5. SHARIF, S. *et al.* 2000. Presence of glutamine at position 74 of pocket 4 in the *BoLA-DR* antigen binding groove is associated with occurrence of clinical mastitis caused by *Staphylococus* species. Vet. Immunol. Immunopathol. **76**: 231–238.
6. APANIUS, V. *et al.* 1997. The nature of selection on the major histocompatibility complex. Crit. Rev. Immunol. **17**: 179–224.

Global Analysis of *Brucella melitensis* Proteomes

CESAR V. MUJER,[a] MARY ANN WAGNER,[a] MICHEL ESCHENBRENNER,[a] TROY HORN,[a] JO ANN KRAYCER,[a] RAJENDRA REDKAR,[b] SUE HAGIUS,[c] PHILIP ELZER,[c] AND VITO G. DELVECCHIO[a]

[a]*Institute of Molecular Biology and Medicine, The University of Scranton, Scranton, Pennsylvania 18510, USA*

[b]*Schott Glass Technologies Inc., Duryea, Pennsylvania 18642, USA*

[c]*Louisiana State University AgCenter, Department of Veterinary Science, Baton Rouge, Louisiana 70803, USA*

ABSTRACT: *Brucella melitensis* is a facultative, intracellular, gram-negative cocco-bacillus that causes Malta fever in humans and brucellosis in animals. There are at least six species in the genus, and the disease is classified as zoonotic because several species infect humans. Using 2-D gel electrophoresis and mass spectrometry, we have initiated (i) a comprehensive mapping and identification of all the expressed proteins of *B. melitensis* virulent strain 16M, and (ii) a comparative study of its proteome with the attentuated vaccinal strain Rev 1. Comprehensive proteome maps of all six *Brucella* species will be generated in order to obtain vital information for vaccine development, identification of pathogenicity islands, and establishment of host specificity and evolutionary relatedness.

KEYWORDS: *Brucella melitensis*; brucellosis; proteomes

INTRODUCTION

Brucella species are pathogenic gram-negative bacteria that cause brucellosis, a chronic infectious disease in humans characterized by undulant fever, arthritic pain, and other neurologic disorders.[1] In domestic animals such as cattle, sheep, and goats, brucellosis frequently causes abortion and sterility.[2] Based on pathogenicity and host preference, six species were identified within the genus: *B. abortus*, *B. canis*, *B. melitensis*, *B. neotomae*, *B. ovis*, and *B. suis*.[3] In addition to the six known species, another strain from marine animals was isolated and tentatively named *B. maris*.[4] Brucellae have the ability to hide and replicate inside macrophages, where they can evade the immune system and other factors in the blood that are capable of killing them.[5]

Address for correspondence: Dr. Vito G. DelVecchio, Institute of Molecular Biology and Medicine, The University of Scranton, Scranton, PA 18510. Voice: 570-941-4817; fax: 570-941-6229.
vimbm@aol.com

Ann. N.Y. Acad. Sci. 969: 97–101 (2002). © 2002 New York Academy of Sciences.

TABLE 1. Annotated proteins of *B. melitensis* 16M and representative list of selected proteins identified on a 2-D gel

Spot	pI	MW (kDa)	Protein Identified
1	5.06	61.2	60 kDa Chaperonin GroEL
2	5.15	59.4	60 kDa Chaperonin GroEL
3	5.15	56.2	60 kDa Chaperonin GroEL
4	5.19	36.8	Leu/Ile/Val-Binding Protein Precursor
5	6.92	57.0	Catalase
6	6.79	35.1	Glyceraldehyde-3-Phosphate Dehydrogenase
7	5.73	33.1	Choloylglycine Hydrolase
8	6.92	31.1	Transporter
9	5.74	29.6	31 kDa Immunogenic Protein Precursor
10	6.44	26.7	LSU ribosomal protein L25P
11	5.52	25.3	DNA Protection During Starvation Protein
12	5.46	23.6	10 kDa Chaperonin GroES
13	5.32	27.5	Periplasmic Oligopeptide-Binding Protein
14	4.65	28.1	D-Ribose-Binding Periplasmic Protein Precursor
15	5.02	28.1	31 kDa Outer-Membrane Immunogenic Protein Precursor
16	4.80	36.5	Sugar-Binding Protein
17	5.08	52.2	Periplasmic Oligopeptide-Binding Protein Precursor

Protein identities were based on tryptic peptide mass fingerprints (monoisotopic masses), searched against the 16M genome using Mascot (Matrix Science).

TABLE 2. Differentially expressed proteins in *B. melitensis* strains 16M vs. Rev 1

Protein	pI	MW (kDa)	Expression level[a]	
1	4.88	34.5	11.9	Decrease [1]
2	5.96	66.5	6.4	
3	6.48	48.8	4.6	
4	5.16	33.7	3.9	
5	6.10	60.4	3.8	
6	6.27	19.3	3.6	
7	5.02	33.0	3.5	
8	5.65	30.0	18.6	Increase [2]
9	4.74	21.2	12.7	
10	5.42	65.5	12.5	
11	5.35	55.0	6.6	
12	5.06	36.9	5.6	
13	5.34	43.0	5.4	
14	5.63	72.1	5.4	
15	5.30	33.9	4.8	
16	5.71	55.9	4.7	

[a]Each value is the volume ratio of matched spots between 16M and Rev 1.
[1]$V_{16M}/V_{Rev\ 1}$; [2]$V_{Rev\ 1}/V_{16M}$

The genome of *B. melitensis* strain 16M (Biotype 1, ATCC 23456) has been sequenced, annotated, and extensively analyzed. The genome is composed of 3.29 mb distributed over two circular chromosomes of 2.11 mb and 1.18 mb and predicted to encode for 2,920 ORFs.[6] More recent annotation of the genome placed the predicted number of ORFs at 3,197. To describe the protein complement of the *B. melitensis* genome, a global proteomics study was conducted using two-dimensional gel electrophoresis for high-resolution protein separation combined with mass spectrometry for protein identification.

Comprehensive mapping and identification of all the expressed proteins were initiated for *B. melitensis* virulent strain 16M and its attenuated vaccine strain Rev 1. Total proteins were first separated by IEF in the first dimension using immobilized pH gradient (IPG) strips with a pH range of 3–10, followed by 10% tricine SDS-PAGE in the second dimension. At this broad pH range, about 500 proteins were visualized on two-dimensional gels (data not shown). This number is significantly below the predicted 3,197 ORFs for this organism. Using overlapping IPG strips with narrow pH ranges (i.e., 3–5, 4.5–5.5, 5–6, 4–7, 6–9, and 6–11), a significantly greater number of protein spots was generated on two-dimensional gels. Thus, at pH 4.5–5.5, more than 400 protein spots were visualized. By systematically "opening up" spots at a narrow pH range and excluding overlaps so that every protein was counted only once, the total number of protein spots detected increased from 500 to 883. Previous studies on *B. melitensis* and other brucellae used only one range of pH, either from 4.7–7.0 or from 3.0–8.0.[7,8]

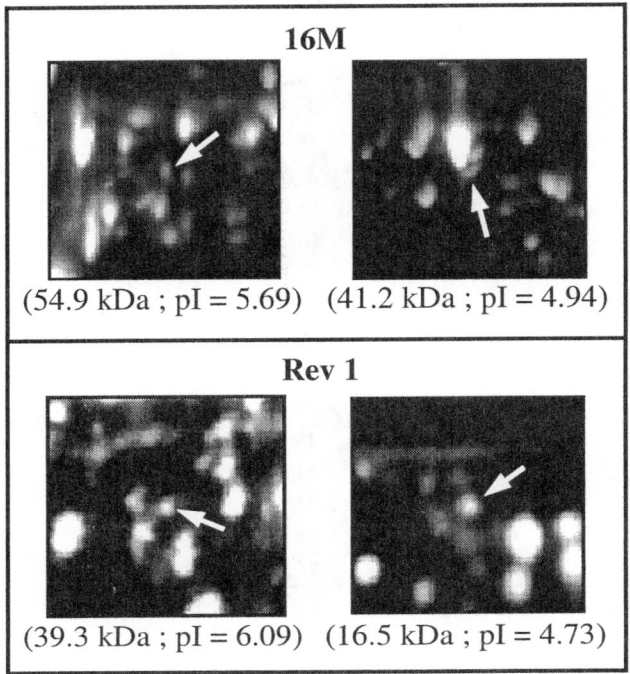

FIGURE 1. Uniquely expressed proteins in *B. melitensis*.

Global identification of *B. melitensis* proteins by MALDI-TOF-MS is currently being undertaken. Peptide mass fingerprint data were searched against the annotated 16M genomic database using the Mascot search engine from Matrix Science. To date, more than 400 distinct protein spots were identified on two-dimensional gels. Some of these proteins are presented in TABLE 1. Identification of the remaining proteins is in progress. Computer-assisted analysis of protein accumulation also indicates that strains 16M and Rev 1 are metabolically distinguishable from each other as shown by the presence of several classes of differentially expressed proteins in each strain. These proteins were grouped into three major classes, namely, uniquely expressed, highly induced, and highly repressed (TABLE 2 and FIG. 1). Identification of these proteins using mass spectrometry is in progress.

REFERENCES

1. CORBEL, J.M. 1997. Brucellosis: an overview. Emerg. Infect. Dis. **2:** 213–221.
2. NICOLETTI, P. 1989. Relationship between animal and human disease. *In* Brucellosis: Clinical and Laboratory Aspects. E.J. Young & M.J. Corbet, Eds.: 41–51. CRC Press, Inc. Boca Raton, FL.
3. CORBEL, M.J. & W.J. BRINLEY-MORGAN. 1984. Genus *Brucella* Meyer and Shaw 1920, 173[AL]. *In* Bergey's Manual of Systematic Bacteriology. N.R. Krieg & J.G. Holt, eds. vol. **1:** 377–388. Williams & Wilkins Co. Baltimore, MD.

4. ROSS, H.M., G. FOSTER, R.J. REID, *et al.* 1994. *Brucella* infection in sea mammals. Vet. Rec. **132:** 359.

5. CORBEIL, L.B., K. BLAU, T.J. INZANA, *et al.* 1988. Killing of *Brucella abortus* by bovine serum. Infect. Immun. **56:** 3251–3261.

6. DELVECCHIO, V.G., R.J. REDKAR, G. PATRA, *et al.* 2001. The *Brucella melitensis* genome sequencing project. Proceedings of the American Society for Microbiology and The Institute for Genomic Research Conference on Microbial Genomes, Monterey, CA, January 28–31, p. 38.

7. TEIXEIRA-GOMES, A.P., A. CLOECKAERT & M.S. ZYGMUNT. 2000. Characterization of heat, oxidative, and acid stress responses in *Brucella melitensis*. Infect. Immun. **68:** 2954–2961.

8. RAFIE-KOLPIN, M., R.C. ESSENBERG & J.H. WYCKOFF, III. 1996. Identification and comparison of macrophage-induced proteins and proteins induced under various stress conditions in *Brucella abortus*. Infect. Immun. **64:** 5274–5283.

Evaluation of *Brucella abortus* Strain RB51 and Strain 19 in Pronghorn Antelope

PHILIP H. ELZER, [a] J. SMITH,[a] T. ROFFE,[b] T. KREEGER,[c] J. EDWARDS,[d] AND D. DAVIS[d]

[a]*Louisiana State University, AgCenter and School of Veterinary Medicine, Baton Rouge, Louisiana 70803, USA*

[b]*USGS, Biological Resources, Bozeman, Montana 59715, USA*

[c]*Wyoming Game and Fish, Laramie, Wyoming 82201, USA*

[d]*Texas A&M University, School of Veterinary Medicine, College Station, Texas 77843, USA*

ABSTRACT: Free-roaming elk and bison in the Greater Yellowstone Area remain the only wildlife reservoirs for *Brucella abortus* in the United States, and the large number of animals and a lack of holding facilities make it unreasonable to individually vaccinate each animal. Therefore, oral delivery is being proposed as a possible option to vaccinate these wild ungulates. One of the main problems associated with oral vaccination is the potential exposure of nontarget species to the vaccines. The purpose of this study was to determine the effects of two *Brucella* vaccines, strain 19 (S19) and the rough strain RB51 (SRB51), in pregnant pronghorn antelope. We conclude that S19 and SRB51 rarely colonize maternal and fetal tissues of pregnant pronghorn and were not associated with fetal death. Oral delivery of either vaccine at this dose appears to be nonhazardous to pregnant pronghorn.

KEYWORDS: *Brucella abortus*; vaccination; pronghorn antelope

INTRODUCTION

A major concern involved with using oral brucellosis vaccines is that nontarget species may inadvertently be exposed to the vaccines and that exposure to these agents could potentially cause reproductive failure in such species. The purpose of this study was to determine if oral vaccination had detrimental effects on reproduction in pronghorn antelope. These nontarget ruminants could possibly be exposed to *Brucella* vaccines (*Brucella abortus* strain 19 or strain RB51)[1–4] used in the eradication and control of brucellosis in elk and bison.

Wild ungulates are susceptible to the infection and disease known as brucellosis. *Brucella abortus* can infect elk (*Cervus elaphus*), and under experimental procedures, elk have transmitted the disease to cattle.[5] Circumstantial evidence indicates that elk have transmitted brucellosis to cattle under natural conditions. The Greater

Address for correspondence: Dr. Philip H. Elzer, LSU Department of Veterinary Science, 111 Dalrymple Building, Baton Rouge, LA 70803, USA. Voice: 225-578-4763; fax: 225-578-4890. pelzer@agctr.lsu.edu

Ann. N.Y. Acad. Sci. 969: 102–105 (2002). © 2002 New York Academy of Sciences.

Yellowstone Area (GYA) contains the largest free-ranging populations of elk and bison (*Bison bison*) in the world. For economic and human health purposes, a cooperative state/federal bovine brucellosis eradication program began in 1934 with the goal of eliminating bovine brucellosis from the United States. The target date for achieving that goal was the end of 1998. The reservoir of brucellosis in wildlife in the GYA creates a conflict with this goal because of the continuing presence of *B. abortus* and the possible risk of brucellosis transmission from wildlife to livestock.[6,7]

The eradication of brucellosis has been addressed in livestock by three methods: (1) depopulation of all animals within a herd upon infection or exposure to *B. abortus* by any member of that herd; (2) test and slaughter within a herd of the individual animals that are infected with the organism; and (3) whole-herd vaccination, which decreases infection and transmission with the eventual elimination of the disease through testing and attrition of infected animals. For either of the first two methods to be employed in the eradication of the disease in the GYA, thousands of elk would have to be slaughtered. It is highly unlikely that the American public, through legal and political opposition, would allow this to occur, even if this action were feasible. Thus, widespread vaccination of elk and bison is probably the only acceptable means of controlling or eliminating wildlife brucellosis from the GYA.

Three primary vaccination methods are currently used for wildlife: (1) ballistic vaccination whereby vaccine is delivered to individual animals by means of a bio-bullet or dart; (2) widespread oral vaccination using baits or treated food distributed within the target animals' environment; or (3) recombinant viruses expressing desired antigens that spread by contagious infection among target animals.

Although successfully used with elk on feedgrounds, there are limitations to ballistic vaccination: (1) individual animals must be located; (2) animals must be approached to within a distance of ≤ 100 feet; and (3) target animals must be successfully struck and inoculated with the vaccine. Oral exposure may address the limitations of ballistic delivery and holds promise for brucellosis vaccination.

Widespread oral vaccination for rabies in foxes (*Vulpes vulpes*) has been developed and successfully implemented in several countries.[8] Oral vaccinations would potentially expose more target animals to the vaccine at a lower cost per animal than would ballistic vaccination. However, successful oral vaccination would require that: (1) the target animal come in contact with the vaccine; (2) the vaccine be ingested by the target animal; (3) the target animal consume a dose sufficient to invoke the desired immune response; and (4) nontarget animals are not adversely affected.

The specific objectives are: (1) to determine the effect of oral vaccination with *B. abortus* strain 19 (S19) in pregnant pronghorn antelope; and (2) to determine the effect of oral vaccination with *B. abortus* strain RB51 (SRB51) in pregnant pronghorn antelope.

To test the hypothesis that "exposure to S19 or SRB51 will not cause any adverse effects on reproduction in pronghorn antelope," the following experimental study was designed.

MATERIALS AND METHODS

Source and Husbandry. Pronghorn antelope were captured with the assistance of the Wyoming Department of Game and Fish. The animals were transported to Texas

A&M University, College Station, Texas. Animals were housed throughout this study at the Texas A&M large animal biocontainment research farm, which is approved for brucellosis research through the USDA and the CDC.

Animals. Ninety pronghorn sexually mature female antelopes were included.

Vaccines. S19 was administered at 1×10^{10} cfu, and SRB51 was administered at 1×10^{10} cfu. These doses were used in accordance with previously published results using the oral vaccination route.[9–12]

Route. Oral vaccination was performed through scarification of the oral mucosa with a wire brush, and the vaccine was placed into the animal's oral cavity. This method for oral vaccination is similar to one the investigators used to orally expose cattle, goats, elk, and bison to *Brucella* vaccines.[9]

Groups. The groups were as follows: (1) saline, 30 animals; (2) S19, 30 animals; and (3) SRB51, 30 animals.

Delivery status was monitored for each animal; and abortions and live and dead births were recorded. Fetuses and dams were necropsied to obtain samples for histology and bacteriology. The following samples were taken: liver, spleen, lung, abomasal fluid, maternal lymph nodes, and the entire reproductive tract.

Owing to unforeseen mortality problems, acute (within 45 days postvaccination) and chronic, the pronghorn antelope were subsequently euthanized throughout the experiment. Acute mortality was due to capture-related problems that included stress, heat, *Pasteurella* pneumonia, and trauma. Foot rot and gram-negative pneumonia contributed to chronic mortality. Despite this, the effects of vaccination on colonization and maintenance of pregnancy were determined.

RESULTS

All of the pronghorns remained pregnant throughout the experiment regardless of vaccine exposure or other health-related problems. Histopathologic examination of the reproductive tracts and lymphoid tissues revealed no *Brucella*-associated lesions in any of the animals. All reproductive tracts appeared healthy and normal.

Tissues were cultured for the presence of the *Brucella* vaccines. Two early gestational animals had positive abomasal cultures; one animal had 3 cfu of SRB51 and another, 2 cfu of S19. Cultures from two animals in mid-gestation were positive for S19; 1 cfu in a fetal liver and 1 cfu from a placenta. There were no *Brucella* culture-positive animals in the saline control group or in any of the late gestational animals.

CONCLUSIONS AND SUMMARY

Oral vaccination with S19 or SRB51 in pregnant pronghorn antelope **did not** cause any abortions, any adverse effects on the reproductive tract, any problems with maintaining pregnancy, and any chronic infections of dam or fetus (no culture-positive animals at late gestation).

SRB51 and S19 rarely colonized maternal or fetal tissues of pregnant pronghorn exposed to the described oral vaccine doses and were not associated with fetal death. Inadvertent oral exposure of pregnant pronghorn antelope to these vaccines appears to pose no threat of infection or abortion.

REFERENCES

1. ENRIGHT, F.M. & P. NICOLETTI. 1994. Vaccination against brucellosis. *In* Proceedings of the National Brucellosis Symposium, Jackson Hole, Wyoming, pp. 222–235.
2. JIMENEZ DE BAGUES, M.P., P.H. ELZER, S.M. JONES, *et al.* 1994. Vaccination with *Brucella abortus* rough mutant RB51 protects BALB/c mice against virulent strains of *B. abortus, melitensis* and *ovis.* Infect. Immun. **62:** 4990–4996.
3. ROOP, R.M., G. JEFFERS, T. BAGCHI, *et al.* 1991. Experimental infection of goat fetuses *in utero* with a stable rough mutant of *B. abortus.* Res. Vet. Sci. **51:** 123–127.
4. SCHURIG, G.G., R.M. ROOP, T. BAGCHI, *et al.* 1991. Biological properties of RB51; a stable rough strain of *Brucella abortus.* Vet. Microbiol. **28:** 171–188.
5. THORNE, E.T., J.K. MORTON, F.M. BLUNT, *et al.* 1978. Brucellosis in elk. II. Clinical effects and means of transmission as determined through artificial infection. J. Wildl. Dis. **14:** 280–284.
6. THORNE, E.T. & J.K. MORTON. 1975. The incidence and importance of brucellosis in elk in northwestern Wyoming. Job Compl. Rep., Fed. Aid in Wildl. Restor., Proj. FW-3-R-21. :12-16. Wyoming Game and Fish Comm. Laramie.
7. DAVIS, D.S. 1990. Brucellosis in wildlife. *In* Animal Brucellosis. K. Nielsen & J.R. Duncan, Eds. :321-334. CRC Press. Boca Raton, FL.
8. WINKLER, W.G. & K. BÖGEL. 1992. Control of rabies in wildlife. Sci. Am. 86–92.
9. ELZER, P.H. *et al.* 1998. Protection against infection and abortion induced by virulent challenge exposure after oral vaccination of cattle with *Brucella abortus* strain RB51. Am. J. Vet. Res. **59:** 1–4.
10. NICOLETTI, P. & F. MILWARD. 1983. Protection by oral administration of *Brucella abortus* strain 19 against an oral challenge exposure with a pathogenic strain of Brucella. Am. J. Vet. Res. **44:** 1641–1643.
11. XIN, X. 1986. Orally administrable brucellosis vaccine: *Brucella suis* strain 2 vaccine. Vaccine **4:** 212–216.
12. HAGIUS, S.D., J.V. WALKER, M.B. FATEMI, *et al.* 1995. Evaluation of *Brucella abortus* strain RB51 as an oral vaccine candidate in swine. Proceedings of the 76th Annual Meeting of the Conference of Research Workers in Animal Diseases, p. 24, Abstr. 139.

Rapid Genotyping of *Bacillus anthracis* Strains by Real-Time Polymerase Chain Reaction

GUY PATRA,[a] LEANNE E. WILLIAMS,[a] YUAN QI,[b] SHARON ROSE,[b] RAJENDRA REDKAR,[c] AND VITO G. DELVECCHIO[a]

[a]*Institute of Molecular Biology and Medicine, The University of Scranton, Scranton, Pennsylvania 18510, USA*

[b]*Biomedical Engineering Graduate Program, University of Texas, Southwestern Medical Center, Dallas, Texas 75390, USA*

[c]*Schott Glass Technologies Inc., Duryea, Pennsylvania 18642, USA*

ABSTRACT: Rapid and accurate identification of *Bacillus anthracis* is critical for patient care as well as outbreak control. We have developed 3 separate PCR-based assays using fluorescence resonance energy transfer (FRET) to detect the presence of pXO1, pXO2 plasmids and a chromosomal marker. A set of amplification primers and probes were used in each assay. The probes were adjacently placed inside the primer sites and were 1-bp apart. The upstream probe was labeled with fluorescein at the 3′ end, and the downstream probe had Cy5 attached at the 5′ end. The probes are included in the PCR reactions and hybridize with the PCR products as they are formed. Binding of probes to PCR products results in transfer of energy from fluorescein to Cy5, resulting in emission from Cy5. Increase in fluorescence, indicating amplification, was monitored in real time on a LightCycler™ LC24. Initial denaturation of target sequences was accomplished at 95°C for 1 min, followed by 28 cycles of denaturation at 95°C for 0 sec, annealing at 58°C for 15 sec, and elongation at 72°C for 5 sec. These assays are specific and can be performed on as little as 25 ng of total DNA or crude cell lysate a from fresh colony. It is thus possible to determine the genotype of *B. anthracis* strains in less than 1 hour.

KEYWORDS: genotyping; *Bacillus anthracis*; polymerase chain reaction

INTRODUCTION

Bacillus anthracis is the causal agent of anthrax, a serious and often fatal infection of livestock and humans, and is one of the most dangerous biological weapons of mass destruction.[1,2] Rapid and accurate identification of *B. anthracis* is critical for patient care as well as outbreak control.

Address for correspondence: Dr. Vito G. DelVecchio, Institute of Molecular Biology and Medicine, The University of Scranton, Scranton, PA 18510. Voice: 570-941-4817; fax: 570-941-6229.

vimbm@aol.com

Ann. N.Y. Acad. Sci. 969: 106–111 (2002). © 2002 New York Academy of Sciences.

MATERIALS AND METHODS

We have developed three separate polymerase chain reaction (PCR)-based assays using fluorescence resonance energy transfer (FRET) assays to detect the presence of pXO1 plasmid, pXO2 plasmid, and a chromosomal marker (*rpoB*). The *rpoB* gene has been used to develop bacterial identification and phylogenetic analysis.[3] A set of amplification primers and FRET probes were used in each assay. The probes were adjacently placed inside the primer sites and were 1 bp apart. The upstream probe was labeled with fluorescein at the 3′ end, and the downstream probe had Cy5 attached at the 5′ end. The probes are added to the PCR reactions and hybridize with the PCR products as they are formed. Binding of probes to PCR products results in transfer of energy from fluorescein to Cy5, resulting in emission from Cy5. Increase in fluorescence indicates an amplification event, which was monitored in real time on a LightCycler™ LC24 (Idaho Technology, Idaho Falls, Idaho). Initial denaturation of target sequences was accomplished at 95°C for 1 minute, followed by 35 cycles of denaturation at 95°C for 0 seconds, annealing at 58°C (pXO1, pXO2) or 63°C (rpoB) for 15 seconds and elongating at 72°C for 5 seconds. These assays are specific and can be performed on as little as 25 ng of total genomic DNA or crude vegetative cell lysate from fresh a colony. Thus, it is possible to characterize the genotype of *B. anthracis* strains in less than 1 hour.

The genomic DNA was extracted according to a method described in detail elsewhere.[4] For this study, 144 *B. anthracis* strains of different geographic origin were used, including 113 (pXO1$^+$/pXO2$^+$), 14 (pXO1$^+$/pXO2$^-$), 11 (pXO1$^-$/pXO2$^+$), and 6 (pXO1$^-$/pXO2$^-$) representing the four genotype combinations. To evaluate assay specificity, 176 related bacilli strains were used including 29 *B. cereus,* 49 *B. thuringiensis*, 73 *Bacillus* sp. Ba813$^+$,[5] a strain each of *B. mycoides*, *B. subtilis*, and *B. megaterium*, and 22 unidentified *Bacillus* species isolates.

The primers were adapted from the multiplex PCR analysis of plasmids pXO1 and pXO2 and chromosomal marker *rpoB* of *B. anthracis*.[6,7] The probes were derived from the *pagA* gene (pXO1), *capC* gene (pXO2), and *rpoB* gene (chromosome) and were designed for the specific detection of all *B. anthracis* genotypes. Upstream and downstream probes were designed to have T_m values higher than those of primers and are separated from each other by one nucleotide (TABLE 1).

The PCR was performed on a LightCycler 24, which is an air thermocycler with a built-in fluorometer. Separate reactions were performed for pXO1, pXO2, and rpoB assays. A 10-μL PCR mixture contained 0.5 μM primers LC23/24 (*pagA* gene), LC57/LC58 (*capC* gene), or rpoBF1/rpoBR1 (*rpoB* gene), 2.5 mM MgCl$_2$, 50 mM KCl, 10 mM Tris-HCl (pH 8.3), upstream probes at 0.2 μM (LCpag1, LCcap1, and BaP1), downstream probes at 0.4 μM (LCpag2, LCcap2, and BaP2), KlenTaq1™ 0.8 U per reaction (Ab Peptides, St Louis, Mo), and 25 ng of bacterial DNA. The PCR cycling was: initial denaturation at 95°C for 1 minute, followed by 35 cycles of denaturation at 95°C for 0 seconds, annealing at 58°C for 15 seconds (pXO1 and pXO2 assays) or 63°C (rpoB assay), and extension at 72°C for 5 seconds. The fluorescence signal was acquired for 100 ms once every cycle at the annealing step, using filter F2/F1. The reaction mixtures were removed from the capillary tubes and visualized by 2% (wt/vol) gel electrophoresis.

TABLE 1. Primers and probes used to detect all genotypes of *Bacillus anthracis* strains

Target[a]	Loci	Primers	Probes	Position[b]	T_m (°C)[c]	Amplicon Length (bp)	Sequence (5' → 3')[d]	Reference
pXO1	*pagA*	LC23		2005–2027	61.2	152	ACTACAGGGGATTTATCTATTCC	This study
M22589		LC24		2135–2156	62.3		ATTGTTACATGATTATCAGCGG	
			LCpag1	2046–2071	70.0		TATTCCATCGGAAAACCAATATTTTC(F)	
			LCpag2	2073–2100	71.1		(Cy5)ATCTGCTATTTGGTCAGGATTTATCAAAA(p)	
pXO2	*capC*	LC57		1605–1622	61.7	263	TCGTTTTTAATCAGCCCG	This study
M24150		LC58		1847–1867	61.4		TGGTAACCCTTGTCTTTGAAT	
			LCcap1	1700–1723	70.5		TTATATGGCCGTAGAAAATTGCG(F)	
			LCcap2	1725–1754	70.4		(Cy5)CAACGCTAATTACAGGTATTTGTTTAAAAC(p)	
rpoB	*rpoB*	rpoBF1		1821–1841	64.6	175	CCACCAACAGTAGAAAATGCC	(7)
L24376		rpoBR1		1973–1995	64.2		AAATTTCACCAGTTTCTGGATCT	
			BaP1	1871–1897	74.4		TCCAAAGGCGTATGATTTAGCAAATGT(F)	
			BaP2	1899–1928	74.1		(Cy5)GGTCGCTACAAGATCAACAAGAAGTTACAC(p)	

[a]GenBank accession no. (M22589, M24150 and L24376).
[b]Based on the target gene accession number (M22589, M24150 and L24376).
[c]Nearest neighbor method.
[d]F, fluorescein; Cy5, cyanine 5; p, phosphate.

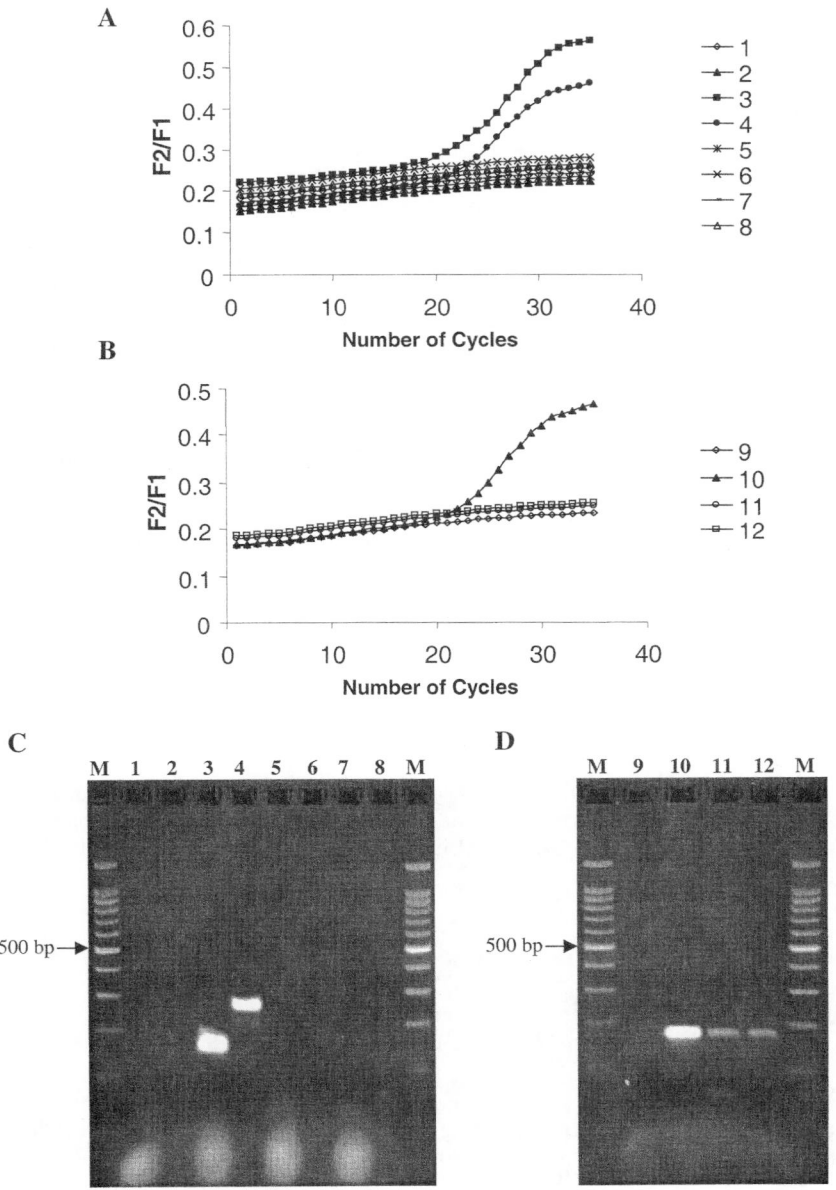

FIGURE 1. Results of pXO1, pXO2, and rpoB FRET-PCR assays. (**A** and **B**) Fluorescence ratio (F2/F1) is plotted against the number of polymerase chain reaction (PCR) cycles. Samples are as follows: 1, negative control pXO1 (no DNA); 2, negative control pXO2 (no DNA); 3, *B. anthracis* RA3 pXO1; 4, *B. anthracis* RA3 pXO2; 5, *B. cereus* 14579 pXO1; 6, *B. cereus* 14579 pXO2; 7, *B. thuringiensis* 10792 pXO1; 8, *B. thuringiensis* 10792 pXO2; 9, negative control rpoB (no DNA); 10, *B. anthracis* RA3 rpoB; 11, *B. cereus* 14579 rpoB; and 12, *B. thuringiensis* 10792 rpoB. (**C** and **D**) Gel electrophoresis of PCR products. *Lanes*, M: 100 bp DNA ladder; samples 1–12 are the same as those in **A** and **B**.

RESULTS AND DISCUSSION

Amplification was monitored on a computer tracking the fluorescence signal ratio of Cy5 fluorescence emission (F2) with a concomitant decrease in fluorescein emission (F1). In general, an increase in fluorescence indicating positive amplification was noted after 17 cycles (~12–14 min), and the assays were accomplished in 20–22 minutes. The 144 *B. anthracis* strains were scored positive for rpoB assay, 127 were detected positive for the pXO1 assay, and 124 were detected positive for the pXO2 assay (data not shown). FIGURE 1 shows the results of FRET-PCR assays on representative *Bacillus* strains. The 176 related *Bacillus* strains were tested negative for pXO1, pXO2, and rpoB FRET-PCR (data not shown), with an exception for rpoB assay for the strain *Bacillus* sp. Ba813 (9594/3).[7] Certain nonspecific PCR products were observed for some reactions (data not shown); however, all of these nonspecific PCR products were not detected in real-time mode because of the specificity of the FRET probes.[8] The assay described is rapid and specific for genotyping of *B. anthracis*. Moreover, the analysis can be performed in a real-time mode without post-PCR gel analysis. The use of the LightCycler not only increases the specificity, but also reduces the time required to accomplish the detection. The assay can be performed on crude vegetative cell lysates in less than 1 hour with minimal sample preparation (data not shown).[7] Moreover, anthrax therapy may become available in the future; at any stage of a *B. anthracis* infection, the course of the disease may be reversed, giving the patient an excellent prognosis.[9] Therefore, these assays are important for rapid and accurate diagnosis of *B. anthracis*.

ACKNOWLEDGMENTS

One of the authors (Y.Q.) was supported by Research Grant DE-FG02-98-ER62592 from the Department of Energy. We thank W. Beyer, R. Bøhm, T.N. Brahmbhatt, J. Burans, J. Ezzel, Z. Liu, M. Mock, and R.J. Zabransky for kindly supplying *Bacillus* strains.

REFERENCES

1. DIXON, T.C. *et al.* 1999. Anthrax. N. Engl. J. Med. **341:** 815–826.
2. ANONYMOUS. 1999. Bioterrorism alleging use of anthrax and interim guidelines for management, United States, 1998. JAMA **281:** 787–789.
3. MOLLET, C., M. DRANCOURT & D. RAOULT. 1997. *rpo*B sequence analysis as a novel basis for bacterial identification. Mol. Microbiol. **26:** 1005–1011.
4. BRUMLIK, M.J. *et al.* 2001. Use of long-range repetitive element polymorphism-PCR to differentiate *Bacillus anthracis* strains. Appl. Environ. Microbiol. **67:** 3021–3028.
5. PATRA, G. *et al.* 1998. Molecular characterization of *Bacillus* strains involved in outbreaks of anthrax in France in 1997. J. Clin. Microbiol. **36:** 3412–3414.
6. RAMISSE, V. *et al.* 1996. Identification and characterization of *Bacillus anthracis* by multiplex PCR analysis of sequences on plasmids pXO1 and pXO2 and chromosomal DNA. FEMS Microbiol. Lett. **145:** 9–16.
7. QI, Y. *et al.* 2001. Utilization of the *rpo*B gene as a specific chromosomal marker for real-time PCR detection of *Bacillus anthracis*. Appl. Environ. Microbiol. **67:** 3720–3727.

8. MORRISON, L.E. & L.M. STOLS. 1993. Sensitive fluorescence-based thermodynamic and kinetic measurements of DNA hybridization in solution. Biochemistry **32:** 3095–3104.

9. SELLMAN, B.R., M. MOUREZ & C.R. JOHN. 2001. Dominant-negative mutants of a toxin subunit: an approach to therapy of anthrax. Science **292:** 695–697.

Basis for the Extraordinary Genetic Stability of Anthrax

JOHNATHAN L. KIEL,[a] JILL E. PARKER,[a] HOMER GIFFORD,[a]
LUCILLE J.V. STRIBLING,[a] JOHN L. ALLS,[b] MARTIN L. MELTZ,[c]
R. PATRICK MCCREARY,[d] AND ERIC A. HOLWITT[e]

[a]Directed Energy Bioeffects Division, Human Effectiveness Directorate,
Air Force Research Laboratory, Brooks Air Force Base, Texas 78235, USA

[b]Veridian, Inc., San Antonio, Texas 78216, USA

[c]Beam Tech, Inc., San Antonio, Texas 78268, USA

[d]Litton/TASC, San Antonio, Texas 78228, USA

[e]Conceptual MindWorks, Inc., San Antonio, Texas 78228, USA

ABSTRACT: Over 500 isolates of anthrax bacillus from around the world represent one of the most genetically homogeneous microbes. There are three possibilities for this genetic stability: (1) anthrax has an extraordinarily high fidelity repair system, (2) genetic damage to anthrax is usually lethal, and/or (3) a highly demanding and selective process exists in its environment that is necessary for the completion of its life cycle. Using probes made from genes selected by growth of an *Escherichia coli* expression vector *Bacillus anthracis* library on hypertrophic high nitrate concentration medium, genes unique to *B. anthracis* were isolated. High nitration conditions generated stable chromosomal mutants that displayed altered morphology and life-cycle progression. Therefore, life-cycle progression connected to nitration, associated with host inflammatory response, selects for mutants that show life-cycle progression tightly coupled to progression of the inflammatory response to anthrax. Significant variation from this coupled progression leads to failure of anthrax to complete its life-cycle at the death of its host.

KEYWORDS: anthrax; *Bacillus anthracis*; genetic stability

INTRODUCTION

Helgason *et al.*[1] have claimed that *Bacillus anthracis*, *B. cereus*, and *B. thuringiensis* are the same species based on the finding that isolates from the same soil location have shown identity in nine chromosomal genes and apparently differed only by plasmid content. Therefore, introduction of plasmids or lysogenic phages carrying the plasmid genes could generate new generations of anthrax bacilli from exist-

Address for correspondence: Dr. Johnathan Kiel, AFRL/HEDB, 2503 Gillingham Drive, Brooks AFB, TX 78235-5101, USA. Voice: 011-210-536-3583; fax: 011-210-536-4716.
Johnathan.Kiel@brooks.af.mil

Ann. N.Y. Acad. Sci. 969: 112–118 (2002). © 2002 New York Academy of Sciences.

ing populations of other bacilli. However, Keim *et al.*[2] have shown that anthrax strains differ primarily by a few duplicated oligonucleotide sequences within the plasmids and genome. Regardless of the extent of genetic variability, the cause of such stability and invariability remains to be determined. This work attempts to determine the metabolic factors that distinguish anthrax bacillus from its close relatives and that determine its unique genetic stability.

MATERIALS AND METHODS

Mutants appeared in a derivative of 3AT growth medium[3] containing 55 g of trypticase soy broth (TSB) base, 12 g potassium nitrate, 100 mg luminol, and 80 mg 3-amino-L-tyrosine HCL per liter of water. The medium was inoculated with spores of the Sterne Strain of *B. anthracis* derived from anthrax spore vaccine (Thraxol-2) manufactured by Mobay Corporation. Fifty microliters of the spore suspension were placed in 5 mL of TSB and preincubated for 2 hours to allow for germination. Fifty microliters of the germinated suspension were added to 100 mL of the 3AT broth medium and allowed to incubate overnight. After 24 hours of growth, the broth cultures were plated onto sheep blood agar and 4X3AT (Beam Tech Corp.) agar plates. After 48 hours of incubation, small colonies were removed and transferred to blood agar for an additional 24 hours of incubation. Spores were produced from the mutant (small colonies) by taking inoculum from solid media or liquid media and transferring it to blood agar plates and incubating at 37°C for 4 days. The spores were harvested from the agar plates with wet sterile cotton-tipped swabs, which were, in turn, placed in sterile water. Using a sterile funnel, vacuum flask, and filter paper, vacuum collection was made of spores passed through the filter paper in the funnel. The filtrate was centrifuged and the button, which contained the pure spores, was collected, Other mutants were generated, selected, and collected in a similar fashion, except that an additional selective agent was applied. Such a mutant, selected in the presence of Cherry gamma bacteriophage, is also reported on here.

An expression library of the chromosomal genes of Sterne strain *B. anthracis* was generated from DNA digested with *BamH*1 endonuclease. The *BamH*1 fragments were cloned into a ZAP expression vector (Stratagene, Inc.) and cloned in *Escherichia coli*. About 50,000 plaque-forming units (pfu; as determined from plates without 3AT) were plated per 3AT medium-containing plates, described above, for a total of six plates. Fewer than 10 plaques were produced per plate of the selective medium out of 50,000 pfus plated. Cloned *B. anthracis* DNA fragments were subjected to polymerase chain reaction (PCR) amplification, sequenced, and confirmed against The Institute for Genetic Research (TIGR) database for the Ames strain of anthrax bacillus. Radiolabeled probes were made from the PCR products and used for Southern blot analysis against *BamH*1 restriction fragments of *Pseudomonas aeruginosa*, *P. stutzeri*, *B. licheniformis*, *B. thuringiensis*, *B. cereus*, *B. globigii* v. *niger*, and *B. anthracis* (Sterne). Primer sets for fragments unique to *B. anthracis* were made from the sequence data. Primers were tested against genomic DNA templates from these same bacilli and pseudomonads.

Table 1. Naturally occurring strains of *Bacillus anthracis* cultured

Isolate	Strain	Genotype	Country	vrrA[a]	vrrB1	vrrB2	vrrC1	vrrC2	CG3	pXO1	pXO2
1	A1.a	1	Italy	313	229	162	613	604	153	123	137
2	A1.b	21	Tanzania	313	229	162	613	604	158	123	137
3	A3.a	43	Turkey	313	229	162	613	532	158	135	141
4	A3.b	60	Germany	301	229	162	583	532	158	129	141
5	A3.c	67	S. Africa	337	229	162	613	532	158	120	135
6	A4	73	China	313	229	162	538	604	158	135	139
7	A4	77	United Kingdom	289	229	153	538	604	158	132	139
8	B2	88	S. Africa	301	256	171	583	532	158	120	143

[a]Variable number tandem repeat sequences (size in base pairs of chromosome) followed by those of plasmids pXO1 and pXO2.

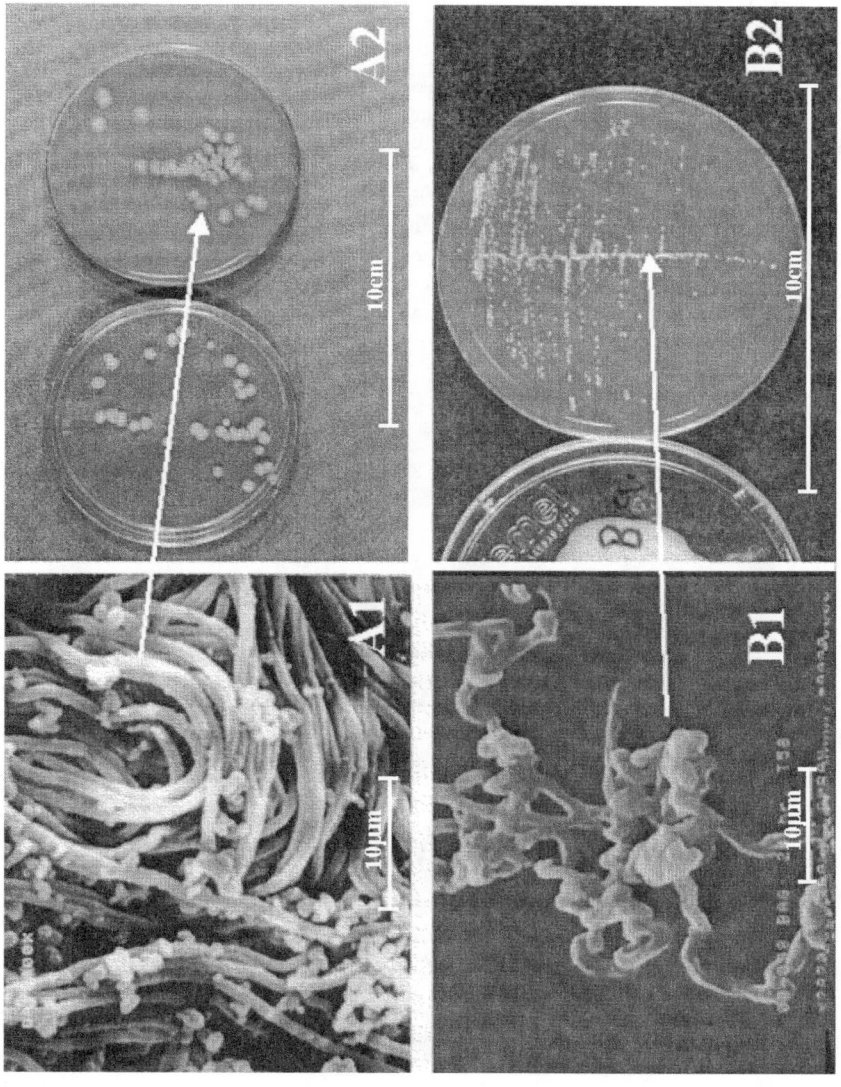

FIGURE 1. Electron micrographs and colony morphology of anthrax and a derived mutant. Typical anthrax "medusa" head (A1, A2). "Curlicue" anthrax mutant (Alls/Gifford) (B1, B2).

RESULTS

The geographic sources and chromosomal and plasmid genetic markers are indicated in TABLE 1. All strains showed penicillin and phage sensitivity by 6 hours of growth. However, the Group B South African strain showed delayed growth when compared to the other strains at 4 hours of cultivation. The Italian A1.a strain showed the slowest growth of the Group A strains. The growth kinetics of the A strains resembled those observed for Sterne, which is in itself an African Group A strain (A6).

Two mutants were isolated from high nitrate hypertrophic 3AT medium. One was a stable Cherry gamma phage-resistant mutant. The other was a microscopic and macroscopic morphologic mutant designated the Alls/Gifford (ag) strain (American Type Culture Collection PTA-3162), or curlicue (FIG. 1). The Alls/Gifford strain did not show growth sensitivity to heat and bicarbonate (carbon dioxide) on 3AT medium as did the Sterne strain.[4] Our attempts to cure ag of its pXO1 plasmid by 10 passages and cultivation over many days at 42°C failed. Alls/Gifford, like Sterne, produced luminescent polymer diazoluminomelanin when grown in 3AT medium,

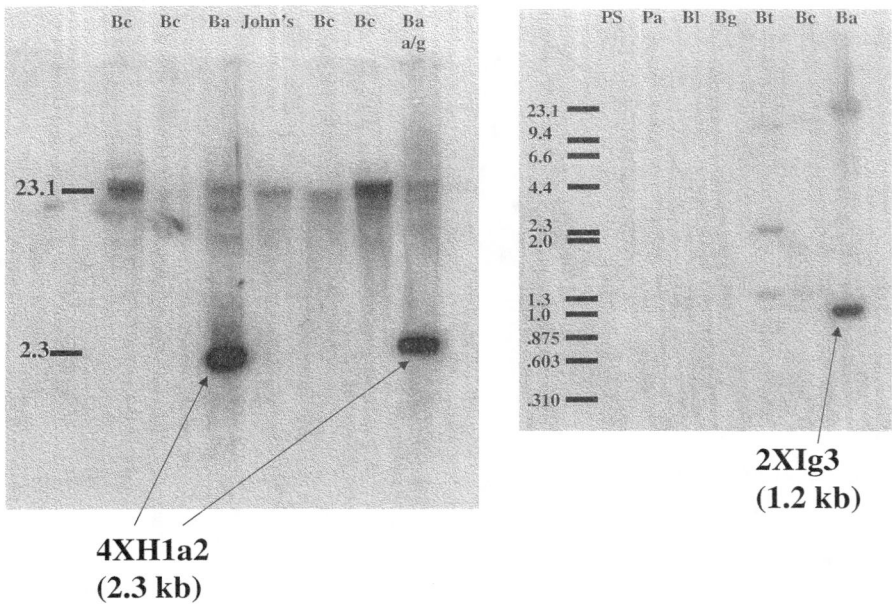

4XH1a2
(2.3 kb)

2XIg3
(1.2 kb)

FIGURE 2. Autoradiographs of responses of endonuclease restriction products to gene probes derived from a library of Sterne strain anthrax selected for on 3AT medium. On the *left,* probe 4XH1a2 applied to *B. cereus* (Bc and John's), *B. anthracis* (Sterne:Ba and Alls/ Gifford: Ba a/g). On the *right,* probe 2XIg3 applied to *P. stutzeri* (PS), *P. aeruginosa* (Pa), *B. licheniformis* (Bl), *B. globigii* v. *niger* (Bg), *B. thuringiensis* (Bt), *B. cereus* (Bc), and *B. anthracis* (Sterne) (Ba). The scales (bars and numbers) represent the location of various sizes of DNA fragments in kilobases on the gel.

was penicillin sensitive, was lysed by Cherry gamma phage, was nonhemolytic, and produced nitrite from nitrate. However, it produced minute pinpoint colonies and grew slowly on all media, uncharacteristic of *Bacillus* spp. (FIG. 1). Phase contrast microscopic examination of Sterne compared to ag in 3AT medium showed that bicarbonate accelerated spore formation in Sterne, but not in ag. In the mutant, nitrate and bicarbonate accelerated the coiling morphology (FIG. 1).

FIGURE 2 shows representative hybridation responses of *P. aeruginosa*, *P. stutzeri*, *B. licheniformis*, *B. cereus*, *B. globigii* v. *niger*, and *B. anthracis* (Sterne and Alls/ Gifford). These genetic samples were probed with gene probes made from clones of the Sterne strain expression library that were selected with hypertrophic 3AT medium. They were designated 8XH2a2, 8XH2b2, 4XH3b3, 4XH3c1, 4XH1a1, 4XH1a2, 2XH4a, 2XH4a1, 2XIg3 (new), 2XIg3 (old), 4XB, 4XC, 4XC1, and 4XD. Eleven of 14 clones were found to be unique to *B. anthracis*. Some proved to be duplicates that, upon sequencing, revealed two unique genes or gene fragments. They are 4XH1a2 and 2XIg3 (old). The 2XH4a1 and 4XC1 are in the same gene fragment. Four others provided a spectrum from reacting with *Bacillus* in general (alpha and beta subunits of *B. subtilis* nitrate reductase) to designating the *B. cereus* group (i.e., 4XH3c1, gamma subunit of *B. subtilis* nitrate reductase, and 8XH2a2). None of the genes or gene fragments selected by the 3AT medium reacted with the pseudomonads, which are also nitrate reductase positive. In general from the Southern blots and polymerase chain reaction results, one can conclude that *B. thuringiensis*, *B. cereus*, and *B. anthracis* are indeed distinct but related species.

CONCLUSIONS

Genetic diversity of *B. anthracis* has been difficult to determine until recently with the discovery of variable number tandem repeat sequences in the genome.[2] Whereas these short sequences are located in transcribed and nontranscribed regions of the genome, in contrast, our probes are for genes or fragments of 1.2–3 kb that are functional in the tolerance of the nitration environment necessary to complete the life cycle of anthrax.[3]

Therefore, they are both subject to genetic damage by nitration[5] and are inviolable because of their necessity for survival of anthrax in the *in vivo* and *ex vivo* environments.[3] The ease with which we produced stable mutants speaks against a high fidelity repair system or uniformly fatal mutations. Therefore, it is our conclusion that environmental factors acting as selective agents play the overwhelming role in maintaining the genetic stability of anthrax.

ACKNOWLEDGMENTS

This work was sponsored in part by the Joint Services Technology Base Program in Chemical and Biological Defense and the Air Force Office of Scientific Research. The statements and opinions expressed here are strictly those of the authors and do not reflect opinion or policy of any agency of the Federal Government of the United States of America. We thank Dr. Martin Hugh-Jones and Dr. Pamela Coker of the LSU Special Pathogens Laboratory for access to their collection of anthrax bacilli strains.

REFERENCES

1. HELGASON, E., O.A. OKSTAD, D.A. CAUGANT, *et al.* 2000. *Bacillus anthracis, Bacillus cereus*, and *Bacillus thuringiensis.* One species on the basis of genetic evidence. Appl. Environ. Microbiol. **66:** 2627–2630.
2. KEIM, P., A.M. KLEVYTSKA, L.B. PRICE, *et al.* 1999. Molecular diversity in *Bacillus anthracis.* J. Appl. Microbiol. **87:** 215–217.
3. KIEL, J.L., J.E. PARKER, J.L. ALLS, *et al.* 2000. Rapid recovery and identification of anthrax bacteria from the environment. Ann. N.Y. Acad. Sci. **916:** 240–252.
4. KIEL, J.L., J.E. PARKER, P.J. MORALES, *et al.* 2000. Pulsed microwave induced bioeffects. IEEE Trans. Plasma Sci. **28:** 161–167.
5. TRETYAKOVA, N.Y., S. BURNEY, B. PAMIR, *et al.* 2000. Peroxynitrite-induced DNA damage in the supF gene: correlation with the mutational spectrum. Mutation Res. **447:** 287–303.

Use of the Mannan Receptor to Selectively Target Vaccine Antigens for Processing and Antigen Presentation through the MHC Class I and Class II Pathways

W.C. DAVIS,[a] R.L. KONZEK,[a] K. HAAS,[b] D.M. ESTES,[b] M.J. HAMILTON,[a] D.R. CALL,[a] V. APOSTOLOPOULOS,[c] AND I.F.C. McKENZIE[c]

[a]Department of Veterinary Microbiology and Pathology, CVM, Washington State University, Pullman, Washington 99164-7040, USA

[b]Department of Veterinary Pathobiology, CVM, University of Missouri, Columbia, Missouri 65211, USA

[c]The Austin Research Institute, Heidelberg 3084, Victoria, Australia

ABSTRACT: Extensive studies have shown that synthetic and recombinant vaccines developed against hemoparasites have not been as effective as whole parasites or crude membrane fractions in eliciting protective immunity. A possible reason is that synthetic vaccines are not being presented in a form that induces the appropriate immune response. We have developed a bovine model system to evaluate the ability of adjuvant compounds to induce an immune response to peptide antigens dominated by a cytokine profile with a Type 1 (cell-mediated) or Type 2 (humoral) bias. In the initial testing of this system, we found that mRNA expression of certain cytokines (interleukin [IL]-1β, IL-6, IL-12, IL-15, GM-CSF, iNOS, and tumor necrosis factor [TNF]-α) is enhanced when monocyte-derived macrophages are stimulated with peptide antigen conjugated with mannan under oxidizing conditions compared to peptide conjugated with reduced mannan. The data suggest this model will be useful in identifying adjuvant systems that selectively modulate the cytokine profile of antigen presenting cells at the time of antigen presentation and the consequent downstream maturation of naïve T cells to effector cells with Type 1 or Type 2 cytokine bias.

KEYWORDS: mannan receptor; vaccine antigens; MHC classification

INTRODUCTION

The cytokine microenvironment present during initiation of an immune response is a primary determinant of the downstream effector response. This includes the presence or absence of specific cytokines, timing of expression of individual cyto-

Address for correspondence: Dr. W.C. Davis, Department of Veterinary Microbiology and Pathology, College of Veterinary Medicine, P.O. 647040, Washington State University Pullman, WA 99164-7040. Voice: 509-335-6051; fax: 509-335-8328.

davisw@mail.vetmed.wsu.edu

Ann. N.Y. Acad. Sci. 969: 119–125 (2002). © 2002 New York Academy of Sciences.

kines, and concentrations of each cytokine at the time of antigen recognition.[13] The cytokine profile of responding naïve T cells is modulated by the cytokines produced by antigen presenting cells (APCs). Depending on the species, the profile of the mature effector cells may or may not be dominated by cytokines associated with a Type 1 or Type 2 immune response. Cytokines are induced by pathogens binding to receptors on APCs. The efficient delivery of antigen to the appropriate receptor, the affinity of the antigen for the receptor, and the specific receptors activated by the pathogen determine the cytokine profile elicited.[11] Although many macrophage receptors are not well characterized, it is known that the mannose receptor is involved in induction of interleukin (IL)-1β, IL-6, IL-12, interferon (IFN)-γ, and GM-CSF.[8] Likewise, lipopolysaccharide induces IL-6, tumor necrosis factor (TNF)-α, and iNOS via its interaction with CD14.[1] The contributions of other macrophage receptors to the cytokine profile induced are unknown, particularly those that recognize oxidized antigen.

Mannan has been investigated extensively for its ability to enhance immune responses in several model systems. Its adjuvant function is thought to stem, at least in part, from an ability to target antigen to cells such as macrophages and dendritic cells with receptors for mannosylated sugars.[14,15,18] Mannan conjugated to peptide antigen under reducing conditions has been found, in mice, to modulate a Type 2 response, whereas peptide antigens conjugated under oxidizing conditions induce strong Type 1 responses with strong cytotoxic T-cell activity.[4,5,12] The study suggests that the redirection of the immune response was a result of a change in the cytokine profile of APCs at the time of antigen presentation. In the current study, we conducted experiments with a mannan-modified peptide to determine if this might be true using a bovine model system. The results show that the cytokine profile of macrophages is altered following uptake of modified antigen.

MATERIALS AND METHODS

A 29-mer peptide (ADSSSAGGQQQESSVSSQSDQASTSSQLG) from *Anaplasma marginale* MSP-1, containing a neutralization-sensitive epitope, was used in the study.[16] It was modified by adding amino acids (KGKGKGKGKG) to the N-terminus to make the peptide more soluble and provide direct conjugation sites for coupling to mannan. Conjugation and preparation of peptide with oxidized and reduced forms mannan were performed as described.[4] Ten-day cultures of monocyte/macrophages were prepared as described.[9] We studied expression of 16 cytokines by reverse transcriptase-polymerase chain reaction (RT-PCR) and RNase protection assay (RPA) to monitor changes that occur in the profile following uptake of conjugated peptides over 8 hours (IL-1β, IL-2, IL-4, IL-6, IL-7, IL-10, 1L-12 p40, IL-13, IL-15, IFN-γ, TNF-α, GM-CSF, TGF-β, and iNOS, with GAPDH as a standard).

RESULTS

As shown in TABLE 1, cytokine message was detectable for some cytokines prior to the addition of peptide conjugates. Initially, IL-1β, IL-7, IL-10, TGF-β, and TNF-α expression from resting macrophages was relatively high, whereas levels of iNOS

TABLE 1. Resting cytokine mRNA profile for bovine monocyte-derived macrophages cultured for 10 days[a]

	Presence		Presence
IL-1β	++	IL-15	−
IL-2[b]	+/−	IL-18	+
IL-4[b]	+/−	GM-CSF	+/−
IL-5	−	IFN-α	−
IL-6	+/−	IFN-γ[b]	+/−
IL-7	++	iNOS	+
IL-10	++	TGF-β	++
IL-12p40	+/−	TNF-α	++
IL-13	−		

[a]These data are a compilation of n = 6 experiments.
[b]Expression of these cytokines is due to lymphocyte contamination in the cultures, primarily γ/δ T cells. This was verified by flow cytometric phenotyping. Cultures contained 90–95% macrophages. − = no expression detected; +/− = expression detected intermittently; + = low to moderate expression; ++ = high expression.

and IL-18 were low, but consistently detectable. Levels of IL-6, IL-12p40, and GM-CSF were detectable by RT-PCR in some cultures, but absent in others. This variability could be due to subtle differences in performing the assay or in total RNA quantitation or to real differences in expression between cultures. Several cytokines were not initially detected in any cultures: IL-5, IL-13, IL-15, and IFN-α. Trace amounts of IL-2, IL-4, and IFN-γ were detected in some cultures (TABLE 1). This expression was thought to originate from the presence of γ/δ T cells in cultures. Flow cytometric phenotyping was performed on all cultures prior to assay and showed that γ/δ T cells were present in all cultures (not shown). All cultures contained 90–95% macrophages (not shown).

Initial experiments with RT-PCR showed that the cytokine mRNA profile of monocyte-derived macrophages changed following stimulation with *A. marginale* oxidized mannan-peptide and reduced mannan-peptide. In particular, IL-6, IL-12, iNOS, and IL-15 showed a consistent trend of higher expression in the oxidized samples compared with the reduced samples at 2, 4, and 8 hours after treatment (FIG. 1).

We used a panel of 13 cytokine RPA probes to assess the cytokine mRNA profile of macrophages stimulated with peptide conjugated with mannan under oxidizing or reducing conditions. As shown in FIGURE 2, graphs 1–7, expression of IL-1β, IL-6, IL-10, IL-12p40, IL-18, and TNF-α was elevated over that of resting macrophages (FIG. 2, graph 8). The general trend that was evident was a higher expression of these cytokine mRNAs in macrophages stimulated with oxidized mannan-peptide. TNF-α mRNA expression increased significantly at 2 hours poststimulation over levels in untreated macrophages and then decreased towards initial levels over the next 6 hours. Expression of TNF-α between the oxidized and reduced treatments at the 2-hour time point was significantly different, as assessed by Student's one-tailed *t* test (*P* <0.02). The difference between treatments was consistent within each experi-

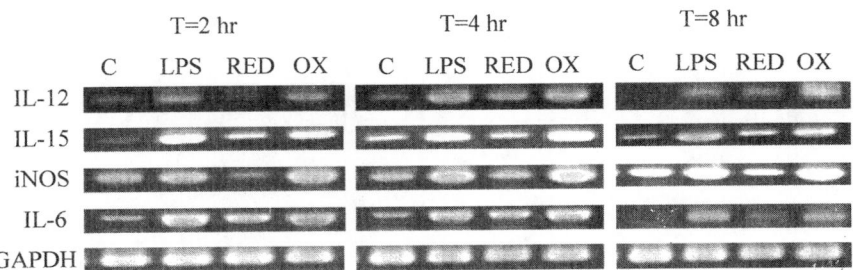

FIGURE 1. Alterations in the profile of cytokine mRNA expressed by monocyte-derived macrophages stimulated with *A. marginale* peptide conjugated with mannan under oxidizing conditions compared with those stimulated with *A. marginale* peptide conjugated with mannan under reducing conditions over 8 hours measured by RT-PCR. Data shown are representative of $n = 6$ experiments. C, nonstimulated control; LPS, macrophages stimulated with 10 µg/mL lipopolysaccharide; RED, macrophages stimulated with 90 µg/mL peptide conjugated with reduced mannan; OX, macrophages stimulated with 90 µg/mL peptide conjugated with oxidized mannan.

ment, even though the difference was statistically insignificant overall. IL-6 and IL-18 expression mimicked the trend of TNF-α, although the magnitude of change of both cytokines was much less. Expression of GM-CSF and IL-12p40 in both treatment groups increased gradually over time; however, the magnitude of expression was greater in the oxidized treated cells. Differences between the treatments was statistically significant only at 4 hours posttreatment ($P < 0.05$); however, the trend of higher expression in the oxidized treated samples was consistently seen in all experiments. IL-10 and IL-1β mRNA expression increased initially over control levels and remained high at consistent levels over time. Expression levels of IL-1β and IL-10 were significantly increased in the oxidized treated cells compared to the reduced treated cells at the 4- and 8-hour time points ($P < 0.05$).

DISCUSSION

These data suggest that the form of the antigen when presented to bovine APCs is important in determining the downstream immune response. Measurable differences occur in the cytokine mRNA profiles of macrophages when stimulated with oxidized mannan-peptides compared to reduced mannan-peptides.

Use of the mannose receptor for uptake and processing of mannosylated antigens by APC has been shown to enhance MHC class II presentation to T cells 200–10,000-fold in cultured human dendritic cells.[6,19] The rapid internalization and concentration of glycosylated antigen allow for more efficient processing and presentation to immune effector cells. In the mouse model, oxidation of mannan-antigen complexes targets antigen to the MHC class I pathway 1,000 times more efficiently than does reduced mannan-antigen. The aldehyde moiety of oxidized mannan is the important determinant in MHC class I targeting.[3] After internalization, oxidized mannan-antigen is rapidly shuttled to the class I pathway via endosomes, resulting

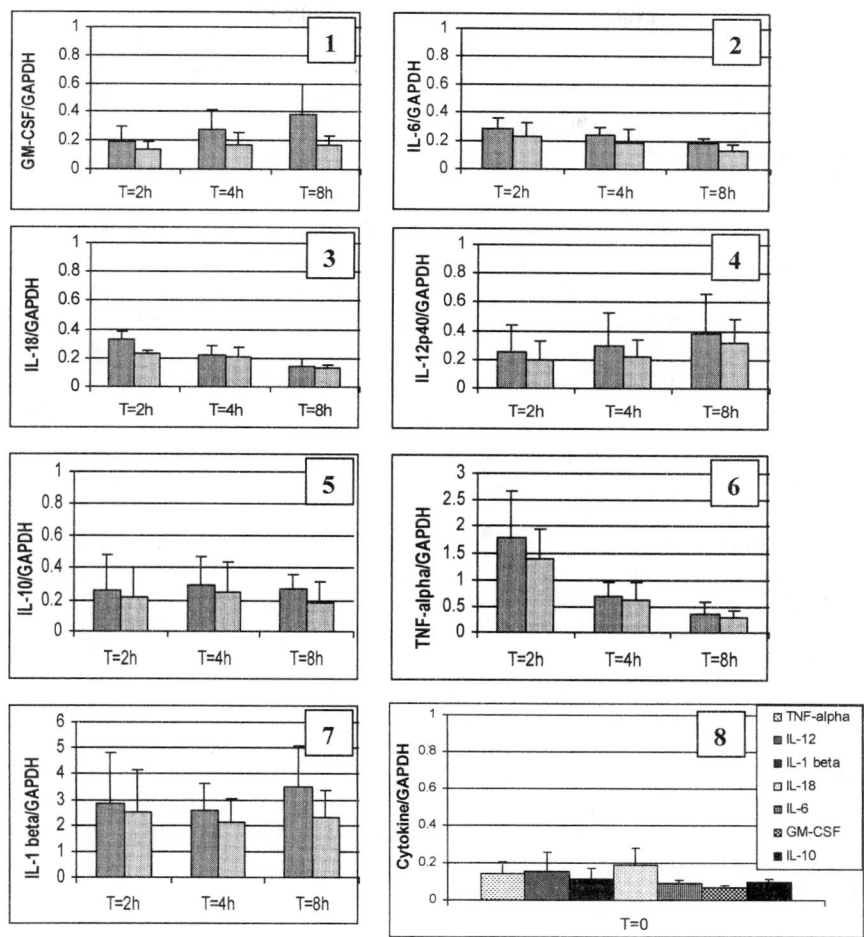

FIGURE 2. Graphs 1–7. Profiles of cytokine mRNA expressed by monocyte-derived macrophages stimulated with *A. marginale* peptide conjugated with oxidized mannan (*dark bars*) compared with those stimulated with *A. marginale* peptide conjugated with reduced mannan (*light bars*) over 8 hours measured by RPA. Graph 8: Resting cytokine mRNA profiles for bovine monocyte-derived macrophages cultured 10 days measured by RPA. Semi-quantitation is by phosphor image analysis using ImageQuant software. Data presented are from three to six replicates for each experiment.

in proteosomal processing and transport to the endoplasmic reticulum, Golgi apparatus, and cell surface.[3] The stimulation of APCs with oxidized mannan-antigen induces high frequency CTL precursors and IL-12 production in the mouse, which can be enhanced when the stimulation is performed in the presence of GM-CSF.[2] This results in secretion of IL-2, IFN-γ, and TNF-α from purified populations of CD4+ and CD8+ T cells.[10]

The importance of the oxidation state in microorganism-induced disease processes has been of recent interest. Oxidation scavenger receptors on macrophages have been identified, but they are not well characterized. Intracellular signaling pathways, such as those mediated by Jun N-terminal kinase and JNK kinase stress and extracellular signal-activated kinase-1, are stimulated by oxidative stressors to regulate expression of cytokine genes.[7,17]

Macrophages play a central role in systemic inflammatory and immune responses because of their wide tissue distribution and their ability to produce large quantities of key inflammatory mediators, such as IL-1β, TNF-α, and iNOS, and immune regulators, such as IL-15, IL-12, and IL-10. These cytokines actively participate in the regulatory pathways responsible for triggering immune responses; however, the relative quantities, timing, and combinations involved in eliciting a desired downstream response have not adequately been shown. Assessing the profile of cytokine mRNAs expressed by macrophages is a beginning step in addressing the value of these cytokines as predictive markers for induction of appropriate immune responses and for monitoring the immunologic status *in vitro*.

Numerous studies have shown the importance of the cytokine microenvironment in which naïve T cells develop on the specific immune response. The changes that we have seen in this system may contribute to a bias in the downstream T-cell response. Additional studies are now under way to perfect the bovine macrophage model to explore the use of mannan to modulate the immune response to candidate vaccines.

ACKNOWLEDGMENTS

This study was supported by grants from the USDA-NRICGP (99-02050) and the College of Veterinary Medicine Animal Health Research Center. The data were presented in part at the International Veterinary Cytokine and Vaccine Conference held in March 16, 2000 at the Tskuba International Congress Center, Tskuba, Ibaraki, Japan.

REFERENCES

1. AMUNA, C.R., T. KAMEI, N. ITO, et al. 1998. Differential regulation of lipopolysaccharide (LPS) activation pathways in mouse macrophages by LPS-binding proteins. J. Immunol. **161:** 2552–2560.
2. APOSTOLOPOULOS, V., N. BARNES, G.A. PIETERSZ & I.F.C. MCKENZIE. 2000. Ex vivo targeting of the macrophage mannose receptor generates anti-tumor CTL responses. Vaccine **18:** 3174–3184.
3. APOSTOLOPOULOS, V., G A. PIETERSZ, S. GORDON, et al. 2000. Aldehyde-mannan antigen complexes target the MHC class I antigen presentation pathway. Eur. J. Immunol. **30:** 1714–1723.
4. APOSTOLOPOULOS, V., G.A. PIETERSZ, B.E. LOVELAND, et al. 1995. Oxidative/reductive conjugation of mannan to antigen selects for T1 or T2 immune responses. Proc. Natl. Acad. Sci.USA **92:** 10128–10132.
5. APOSTOLOPOULOS, V., G.A. PIETERSZ & I.F.C. MCKENZIE. 1996. Cell-mediated immune responses to MUC1 fusion protein coupled to mannan. Vaccine **14:** 930–938.
6. ENGERING, A.J., M. CELLA, D. FLUITSMA, et al. 1997. The mannose receptor functions as a high capacity and broad specificity antigen receptor in human dendritic cells. Eur. J. Immunol. **27:** 2417–2425.

7. FOLETTA, V.C., D.H. SEGAL & D.R. COHEN. 1998. Transcriptional regulation in the immune response system: all roads lead to AP1. J. Leukocyte Biol. **63:** 139–152.
8. FRASER, I.P., H. KOZIEL & R.A.B. EZEKOWITZ. 1998. The serum mannose–binding protein and the macrophage mannose receptor are pattern recognition molecules that link innate and adaptive immunity. Semin. Immunol. **10:** 363–372.
9. GOFF, W.L., K. O'ROURKE, W.C. JOHNSON, _et al._ 1998. The role of IL-10 in iNOS and cytokine mRNA expression during in vitro differentiation of bovine mononuclear phagocytes. J. Interferon & Cytokine Res. **18:** 139–149.
10. LEES, C.J., V. APOSTOLOPOULOS, B. ACRES, _et al._ 2000. The effect of T1 and T2 cytokines on the cytotoxic T cell response to mannan-MUC1. Cancer Immunol. Immunother. **48:** 644–652.
11. LONDON, C.A., A.K. ABBAS & A. KELSO. 1998. Helper T cell subsets: heterogeneity, functions and development. Vet. Immunol. Immunopathol. **63:** 37–44.
12. MCKENZIE, I.F.C., V. APOSTOLOPOULOS, C. LEES, _et al._ 1998. Oxidised mannan antigen conjugates preferentially stimulate T1 type immune responses, Vet. Immunol. Immunopathol. **63:** 185–190.
13. MEDZHITOV, R. & C.A. JANEWAY. 1998. Innate immune recognition and control of adaptive immune responses. Semin. Immunol. **10:** 351–353.
14. OHISHI K., H. KABEYA, H. AMANUMA & M. ONUMA. 1996. Induction of bovine leukaemia virus Env-specific Th-1 type immunity in mice by vaccination with short synthesized peptide-liposome, Vaccine **14:** 1143–1148.
15. OHISHI, K., H. KABEYA, H. AMANUMA & M. ONUMA. 1997. Peptide-based bovine leukemia virus (BLV) vaccine that induces BLV-Env specific Th-1 type immunity. Leukemia **11** (Suppl.): 223–226.
16. PALMER, G.H., S.D. WAGHELA, A.F. BARBET, _et al._ 1987. Characterization of a neutralization-sensitive epitope on the Am 105 surface protein of _Anaplasma marginale._ Int. J. Parasitol. **17:** 1279–1285.
17. PROCYK, K.J., M.R. RIPPO, R. TESTI, _et al._ 1999. Distinct mechanisms target stress and extracellular signal-activated kinase-1 and Jun N-terminal kinase during infection of macrophages with Salmonella. J. Immunol. **163:** 4924–4930.
18. SUGIMOTO, M., K. OHISHI, M. FUKASAWA, _et al._ 1995. Oliogomannose-coated liposomes as an adjuvant for the induction of cell-mediated immunity. FEBS Lett. **363:** 53–56.
19. TAN, M.C., A.M. MOMMAAS, J.W. DRIJFHOUT, _et al._ 1997. Mannose receptor-mediated uptake of antigens strongly enhances HLA class II-restricted antigen presentation by cultured dendritic cells. Eur. J. Immunol. **27:** 2426–2435.

IFN-γ As an Indicator of Successful Immunization of Goats Vaccinated with a Killed *Cowdria ruminantium* Vaccine

I. ESTEVES, A. BENSAID, D. MARTINEZ, AND P. TOTTE

CIRAD-EMVT, Petit-Bourg, Guadeloupe, France (French West Indies)

ABSTRACT: *Cowdria ruminantium*-induced production of IFN-γ was measured by ELISA on a weekly basis during the course of vaccination with killed organisms emulsified in ISA50. Upon challenge, all (3/3) vaccinated animals that gave the lowest IFN-γ response died of peracute cowdriosis. On the other hand, only one of three animals showing high IFN-γ responses to vaccination died, but with a delay of 4 days in comparison with naïve controls. Thus, there seems to be a threshold level of IFN-γ below which the probability for vaccinated animals to survive a lethal challenge is very low. During challenge, a much lower, but still physiologically meaningful production of IFN-γ was detected using the 24-hour whole blood assay on day 5 after infection in animals controlling the infection. In contrast, IFN-γ production was absent or negligible in naïve and vaccinated animals that died within 8–10 days after infection. Although these results need to be validated on a larger number of animals, they strongly suggest that IFN-γ is a useful indicator of protective immunity in animals immunized with killed *Cowdria*.

KEYWORDS: gamma interferon; immunization; *Cowdria ruminantium*; vaccine

INTRODUCTION

Cowdria ruminantium is a tick-transmitted intracellular ehrlichial bacterium that causes heartwater, an economically important infectious disease of ruminants in sub-Saharan Africa and on certain Caribbean islands.[1] Several observations underlie the important role of gamma interferon (IFN-γ) in resistance against obligate intracellular organisms including *C. ruminantium*-related members of the order Rickettsiales.[2] This cytokine is a very potent inhibitor of *C. ruminantium* growth in endothelial cells *in vitro*.[3] *In vivo,* pretreatment with recombinant IFN-γ protects mice against *C. ruminantium* infection.[4] IFN-γ has several other positive effects on immune responses, which were recently reviewed.[5] However, despite these observations, no direct correlation between survival and IFN-γ production has been demonstrated. In this study, we analyzed for the first time the kinetics of IFN-γ production in goats during vaccination with killed *C. ruminantium* and during challenge.

Address for correspondence: I. Esteves, CIRAD-EMVT, Domaine Duclos 97170 Petit-Bourg, Guadeloupe, France. Voice: 0590 25 54 44; fax: 0590 94 03 96.
tourais.esteves@cirad.fr

Ann. N.Y. Acad. Sci. 969: 126–130 (2002). © 2002 New York Academy of Sciences.

TABLE 1. Vaccination protocol of experimental animals

Group	Weeks	Dose (μg) /goat	Adjuvant
I	0	40	ISA50
	6	40	ISA50
	11	100	ISA50
II	0	40	ISA50
	6	40	ISA50
	18	100	CFA
	29	300	IFA

MATERIALS AND METHODS

Immunization and Challenge of Experimental Animals

Six age-matched Creole goats from Les Saintes, a heartwater-free island, were used in this study. All animals were immunized by subcutaneous inoculation of killed elementary bodies of *C. ruminantium* (Gardel strain) cultured in bovine umbilical endothelial cells, as described previously.[6] Six goats received 40 μg of *C. ruminantium* emulsified in Montanide ISA50 (ISA50) adjuvant, followed 6 weeks later by a similar inoculation. Three of these animals (group I) received 100 μg in ISA50 at week 11. The other three goats (group II) received 100 μg of *C. ruminantium* emulsified in complete Freund's adjuvant (CFA) at week 18 and another 300 μg in incomplete Freund's adjuvant (IFA) at week 23. The vaccination protocols are shown in TABLE 1. The challenge was done with culture-derived *C. ruminantium* elementary bodies 6 months and 3 months after the last inoculation for groups I and II, respectively. Two control animals were also inoculated in parallel.

IFN-γ Assays

IFN-γ was measured by ELISA (Bovigam CSL) in supernatant obtained by two different methods: whole blood stimulated 24 hours and peripheral blood mononuclear cells (PBMCs) stimulated 4 days *in vitro* in the presence or absence of *C. ruminantium* antigens. Then 200 μL of blood were stimulated with 20 μL of antigen at a final concentration of 5 μg/mL in 96-well flat-bottomed plates. Fresh PBMCs were seeded at a density of 3×10^5 cells/well in 96-well flat-bottomed plates in a final volume of 200 μL of RPMI medium containing 10% fetal bovine serum, 5×10^{-5} 2-mercaptoethanol, 100 U/mL penicillin, 100 μg/mL streptomycin, 2 mM L-glutamine, and *C. ruminantium* antigen at 1 μg/mL. The assay was conducted on a weekly basis after vaccination and every 2 days after challenge. Results were expressed in percentage of the kit positive control given by the following formula: % Positive = 100 × [(Sample OD–Negative OD)/(Positive OD–Negative OD)], where OD is the optical density at 450 nm. Positive (± 6 U/mL) and negative controls were given with the kit. Results are means of duplicates ± standard deviation (SD) and were considered significant only if above background (medium alone without antigen) + 3 × SD.

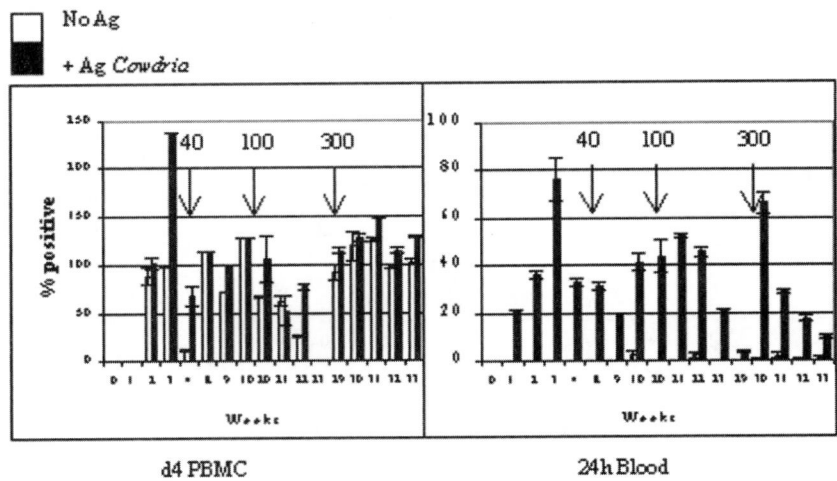

FIGURE 1. IFN-γ production during vaccination. → Booster injection and dose (μg).

RESULTS

Kinetics of IFN-γ Production during Vaccination

We chose to vaccinate animals with low doses of antigen (40 μg) first to investigate if a booster injection would increase IFN-γ production. Results are shown in FIGURE 1 for one animal of group II. (Others showed a similar pattern.) In both groups, there was no IFN-γ production before vaccination, and a peak was observed at week 2 or 3 followed by a rapid decline. IFN-γ production in response to *C. ruminantium* was always higher in 4-day supernatant from PBMCs than in 24-hour whole blood. However, the background was also higher with PBMCs, especially after booster injections. Booster injections did increase IFN-γ levels, but only in group II animals and never above the level observed after the first injection.

Comparison between IFN-γ Production during Vaccination and Survival from a Lethal Challenge

The challenge was very strong because control animals died in 8 days (TABLE 2) without showing clinical signs other than fever (i.e., acute cowdriosis). Postmortem analysis revealed hydropericardium in all dead animals. In group I, the only animal that survived was also the best IFN-γ producer (IFN-γ production without background). In group II, the best producer of IFN-γ died, but 4 days after the controls; however, this animal was operated for an abdominal hernia 2 weeks before challenge.

TABLE 2. IFN-γ production during vaccination and challenge with *Cowdria ruminantium*

Animals	IFN-γ production[a]					Challenge outcome		
	During vaccination	During challenge[b]				Days before death	Incubation period (days)	Maximal temperature (°C)
		d0	d2	d5	d8			
Naïve Controls								
9915	—	0	0	0	—	8	6	41.3
9919	—	0	3	0	—	8	7	39.5
Group I								
9903	0	0	0	1	1	10	7	41.3
9905	51	0	0	7	0	Survival	6	41.3
9911	22	0	0	0	3	9	7	40.5
Group II								
9906	187	3	0	4	2	12	7	41.4
9908	76	22	2	9	0	Survival	6	41.9
95206	27	0	0	0	1	9	8	40.8

[a] As measured by the whole blood assay and given in % of positive above background. Only peak production during vaccination is shown.
[b] Days after challenge.

Comparison between IFN-γ Production during Lethal Challenge and Survival

Just before challenge, only recently vaccinated goats (group II) produced IFN-γ. After challenge, the two naïve controls did not produce IFN-γ, whereas low production was detected in some vaccinated animals on day 5. The two animals that survived are also those that produced the highest levels of IFN-γ. Animal 9906 that died on day 12 produced more IFN-γ than did those that died on days 9 and 10.

DISCUSSION

Although 4-day PBMC cultures gave higher IFN-γ titers that did 24-hour whole blood assays, the former method is hampered by high background (response in the absence of *C. ruminantium* antigens). In all animals, the highest IFN-γ production was observed 2 or 3 weeks after the first injection and was not augmented by booster injections. Upon challenge, all three vaccinated animals that showed the lowest IFN-γ response to vaccination died of peracute cowdriosis, whereas only one of three animals showing high IFN-γ responses died, but with a delay of 4 days in comparison with controls. Thus, there appears to be a threshold level of IFN-γ produced during vaccination below which animals do not survive challenge and above which most animals are protected. During challenge, IFN-γ levels also correlate well with survival. It should be noted that although the production was very low, it is nevertheless biologically significant, because as little as 0.1 U/mL of recombinant IFN-γ (i.e., 2% of positive in our test) has been shown to reduce *C. ruminantium* growth by 40% *in vitro* in goat endothelial cells.[3] Our data confirm and extend other studies in which 81% (13/16) of cattle and 100% of sheep (*n* = 3) that were immunized by the same method and that produced IFN-γ in response to *C. ruminantium* antigens survived subsequent challenge (C. Kelly & K. Sumption, personal communication). All together, these results suggest that IFN-γ is a useful indicator of protective immunity in animals vaccinated with killed *C. ruminantium*. This warrants evaluation of the whole blood IFN-γ test in vaccination trials to see if it can limit losses encountered with highly valuable and susceptible exotic breeds. Moreover, these results further support the strategy aimed at identifying IFN-γ–inducing proteins of *C. ruminantium* for evaluation as potential candidate vaccine antigens.

ACKNOWLEDGMENT

This work received support from the European Union (INCO-DC Program) under contract IC18-CT95-0008. I. Esteves is supported by a fellowship from the Praxis XXI program of the European Union.

REFERENCES

1. CAMUS, E. *et al.* 1996. Heartwater: A Review. Office International des Epizooties. Paris, France.
2. BYRNE, G.I. & J. TURCO. 1988. Interferon and nonviral pathogens. *In* Immunology Series. G.I. Byrne & J. Turco, Eds. Vol. 42. Marcel Dekker. New York-Basel.
3. TOTTÉ, P. *et al.* 1996. Recombinant bovine interferon gamma inhibits the growth of *Cowdria ruminantium* but fails to induce major histocompatibility complex class II following infection of endothelial cells. Vet. Immunol. Immunopathol. **53:** 61–71.
4. TOTTÉ, P. *et al.* 1994. Protection against *Cowdria ruminantium* infection in mice with gamma interferon produced in animal cells. *In* Animal Cell Technology: Basic and Applied Aspects. vol. **6:** 595–599. Kluwer Academic Publishers.
5. TOTTÉ, P. *et al.* 1999. Immune responses to *Cowdria ruminantium* infections. Parasitol. Today **15:** 286–290.
6. MARTINEZ, D. *et al.* 1994. Protection of goats against heartwater is acquired by immunisation with inactivated elementary bodies of *Cowdria ruminantium*. Vet. Immunol. Immunopathol. **41:** 153–163.

Major Outer Membrane Proteins of *Ehrlichia ruminantium* Encoded by a Multigene Family

H. VAN HEERDEN, N.E. COLLINS, M.T.E.P. ALLSOPP, AND B.A. ALLSOPP

Onderstepoort Veterinary Institute, Onderstepoort 0110, Pretoria, South Africa

ABSTRACT: Immune responses of infected animals and humans have been reported to be directed against variable outer membrane proteins of *Ehrlichia* species that are encoded by polymorphic multigene families. In *Ehrlichia* (= *Cowdria*) *ruminantium*, two immunodominant proteins have been identified, namely major antigenic protein 1 (MAP1) and open reading frame 2 (ORF2). The aim of the present study was to identify additional *map*1-like genes in the *E. ruminantium* genome. A 12 kb clone that hybridized with the *map*1 probe was amplified using long template PCR. The PCR product was partially digested, cloned, and sequenced. Four *map*1-like genes are located in tandem, namely *map*1-1 (*orf*2) and *map*1-2 upstream of *map*1 as well as *map*1+1 downstream of *map*1. A large ORF (2.4 kb) at the 3' end is homologous to *secA* genes of other organisms. The sequence data in this study support other findings that outer membrane proteins are located in tandem and are encoded by a polymorphic multigene family.

KEYWORDS: *Ehrlichia ruminantium*; proteins; multigene family; outer membranes

INTRODUCTION

Ehrlichia (Cowdria) ruminantium is an obligate intracellular parasite causing heartwater in ruminants. This disease is endemic throughout sub-Saharan Africa[1] and certain Caribbean islands.[2,3] Heartwater is transmitted by ticks of the genus *Amblyomma*. Phylogenetic studies based on 16S ribosomal DNA and outer membrane proteins sequence comparisons have revealed a close relation amongst *E. ruminantium, E. chaffeensis,* and *E. canis.*[4,5] Outer membrane protein genes that have been identified in these organisms include the major antigenic protein 1 (MAP1) of *E. ruminantium*[6,7] and the 28 kDa protein (p28) found in *E. canis* and *E. chaffeensis.*[8–10] These outer membrane proteins are encoded by polymorphic multigene families. Dominant immune responses have been observed in infected animals and humans against the variable outer membrane proteins of *Ehrlichia* species. Recently, a second *E. ruminantium map*1-like gene (*map*1-1 = *orf*2) was located upstream of *map*1.[7] A partial sequence of a third member of the multigene family has been iden-

Address for correspondence: H. van Heerden, Onderstepoort Veterinary Institute, Private Bag X5, Onderstepoort 0110, Pretoria, South Africa.
henriett@moon.ovi.ac.za

Ann. N.Y. Acad. Sci. 969: 131–134 (2002). © 2002 New York Academy of Sciences.

tified upstream of *map*1-1 (= *orf*3).[7] The aim of this study was to identify additional members of the *map*1 multigene family in tandem in the *E. ruminantium* genome.

MATERIALS AND METHODS

A large insert library in LambdaGEM11 was constructed at Onderstepoort Veterinary Institute (Private Bag X5, Onderstepoort 0110), South Africa, by K.A. Brayton using genomic DNA of the Welgevonden strain of *E. ruminantium*. This large insert library was screened with a *map*1 probe[11] and recombinant lambda DNA from clones, which hybridized with the *map*1, probe was prepared, as described by the manufacturers (Promega Corp.). A clone that hybridized with the *map*1 probe was selected and amplified using the primers T7GEM11 (5′CTAATACGACTCACTATAGG3′) and SP6GEM11 (5′CCATTTAGGTGACAC-TATAG3′). The PCRs were performed in 1X LA PCR buffer II, 2.5 mM MgCl$_2$, 0.4 mM of each dNTP, 0.4 μM of each primer, 0.1 U TaKaRa LA *Taq* polymerase, and 1 μL DNA. The reaction conditions were: 2 min of initial denaturing at 94°C, followed by 10 cycles of 10 sec at 94°C, 30 seconds at 52°C, and 15 minutes at 68°C, 15 cycles of 10 sec at 94°C, 30 sec at 52°C, and 15 min at 68°C, with 20-sec increases per cycle with a final extension of 68°C for 7 minutes.

The PCR product was partially digested with *Alu*1 and *Sau*3A (Roche) for 15 minutes at 37°C. Fill-in reaction was performed with the Klenow fill-in kit (Stratagene) to prepare digested PCR products for insertion into a plasmid vector, pUC18, that was cut with *Sma*1 and dephophorylated.[12] The resulting blunt-ended PCR products were purified with a Concert PCR purification kit (Life Technologies), ligated into the pUC18 vector, and transformed into XL-1 Blue MRF′ (Stratagene) cells. Recombinants were selected on LB-ampicillin (100 μg/mL). The plasmids were extracted from individual cultures using a high pure plasmid isolation kit (Roche). Both strands of the plasmids containing inserts were sequenced using the BigDye terminator cycle sequencing kit (Perkin Elmer Applied Biosystems). The sequenced products were analyzed using the Staden package.[13]

RESULTS AND DISCUSSION

Two clones from the *E. ruminantium* LambdaGEM11 library were found that hybridized with the *map*1 probe. One clone was selected, and a 12-kb PCR product was obtained using TaKaRa LA *Taq*. Sequencing analyses of subcloned PCR product demonstrated that five open reading frames, including *map*1, are located in tandem in the genome (FIG. 1). Two of these open reading frames (ORFs) were previously identified as *map*1 and *map*1-1 (*orf*2).[7] In the present study, additional *map*1-like genes were found in tandem with *map*1 and *map*1-1. Upstream of *map*1 (873 bp), two ORFs were found that included the previously characterized *map*1-1 (*orf*2, 849 bp) and *map*1-2 (861 bp). However, the starting codon of *map*1-2 is not present and needs to be identified with genome walking. *Map*1-2 ends 1,390 bp upstream of the *map*1-1 gene (FIG. 1). Another *map*1-like gene designated *map*1+1 consisting of 858 bp was found 1,607 bp downstream of *map*1. Of the four *map*1-like genes, only *map*1+1 was orientated on the complementary strand. The finding of four *map*1-like

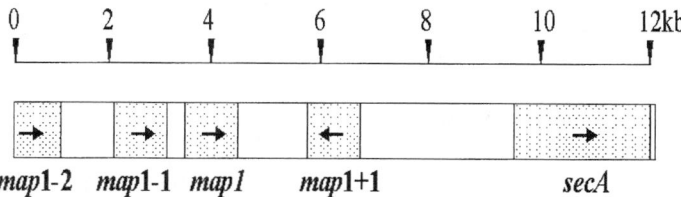

FIGURE 1. Arrangement of *map*1-2, *map*1-1, *map*1, *map*1+1, and *SecA* genes in a 12-kb clone of *C. ruminantium* (Welgevonden), with the direction of transcription 5′ to 3′ indicated by *arrows* in each ORF.

members in tandem in the *E. ruminantium* genome verifies that *map*1 is a member of an outer membrane protein multigene family.

The fifth ORF identified in the 12-kb clone is a large ORF of 2.4 kb at the 3′ end, which is homologous to *secA* genes of other organisms. SecA is part of a multisubunit membrane-bound enzyme responsible for translocation of proteins. This ORF starts 2,763 bp downstream from the stop codon of *map*1+1 (FIG. 1), suggesting that *map*1+1 may be the last of the tandemly arranged *map*1-like genes.

Database searches revealed that *map*1-1 and *map*1-2 are more closely related to *p28-2* (E value in Blast database searches of e-121) and *p28-11* (E value in Blast database searches of 7e-56) genes of *E. canis* and *E. chaffeensis*, respectively, than to *map*1 of *E. ruminantium*. The downstream member *map*1+1 was related to the *p28-20* gene of *E. chaffeensis* (E value in Blast database searches of 2e-98). The *E. ruminantium* MAP1-like proteins are homologous to *E. chaffeensis* and *E. canis* P28 proteins, which are also encoded by multigene families.[8–10] Multigene families might be involved in mechanisms used by these related organisms to avoid the host immune system.

REFERENCES

1. UILENBERG, G. 1983. Heartwater (*Cowdria ruminantium* infection): current status. Adv. Vet. Sci. Comp. Med. **27:** 427–480.
2. PERREAU, P. *et al.* 1980. Existence de la cowdriose (heartwater) a *Cowdria ruminantium* chez les ruminants des Antilles Françaises (La Guadeloupe) et des Mascareignes (La Reunion et Ile Maurice). Rev. Elev. Med. Vet. Pays Trop. **33:** 21–22.
3. BURRIDGE, M.J. 1985. Heartwater invades the Caribbean. Parasitol. Today **1:** 1–3.
4. DAME, J.B. *et al.* 1992. Phylogenetic relationship of *Cowdria ruminantium*, agent of heartwater, to *Anaplasma marginale* and other members of the order Rickettsiales determined on the basis of the 16S rRNA sequence. Int. J. Syst. Bacteriol. **42:** 270–274.
5. VAN VLIET, A.H.M. *et al.* 1992. Phylogenetic position of *Cowdria ruminantium* (Rickettsiales) determined by analysis of amplified 16S ribosomal DNA sequences. Int. J. Syst. Bacteriol. **42:** 494–498.
6. VAN VLIET, A.H.M. *et al.* 1994. Molecular cloning, sequencing analysis, and expression of the gene encoding the immunodominant 32-kilodalton protein of *Cowdria ruminantium*. Infect. Immun. **62:** 1451–1456.
7. SULSONA, C.R. *et al.* 1999. The *map1* gene of *Cowdria ruminantium* is a member of a multigene family containing both conserved and variable genes. Biochem. Biophys. Res. Commun. **257:** 300–305.

8. OHASHI, N. *et al.* 1998. Immunodominant major outer membrane proteins of *Ehrlichia chaffeensis* are encoded by a polymorphic multigene family. Infect. Immun. **66:** 132–139.

9. REDDY, G.R. *et al.* 1998. Molecular characterization of a 28 kDa surface antigen gene family of the tribe Ehrlichiene. Biochem. Biophys. Res. Commun. **47:** 636–643.

10. YU, J.-X. *et al.* 2000. Characterization of the complete transcriptionally active *Ehrlichia chaffeensis* 28 kDa outer membrane protein multigene family. Gene. **248:** 59–68.

11. ALLSOPP, M.T.E.P. *et al.* 1999. Evaluation of the 16S, *map1* and pCS20 probes for detection of *Cowdria* and *Ehrlichia* species. Epidemiol. Infect. **122:** 323–328.

12. SAMBROOK, J. *et al.* 1989. Molecular Cloning: a Laboratory Manual, 2nd edit. Cold Springs Harbor Laboratories. Cold Springs Harbor, NY.

13. BONFIELD, J.K. *et al.* 1995. A new DNA sequence assembly program. Nucleic Acids Res. **23:** 4992–4999.

Cowdria ruminantium Antigens of around 15 kDa Are Potent Inducers of IFN-γ

N. GUNTER,[a] I. ESTEVES,[b] Y. KANDASSAMY,[b] D. MARTINEZ,[b] A. BENSAID,[b] M. VAN KLEEF,[a] D. DU PLESSIS,[a] AND P. TOTTE[b]

[a]*Department of Immunology, Onderstepoort Veterinary Institute, Onderstepoort, Republic of South Africa*

[b]*CIRAD-EMVT, Guadeloupe, French West Indies*

ABSTRACT: Cellular responses induced in two Creole goats by vaccination with killed *Cowdria ruminantium* (*Cowdria*) were confirmed by IFN-γ production and interleukin-2 receptor (IL-2R) expression. Both CD4[+] and CD8[+] but not WC1[+] T cells showed a substantial increase in cell surface expression of IL-2R molecules in response to whole *Cowdria* lysate. *Cowdria* (Welgevonden strain) proteins were fractionated using continuous-flow electrophoresis and tested for their ability to induce IFN-γ production by PBMC collected three weeks after the first inoculation and one week after the booster injection. Pooled fractions of around 15, 22, and 24 kDa were found to induce significant IFN-γ production in both vaccinated animals on one of the two occasions. Antigens of around 15 kDa induced substantially higher IFN-γ production than any other fractions in both animals. These pilot experiments pave the way towards the identification of proteins/genes that have potential for the development of a recombinant vaccine against heartwater.

KEYWORDS: *Cowdria ruminantium*; recombinant vaccine against heartwater; interferon-gamma production

INTRODUCTION

Cowdria ruminantium is a tick-transmitted obligate intracellular bacterium that preferentially invades vascular endothelial cells, causing an often fatal disease in wild and domestic ruminants of sub-Saharan Africa and several islands in the Caribbean.[1] Control of the pathogen can be achieved through immunization, but available vaccines are expensive to produce, and this has drastically limited their use, especially within small-scale farming communities. There is general agreement that a recombinant vaccine produced by genetically engineered live vectors would be the most practical and affordable solution. In order to achieve this goal, genes of *Cowdria* that are capable of stimulating protective immunity need to be identified and cloned into appropriate vectors. Protective immunity is believed to be predominantly cell mediated, with a pivotal role for IFN-γ.[2] Therefore, we have adopted a strategy

Address for correspondence: P. Totte, Ph.D., CIRAD-EMVT, Domaine Duclos, 97170 Petit-Bourg, Guadeloupe (France). Voice: 590-25-54-42; fax: 590-94-03-96.
philippe.totte@cirad.fr

Ann. N.Y. Acad. Sci. 969: 135–140 (2002). © 2002 New York Academy of Sciences.

of identifying interferon (IFN)-γ–inducing proteins of *Cowdria* for evaluation as a potential candidate vaccine.

Previous results have indicated that *Cowdria* antigens separated by gel filtration combined with fast-performance liquid chromatography (FPLC) and capable of inducing IFN-γ production by immune bovine CD4[+] T cell lines reside in the 22–32-kDa molecular size range.[3] However, FPLC is limited to the use of soluble proteins and by the presence of numerous protein bands in many of the antigenic fractions when analyzed by SDS-PAGE. Here, we report on the use of continuous-flow electrophoresis (CFE) to further fractionate *Cowdria* proteins and show that antigens of around 15 kDa induce substantial IFN-γ production by PBMC obtained from goats immunized with killed *Cowdria* organisms.

MATERIALS AND METHODS

Experimental Animals and Immunization

Age-matched Creole goats from Les Saintes Islands, a heartwater-free region of the Caribbean, were used in this study. Two animals were immunized as described previously[4] by subcutaneous injection of 200 μg of killed *Cowdria* (Welgevonden strain) in ISA50 (Seppic, France) followed one month later by a second inoculation. In the same manner, two additional goats received PBS in ISA50 as a control group.

Cowdria *Cultivation and Antigen Preparation*

Cowdria ruminantium (Welgevonden strain) was purified from supernatants of infected bovine umbilical endothelial cells (BUEC) as previously described.[5] Briefly, when 70–80% lysis of the monolayer occurred, the supernatant was collected and cell debris removed by centrifugation at $1000 \times g$ for 10 min. The supernatant was further centrifuged at $14,000 \times g$ for 30 min; and, after one wash in PBS, purified organisms were killed by freeze-thawing 5 times in liquid nitrogen, resuspended in PBS, and stored at −20 °C until use. Lysates of uninfected BUEC (CellAg) were also prepared for control purposes. The protein content was determined by the Bradford method (Pierce). All preparations were used in *in vitro* assays at a final concentration of 1 μg/mL.

Flow Cytometry

Cell surface expression of interleukin-2 receptor (IL-2R) on T lymphocyte subsets was analyzed by two-color immunofluorescence staining using specific monoclonal antibodies (mAb) against the α chain of bovine IL-2R (mAb CACT116A), CD4 (GC50), CD8 (7C2), and WC1 (CC15), which is found on γδTCR[+] T cells. Samples were analyzed on a fluorescence-activated cell sorter (FACScalibur, Becton Dickinson, San Jose, CA). Results are expressed as the percentage increase in the number of IL-2R molecules per cell given by the mean intensity of fluorescence (MIF) of mAb CACT116A. Standard deviation of means of quadruplicate tests never exceeded 20%. Therefore, percentage increases above 20% were considered as significant.

IFN-γ Assay

A capture ELISA kit (CSL, Australia) was used to detect IFN-γ in culture supernatants. Results are expressed as percent of the kit positive control, which corresponds to 6 U/mL. Only values > the mean + 3SD of the no-antigen control were considered as significant. For assays with Prep-Cell fractions, 20 μL of each pooled fraction was added to 3×10^5 PBMC/well in 96-well flat-bottomed plates in a final volume of 200 μL. IFN-γ assays were performed on day-4 supernatants.

Continuous Flow Electrophoresis

Separation of 10 mg of purified *Cowdria* organisms was performed on a Prep-Cell apparatus (Bio-Rad) as described previously.[6] Briefly, solubilized *Cowdria* proteins were electrophoresed under reducing conditions on a 15% acrylamide cylindrical gel. A total of 108 fractions were collected after elution, precipitated in ice-cold acetone, washed in ethanol, resuspended in PBS, and stored at −70° C. Every 6 frac-

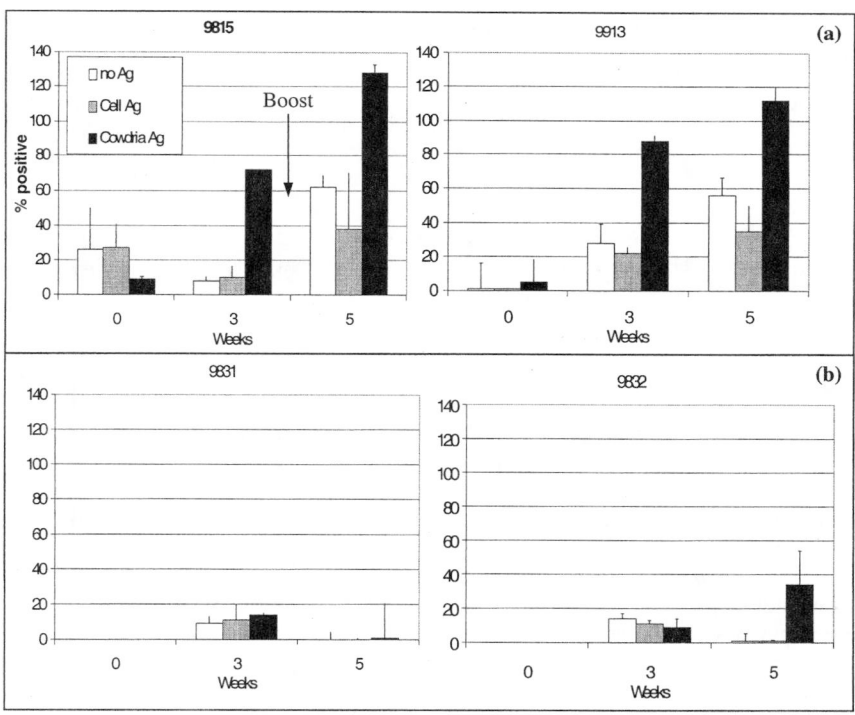

FIGURE 1. IFN-γ production in goats during vaccination with killed *Cowdria* **(a)** and in controls that received adjuvant alone **(b)**. IFN-γ was measured by ELISA in day 4 supernatants of PBMC incubated with medium alone (noAg), a lysate from uninfected endothelial cells (CellAg), and a lysate from *Cowdria ruminantium* (CowdriaAg). Results are means of duplicates + SD.

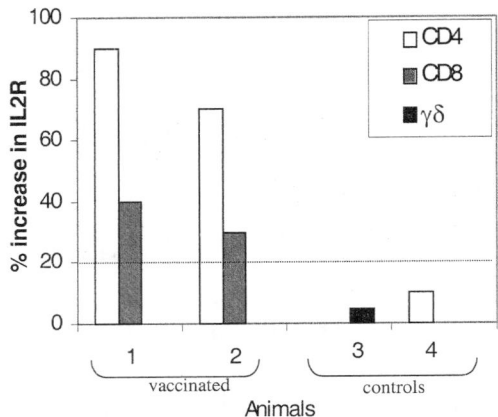

FIGURE 2. *Cowdria*-induced IL-2R expression on T lymphocyte subsets three weeks after vaccination. IL-2R expression on CD4+, CD8+, and WC1+ T cells in response to *Cowdria* Ags was measured by flow cytometry after 4 days of culture of PBMC. Results are expressed in percent increase in the mean intensity of fluorescence, which is an estimation of the number of IL-2R molecules per cell. Activation induced by Ags prepared from uninfected endothelial cells was deducted to show only the net effect of *Cowdria*. Only percentages above the *dotted line* were considered as significant (see MATERIALS AND METHODS for reproducibility of flow cytometry).

tions were pooled before use in IFN-γ assays. The content of each pool was analyzed by SDS-PAGE after silver staining of the gel.

RESULTS AND DISCUSSION

Three weeks after vaccination, PBMC from two vaccinated goats but not naive controls produced substantial amounts of IFN-γ in response to *Cowdria* Ags (FIG. 1). This *Cowdria*-induced production of IFN-γ was confirmed one week after the booster injection despite high background responses. Surprisingly, at that time, PBMC of one of the controls produced a small but significant amount of IFN-γ and only in response to *Cowdria* Ags (FIG. 1b). This is not likely to be due to a sudden exposure to the pathogen since antibody titers to *Cowdria* did not increase throughout the experiment (data not shown). On the other hand, it has been shown previously that oil-based adjuvant can induce rapid but short-term cellular responses, including IFN-γ production, in the absence of antigen.[7] Since we could not exclude that part of the IFN-γ produced by immune PBMC at week five was due to an adjuvant effect, we decided to also use PBMC from animal #9832 to screen CFE fractions.

Vaccination with killed *Cowdria* induced the activation of CD4+ and to a lesser extent CD8+ T cells, as shown by the increased expression of IL-2R on these cells after antigenic recall *in vitro* (FIG. 2). These results are consistent with an involvement of these cells in the production of IFN-γ.

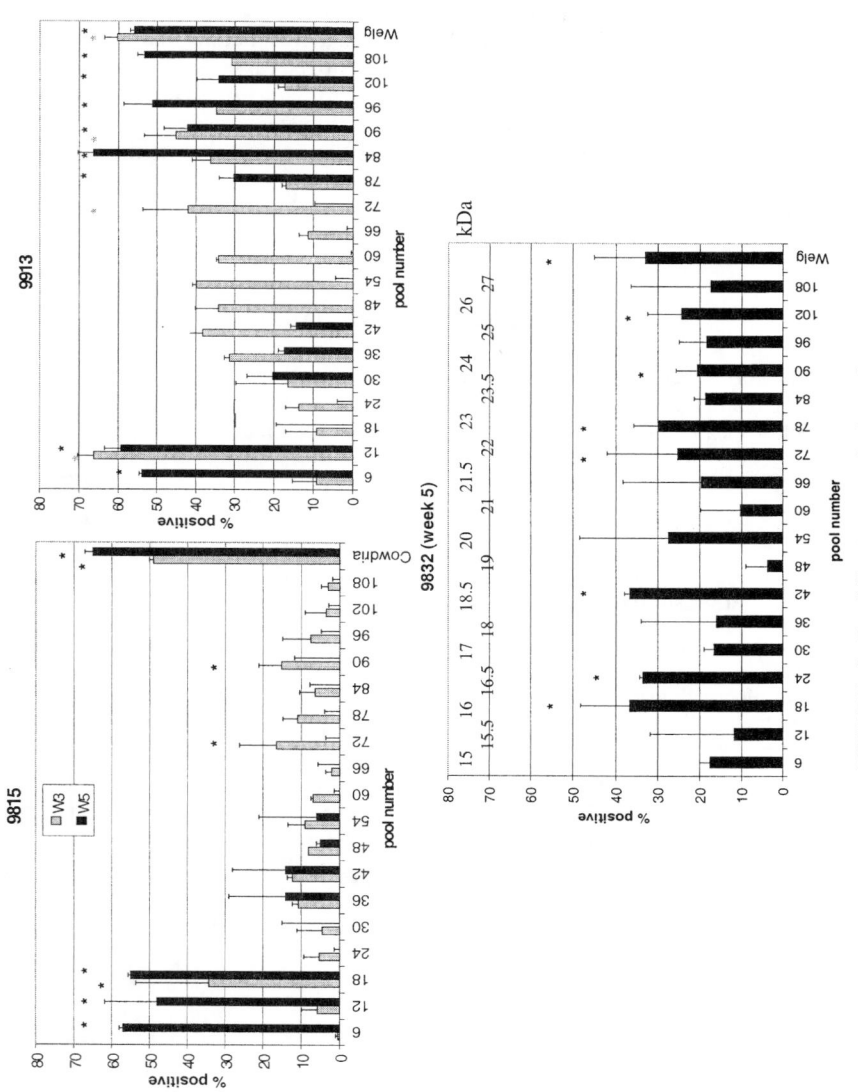

FIGURE 3. *See following page for legend.*

In an attempt to identify which proteins are involved in the production of IFN-γ, *Cowdria* antigens were fractionated by CFE and incubated with immune PBMC on two occasions after vaccination. At week three, only pools 72 and 90, corresponding to 22 and 24 kDa, respectively, induced IFN-γ in both vaccinated animals (FIG. 3). After the booster injection, PBMC from both vaccinated animals but not the naive control (#9832) reacted strongly to pools 6 and 12, corresponding to around 15 kDa.

In conclusion, we show here that the use of sensitized PBMC combined with CFE fractionation permits rapid and simple screening for *Cowdria* proteins that trigger the synthesis of IFN-γ by immune lymphocytes. However, precise definition of the molecular weight of these proteins will require careful analysis of the content of each fraction before pooling in order to limit overlapping. Nonetheless, these preliminary data already suggest that *Cowdria* antigens of around 15 kDa are potent inducers of IFN-γ.

ACKNOWLEDGMENTS

This work received support from the South African Foundation for Research Development and the French Ministry of Foreign Affairs. It also benefited from the help of the European Union (INCO-DC program) under Contract No. IC18-CT95-0008.

REFERENCES

1. CAMUS, E. *et al.* 1996. Heartwater, a review. Office International des Epizooties, Paris.
2. TOTTÉ, P. *et al.* 1999. Immune responses to *Cowdria ruminantium* infections. Parasitol. Today **15:** 286–290.
3. TOTTÉ, P. *et al.* 1999. Bovine CD4+ T–cell lines reactive with soluble and membrane antigens of *Cowdria ruminantium*. Vet. Immunol. Immunopathol. **70:** 269–276.
4. MARTINEZ, D. *et al.* 1994. Protection of goats against heartwater is acquired by immunisation with inactivated elementary bodies of *Cowdria ruminantium*. Vet. Immunol. Immunopathol. **41:** 153–163.
5. BEZUIDENHOUT, J.D., C.L. PATTERSON & B.J.H. BARNARD. 1985. *In vitro* cultivation of *Cowdria ruminantium*. Onderstepoort J. Vet. Res. **52:** 113–120.
6. VAN KLEEF, M. *et al.* 2000. Identification of *Cowdria ruminantium* antigens that stimulate proliferation of lymphocytes from cattle immunized by infection and treatment or with inactivated organisms. Infect. Immun. **68:** 603–614.
7. EMERY, D.L., J.S. ROTHEL & P.R. WOOD. 1990. Influence of antigens and adjuvants on the production of gamma-interferon and antibody by ovine lymphocytes. Immunol. Cell. Biol. **68:** 127–136.

FIGURE 3. IFN-γ production by PBMC in response to pooled Prep-Cell fractions of *Cowdria ruminantium* antigens. Each pool is made of 6 fractions. PBMC were collected 3 weeks (w3) after vaccination and 1 week after the booster injection (w5). Results are expressed as percent of the kit positive above background (medium only). Each pool that induces a significant production (above medium + 3 SD) is marked with an *asterisk*. Results are mean of duplicates + SD. An estimation of the molecular weight of each pool is given on the last graph in kDa.

Amino Acid Content of Cell Cultures Infected with *Cowdria ruminantium* Propagated in a Protein-free Medium

A.I. JOSEMANS AND E. ZWEYGARTH

Onderstepoort Veterinary Institute, Onderstepoort 0110, Pretoria, South Africa

ABSTRACT: The *in vitro* culture of *Cowdria ruminantium*, the causative agent of heartwater in domestic ruminants, was first achieved in 1985. Culture media were usually supplemented with serum and tryptose phosphate broth, both undefined components, contributing to great variability. Recently, we reported about the propagation of stocks of *C. ruminantium* in a protein-free culture medium referred to as SFMC-23, which is chemically fully defined. To clarify whether the amino acid composition in SFMC-23 is adequate for the *in vitro* propagation of *Cowdria*, the Welgevonden stock was propagated in SFMC-23 medium. After a 3-day culture period, samples were taken from uninfected and infected bovine endothelial cell cultures. They were analyzed for free amino acids by the Pico Taq reversed-phase HPLC precolumn derivatization method. Eighteen different amino acids were examined. A considerable decrease in concentration was observed with proline (29%) and glutamine (62%). Further dramatic changes were observed with amino acids which accumulated in the culture medium: aspartic acid, serine, asparagine, tryptophane, glycine, and alanine. The concentration of alanine increased by approximately 660%. The concentrations of all other amino acids analyzed remained within a 25% range, either increasing or decreasing. These results suggest that only glutamine may run short during *in vitro* cultivation. It seems more likely that accumulation of various amino acids may impact negatively on long-term *Cowdria* propagation.

KEYWORDS: *Cowdria ruminantium*; amino acid utilization of *C. ruminantium*; metabolic processes of *C. ruminantium*

Heartwater is a rickettsial disease of ruminants caused by *Cowdria ruminantium*. It is prevalent in sub-Saharan Africa, some islands off its eastern and western coasts,[1] and in the Caribbean.[2,3] It is transmitted by ixodid ticks of the genus *Amblyomma* and is often fatal. The *in vitro* culture of *C. ruminantium* was first achieved by Bezuidenhout, Paterson, and Barnard.[4] Today, the majority of heartwater research is based on culture-produced organisms.[5] However, the production of *C. ruminantium in vitro* in a consistent fashion remains difficult to achieve. Recent advances have

Address for correspondence: A.I. Josemans, Onderstepoort Veterinary Institute, Private Bag X5, Onderstepoort 0110, Pretoria, South Africa. Voice: +27 12 5299411; fax: +27 12 5299434.
Antoinettm@moon.ovi.ac.za

Ann. N.Y. Acad. Sci. 969: 141–146 (2002). © 2002 New York Academy of Sciences.

been made towards culture in a completely chemically defined protein-free medium. *C. ruminantium* has been grown in serum-free media, supplemented with bovine lipoproteins and transferrin.[6] These two components were replaced with chemically defined lipids and protein-free iron complexes.[7] The replacement of undefined components has enabled us, in this study, to determine the amino acid utilization of *C. ruminantium*, to identify substrate deficiencies, and to gain an insight into the metabolic processes of the organism.

MATERIALS AND METHODS

The Welgevonden stock of *C. ruminantium*[8] was grown in a continuous bovine aorta endothelial cell line, BA886.[9] These cells were initially screened for the absence of mycoplasma contaminants by staining with bis-benzamide (Hoechst 33258) and examination under the fluorescence microscope. The mycoplasma-free status of the cells and the *Cowdria* cultures were confirmed by means of a mycoplasma-specific polymerase chain reaction (PCR) test.[10] Cultures were propagated as previously described[11] with minor modifications. Uninfected cells were propagated at 37 °C as monolayers in medium consisting of Dulbecco's modified Eagles medium nutrient mixture F-12 Ham (Sigma, St. Louis, MO) with additives as previously described.[7] Infected cultures of *C. ruminantium* were propagated in a protein-free medium referred to as "serum-free medium for *Cowdria* No. 23" (SFMC-23).[7] The amino acid concentrations in the medium were determined before and after a 3-day cultivation period, on a Waters Automated Analyzer (Millipore Corp.) using Pico-Tag phenyl isothiocyanate (PTC) pre-derivatization methodology.[12] Fresh medium (3 samples), infected culture supernatants (9 samples), and uninfected culture supernatants (3 samples) were analyzed for 18 different amino acids. Amino acid concentrations in 3-day culture supernatants were expressed as percentages of concentrations in the original medium (TABLE 1).

RESULTS AND DISCUSSION

The average amino acid concentrations are shown in FIGURE 1, while the magnitude of changes are summarized in TABLE 1. Glutamine was the amino acid that was most markedly depleted in both infected and uninfected cultures, by 62% and 53%, respectively. In mammalian cell cultures glutamine is not used directly for protein synthesis, but is metabolized into glutamic acid, aspartic acid, asparagine, and proline, and to a lesser degree into serine and alanine.[13] All these metabolites were increased in uninfected cultures, except for glutamic acid, which was consumed by the BA886 cells. The largest increase in uninfected cultures was found for alanine (1047%), while a slightly lower increase for alanine (761%) was observed in *Cowdria*-infected cultures. Assuming that the host cell metabolism is not grossly disrupted until close to the time of release of the elementary bodies, amino acids from the host cells released into the medium can be used by *Cowdria* organisms. Thus, in our experiments the concentration of proline in the supernatant was 64% lower in infected than in uninfected cultures after 3 days, indicating that there must have been a large consumption of this amino acid by the *Cowdria* organisms. Similar results

TABLE 1. Concentrations of 18 amino acids in SFMC-23 medium and after 3 days in BA866 cell cultures and *Cowdria*-infected cultures

	A	B		C	
Amino acid	Concentration in SFMC-23 mM/mL	Concentration after 3 days in uninfected culture as % of A	Change vs. A	Concentration after 3 days in infected culture as % of A	Change vs. B %
Glycine	0.267	**190**[a]	↑	**317**	**+67**
Aspartic Acid	0.056	**150**	↑	**166**	+11
Alanine	0.049	**1047**	↑	**761**	**−27**
Proline	0.098	**198**	↑	**71**	**−64**
Tryptophan	0.034	**191**	↑	**132**	**−31**
Asparagine	0.039	**182**	↑	**159**	−13
Serine	0.151	**178**	↑	**166**	−7
Threonine	0.247	114	↑	112	−1
Glutamic Acid	0.600	**55**	↓	101	**+84**
Phenylalanine	0.188	86	→	87	+2
Tyrosine	0.222	82	→	83	+1
Methionine	0.104	82	→	83	+1
Lysine	0.441	79	→	83	+5
Leucine	0.442	77	→	79	+2
Glutamine	5.145	**47**	↓	**38**	−19
Arginine	0.623	96	→	94	−2
Valine	0.445	81	→	81	−1
Isoleucine	0.401	76	↓	75	−1

[a]changes in concentration > 25% in bold.

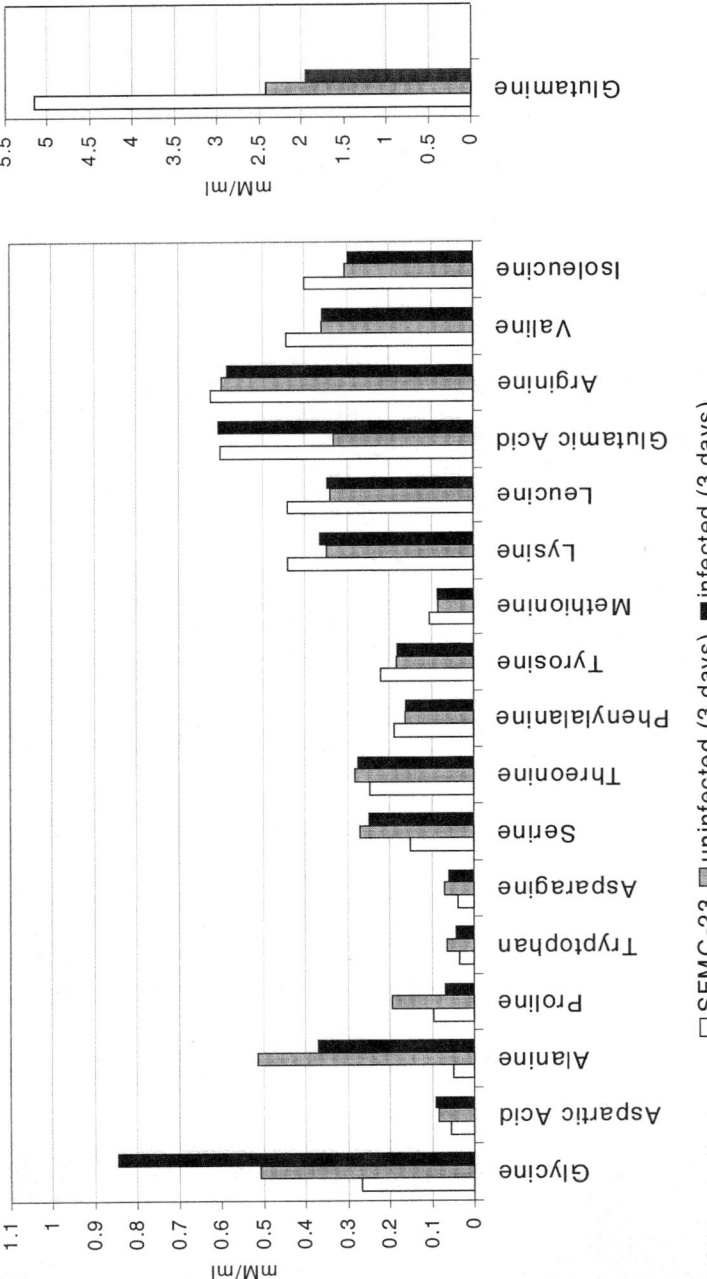

FIGURE 1. Average amino acid concentrations in serum-free medium and in supernatant of *Cowdria*-infected cultures and uninfected controls.

were found with alanine and tryptophan, which were consumed at a lower rate. In another study[14] it was found that *C. ruminantium* in serum-containing cultures consumed proline at a similar rate to that described here. Another rickettsia, *Rickettsia prowazekii*, appears to require proline for growth as maximal rickettsial growth occurred only in host cells with an intracellular proline pool of 1 mM or greater.[15]

Neitz and Yunker[14] found that within 2 days arginine was almost completely depleted both in infected and uninfected cultures in a serum-containing medium. They concluded that their medium (Glasgow's MEM) might have been deficient in arginine. In contrast, in our cultures only 4% or 6% of the initial arginine was consumed in uninfected and infected cultures, respectively. A possible explanation for this discrepancy may lie in the work of Capiaumont *et al.*,[16] who suggested that if the arginine in a culture medium is suddenly completely consumed after 2 or 3 days, there is probably mycoplasma contamination.

These results suggest that the concentrations of glutamine and proline may be limiting during *in vitro* cultivation. It also seems likely that the accumulation of various amino acids or metabolic by-products in the medium could have a negative impact on long-term *Cowdria* propagation.

ACKNOWLEDGMENTS

We thank Dr. B. A. Allsopp for helpful comments on the manuscript. This research was supported by the Agricultural Research Council of South Africa and the European Union (Cowdriosis Network), Grant No. IC18-CT95-0008 (DG12-SNRD).

REFERENCES

1. UILENBERG, G. 1983. Heartwater (*Cowdria ruminantium* infection): current status. Adv. Vet. Sci. Comp. Med. **27:** 427–480.
2. PERREAU, P., P.C. MOREL, N. BARRÉ & P. DURAND. 1980. Existence de la cowdriose (heartwater) à *Cowdria ruminantium* chez les ruminants des Antilles françaises (La Guadeloupe) et des Mascareignes (La Reunion et île Maurice). Rev. Elev. Méd. Vét. Pays Trop. **33:** 21–22.
3. BIRNIE, E.F., M.J. BURRIDGE, E. CAMUS & N. BARRÉ. 1984. Heartwater in the Caribbean: isolation of *Cowdria ruminantium* from Antigua. Vet. Rec. **116:** 121–123.
4. BEZUIDENHOUT, J.D., C.L. PATERSON & B.J.H. BARNARD. 1985. *In vitro* cultivation of *Cowdria ruminantium*. Onderstepoort J. Vet. Res. **52:** 113–120.
5. YUNKER, C.E. 1995. Current status of *in vitro* cultivation of *Cowdria ruminantium*. Vet. Parasitol. **57:** 205–211.
6. ZWEYGARTH, E., A.I. JOSEMANS & E. HORN. 1998. Serum-free media for the *in vitro* cultivation of *Cowdria ruminantium*. Ann. N.Y. Acad. Sci. **849:** 307–312.
7. ZWEYGARTH, E. & A.I. JOSEMANS. 2001. A chemically defined medium for the growth of *Cowdria ruminantium*. Onderstepoort J. Vet. Res. **68:** 37–40.
8. DU PLESSIS, J.L. 1985. A method for determining the *Cowdria ruminantium* infection rate of *Amblyomma hebraeum*: effects in mice injected with tick homogenates. Onderstepoort J. Vet. Res. **52:** 55–61.
9. YUNKER, C.E., B. BYROM & S. SEMU. 1988. Cultivation of *Cowdria ruminantium* in bovine vascular endothelial cells. Kenya Vet. **12:** 12–16.
10. VAN KUPPEVELD, F.J.M., K.-E. JOHANSSON, J.M.D. GALAMA, *et al.* 1994. Detection of Mycoplasma contamination in cell cultures by a Mycoplasma group-specific PCR. Appl. Environ. Microbiol. **60:** 149–152.

11. ZWEYGARTH, E., S.W. VOGEL, A.I. JOSEMANS & E. HORN. 1997. *In vitro* isolation and cultivation of *Cowdria ruminantium* under serum-free culture conditions. Res. Vet. Sci. **63:** 161–164.
12. BIDINGMEYER, B.A., S.A. COHEN & T.L. TARVIN. 1984. Rapid analysis of amino acids using pre-column derivatization. J. Chromogr. **336:** 93–104.
13. EAGLE, H. 1959. Amino acid metabolism in mammalian cell cultures. Science **130:** 432–437.
14. NEITZ, A.W.H. & C.E. YUNKER. 1996. Amino acid and protein depletion in medium of cell cultures infected with *Cowdria ruminantium*. Ann. N.Y. Acad. Sci. **791:** 24–34.
15. AUSTIN, F.E. & H.H. WINKLER. 1988. Proline incorporation into protein by *Rickettsia prowazekii* during growth in Chinese hamster ovary (CHO-K1) cells. Infect. Immun. **56:** 3167–3172.
16. CAPIAUMONT, J., C. LEGRAND, B. DOUSSET, *et al.* 1995. Arginine consumption as a monitor of mycoplasma infection of cultured cells. In Vitro Cell. Dev. Biol. **31:** 497–498.

Sequencing of a 15-kb *Ehrlichia ruminantium* Clone and Evaluation of the *cpg*1 Open Reading Frame for Protection against Heartwater

ELMARIÉ LOUW,[a] K.A. BRAYTON,[b] N.E. COLLINS,[a] A. PRETORIUS,[a] F. VAN STRIJP,[a] AND B.A. ALLSOPP[a]

[a]*Molecular Biology Section, Onderstepoort Veterinary Institute, Pretoria, South Africa*

[b]*Department. of Veterinary Microbiology and Pathology, Washington State University, Pullman, Washington 99164-7040, USA*

ABSTRACT: A 1.2 kb polymorphic fragment from the Gardel isolate of *Ehrlichia* (formerly *Cowdria*) ruminantium was used to isolate a 15kb clone from the *E. ruminantium* Welgevonden LambdaGEM-11 library. This clone, WL2EL1, was subcloned and sequenced. Eight open reading frames (ORFs) were identified. The ORF in WL2EL1 which contained the Welgevonden homologue of the 1.2 kb polymorphic fragment was designated *Cowdria* polymorphic gene 1 (*cpg*1). The *cpg*1 ORF was cloned into pCMViUB, a genetic vaccine vector. Mice and sheep were immunized with pCMViUB/*cpg*1 by intramuscular injection and gene gun inoculation. Although all of the immunized mice died, there was a trend for mice that received larger amounts of pCMViUB/*cpg*1 DNA to survive longer. Four out of five sheep immunized with the construct survived lethal challenge.

KEYWORDS: *Ehrlichia ruminantium*; recombinant vaccine against *E. ruminantium*; *cpg*1 gene

Ehrlichia (formerly *Cowdria*) *ruminantium* is an obligate intracellular *Rickettsia* that causes heartwater in ruminants, a major constraint to livestock production in sub-Saharan Africa.[1] The existing vaccine is difficult to manufacture, distribute, and administer and cannot be used in nonendemic areas, because it contains viable organisms.[2] A recombinant vaccine would be the ideal solution, and we are in the process of identifying potential vaccine candidates. As partial, or total, lack of cross-protection between isolates has been shown for heartwater-infected animals,[3] this suggests that the genes responsible for eliciting an immune response differ between isolates. Thus, the genes that encode good vaccine candidates are likely to be polymorphic.[4] We have cloned the genomic region encoding the polymorphic *cpg*1 gene from the Welgevonden strain of *E. ruminantium* and used this open reading frame (ORF) to test for protection from lethal *E. ruminatium* challenge in mice and sheep.

Address for correspondence: Elmarié Louw, Molecular Biology Section, Onderstepoort Veterinary Institute, Pretoria, South Africa. Voice: 012-5299 280; fax: 012-5299 431. elmarie@moon.ovi.ac.za

Ann. N.Y. Acad. Sci. 969: 147–150 (2002). © 2002 New York Academy of Sciences.

METHODS

A 1.2-kb fragment amplified from the *E. ruminantium* Gardel isolate by random amplified polymorphic DNA (RAPD)[5] was used to select a 15-kb clone (WL2EL1) from the LambdaGEM-11 *E. ruminantium* Welgevonden library.[6] The WL2EL1 insert was amplified by long-template PCR, and nebulized fragments of the insert were cloned and sequenced to produce a contig of 15 kb containing the full-length *cpg*1 gene.

The *cpg*1 gene was cloned directionally into pCMViUB, a genetic vaccine vector (S.A. Johnston, University of Texas Southwestern Medical Center, personal communication). Three groups of 10 C57BL/6J mice were immunized with pCMViUB/*cpg*1 by intramuscular (IM) injection (12.5 µg, 25 µg, and 100 µg) and gene gun[7] inoculation (0.5 µg, 1 µg, and 4 µg). Additionally, five sheep were immunized with pCMViUB/*cpg*1 by IM (200 µg) and GG (20 µg) inoculation. Empty vector served as a negative control. The mice and sheep were immunized three times at three-week intervals and challenged five weeks after the third inoculation with a lethal dose of *E. ruminantium*. Western blot analyses were performed on sera collected from the mice before immunization and before challenge. Western blot analyses of sheep sera are in progress. Lymphocyte proliferation assays were performed on peripheral blood mononuclear cells (PBMC) collected from sheep before immunization and one week before challenge. Cells were stimulated by *E. ruminantium* lysate (positive antigen) and uninfected bovine endothelial cell lysate (negative antigen). On day three of the culture period, proliferation was estimated by measurement of [^{3}H] thymidine uptake. Results are expressed as stimulation index (SI: counts per minute [cpm] of positive antigen divided by cpm of negative antigen) averaged from triplicate plates.

RESULTS AND DISCUSSION

The WL2EL1 phage clone is 14,950 bp with a GC content of 28.5%; it contains eight ORFs larger than 100 amino acids. Results of a PSI-BLAST[8] search with the deduced amino acid sequence of each ORF is shown in TABLE 1, showing that few of these ORFs have known functions. Results of the challenge experiment show that none of the mice survived lethal *E. ruminantium* challenge; however, mice that received larger amounts of pCMViUB/*cpg*1 DNA survived longer (FIG. 1).

The pCMViUB/*cpg*1 construct should express CPG1 fused to ubiquitin *in vivo*, targeting CPG1 to the proteasome, and therefore favoring a cellular immune response.[9] We tested for a humoral response by Western blot using sera from the immunized mice against *E. ruminantium* endothelial cell culture extracts and found a *E. ruminantium* protein band of approximately 84 kDa, the size predicted by the open reading frame, in 1 out of 30 mice immunized with pCMViUB/*cpg*1. The virtual absence of a humoral immune response suggests that a cellular response might have been favored in these mice, which is essential for long-lasting protection against heartwater.[10] However, this result demonstrates that CPG1 is expressed in bovine endothelial cell culture.

One of the sheep inoculated with pCMViUB/*cpg*1 and all the sheep inoculated with pCMViUB developed severe heartwater signs upon challenge and required

TABLE 1. Open reading frames (ORFs) greater than 300 base in length were translated and used in a PSI-BLAST[8] search for homologies with existing proteins

ORFs	ORF Length	Closest Homologies
ORF1	585 bp (194 aa)	ABC-transporter ATP-binding protein (*Bacillus halodurans*)
ORF2	528 bp (175 aa)	Hypothetical protein (*Wolbachia*)
ORF3	666 bp (221 aa)	Hypothetical protein RP490 (*Rickettsia prowazekii*)
ORF4	759 bp (252 aa)	Biotin-protein ligase (birA) RP533 (*Rickettsia prowazekii*)
*Cpg*1	2424 bp (807 aa)	None
ORF5	918 bp (305 aa)	None
ORF6	2496 bp (831 aa)	None
ORF7	1119 bp (372 aa)	None

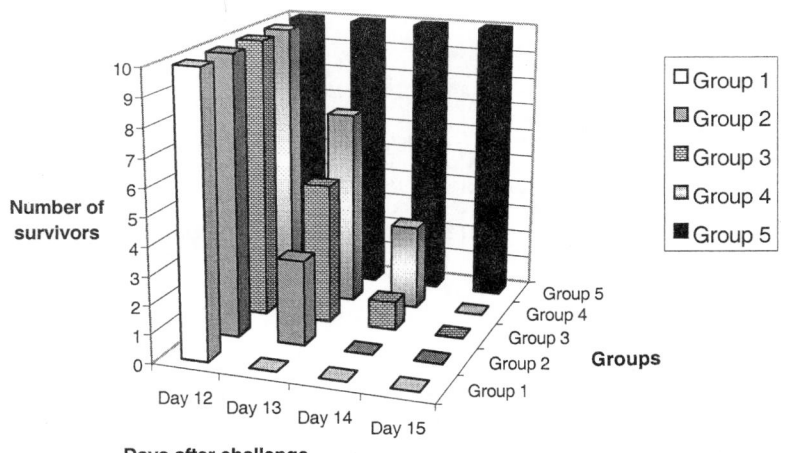

FIGURE 1. Variation in survival of immunized mice. *Group 1*: Negative control, pCMViUB immunized; *Group2*: pCMViUB/cpg1, 12.5 μg IM and 0.5 μg GG; *Group 3*: pCMViUB/cpg1, 25 μg IM and 1 μg GG; *Group 4*: pCMViUB/cpg1, 100 μg IM and 4 μg GG; *Group 5*: Positive control, infected and treated.

treatment.[11] The challenge dose was 10 LD_{50}. Four of the sheep were protected from a lethal challenge, and further, proliferation assays showed positive results (stimulation index > 2) for three of the pCMViUB/*cpg*1-inoculated sheep (TABLE 2), indicating that a memory T lymphocyte response was present. This and other experiments in our laboratory (Collins *et al.*, unpublished results) demonstrate that constructs that are not protective in mice do elicit protection in the target animal, suggesting that mice may not be a good model system for heartwater studies. These experiments demonstrate that *cpg*1 is able to induce a cellular immune response capable of protecting the target animal from clinical heartwater, and therefore this gene (product) is a potential vaccine candidate against heartwater.

TABLE 2. Proliferative response (Stimulation Index, SI)) of PBMC collected from sheep before and after immunization

Sheep (pCMViUB)	SI before immunization	SI after immunization	Sheep (pCMViUB/*cpg*1)	SI before immunization	SI after immunization
1	0.89 ± 0.05	1.30 ± 0.05	1	0.54 ± 0.54	4.32 ± 0.95
2	0.98 ± 0.24	1.20 ± 0.39	2	0.78 ± 0.07	1.76 ± 0.10
3	1.13 ± 0.22	1.24 ± 0.31	3	0.91 ± 0.29	2.06 ± 0.35
4	1.26 ± 0.48	1.11 ± 0.25	4	0.46 ± 0.25	3.11 ± 0.91
5	0.81 ± 0.18	0.94 ± 0.16	5	0.82 ± 0.30	1.87 ± 0.93

ACKNOWLEDGMENT

I would like to acknowledge Albert Bensaid for supplying the 1.2-kb fragment used for screening the library.

REFERENCES

1. UILENBERG, G. 1983. Heartwater (*Cowdria ruminantium*): current status. Adv. Vet. Sci. Comp. Med. **27:** 427–480.
2. OBEREM, P.T. & J.D. BEZUIDENHOUT. 1987. The production of heartwater vaccine. Onderstepoort J. Vet. Res. **54:** 485–488
3. DU PLESSIS, J.L. *et al.* 1989. The heterogenicity of *Cowdria ruminantium* stocks: cross-immunity and serology in sheep and pathogenicity to mice. Onderstepoort J. Vet. Res. **56:** 195–201.
4. TOTTÉ, P. *et al.* 1999. Immune responses to *Cowdria ruminantium* infections. Parasitol. Today **15:** 286–290.
5. PEREZ, J. *et al.* 1997. Detection of genomic polymorphisms among isolates of the intracellular bacterium *Cowdria ruminantium* by random amplified polymorphic DNA and Southern blotting. FEMS Microbiol. Lett. **154:** 73–79.
6. DE VILLIERS, E.P. 2001. Genome analysis of *Cowdria ruminantium*. Ph.D thesis. University of Utrecht, the Netherlands.
7. BRAYTON, K.A., *et al.* 1997. Development of the OPgun™ for bombardment of animal tissues. Onderstepoort J. Vet. Res. **64:** 153–156.
8. ALTSCHUL, S.F. *et al.* 1997. Gapped BLAST and PSI-BLAST: a new generation of protein database search programs. Nucleic Acids Res. **25:** 3389–3402.
9. DELOGU, G. *et al.* 2000. DNA Vaccination against tuberculosis: expression of a ubiquitin-conjugated tuberculosis protein enhances antimycobacterial immunity. Infect. Immun. **68:** 3097–3102.
10. STEWART, C.G. 1987. Specific immunity in mice to heartwater. Onderstepoort J. Vet. Res. **54:** 343–344.
11. VAN DE PYPEKAMP, H.E. & L. PROZESKY. 1987. Heartwater. An overview of the clinical signs, susceptibility and differential diagnoses of the disease in domestic ruminants. Onderstepoort J. Vet. Res. **54:** 263–266.

Genetic Immunization with *Ehrlichia ruminantium* GroEL and GroES Homologues

ALRI PRETORIUS,[a] F. VAN STRIJP,[a] K.A. BRAYTON,[b] N.E. COLLINS,[a] AND B.A. ALLSOPP[a]

[a]*Molecular Biology Section, Onderstepoort Veterinary Institute, Pretoria, South Africa*

[b]*Department of Veterinary Microbiology and Pathology, Washington State University, Pullman, Washington 99164-7040, USA*

ABSTRACT: *Ehrlichia ruminantium* GroEL and GroES genes were amplified from *E. ruminantium* Welgevonden genomic DNA and were cloned into genetic vaccine and *Salmonella* expression vectors. These constructs were used to inoculate Balb/c and C57BL/6J mice. Both GroEL and GroES induced low levels of protection in Balb/c and C57BL/6J mice immunized with the *Salmonella* expression vectors. None of the mice inoculated with the genetic vaccine survived. Immunological memory was also tested in these mice and a correlation between splenocyte proliferation and the survival rate was observed.

KEYWORDS: *Ehrlichia ruminantium* GroEl/ES gene homologues; recombinant vaccine against *Ehrlichia ruminantium*; GroEL; GroES

The chaperonin GroEL is a 60-kDa heat shock protein that, together with its cochaperonin GroES, assists in protein processing and assembly.[1] Bacterial heat shock proteins were shown to be important immunogens that stimulate both T and B cells and can directly induce cytokine secretion in macrophages.[2] In addition, intracellular bacteria have been shown to secrete GroEL proteins into the host cytoplasm.[3] This exposure to host immune mechanisms could play a role in the induction of a protective immune response to the invading pathogen. The *Ehrlichia ruminantium* GroEL/ES gene homologues[4] were used to immunize mice by genetic immunization[5] and bivalent *Salmonella* immunization to test their suitability as recombinant vaccine candidates.

METHODS

Cloning of groEL and groES

GroEL and GroES genes were PCR amplified from *E. ruminantium* (Welgevonden) genomic DNA. The amplification products were cloned directionally into the

Address for correspondence: Alri Pretorius, Molecular Biology Section, Onderstepoort Veterinary Institute, Pretoria, South Africa. Voice: +27 12-5299214; fax: +27 12-5299431.
Alri@moon.ovi.ac.za

Ann. N.Y. Acad. Sci. 969: 151–154 (2002). © 2002 New York Academy of Sciences.

eukaryotic pCMVi ubiquitin expression vector (S. A. Johnston, University of Texas, Southwestern Medical Center, personal communication) and into a *Salmonella* expression system using the high copy number pYA3334 expression vector.[6] To confirm the presence of the groELS genes, and appropriate reading frame, the plasmids were sequenced. Expression of the gene products was confirmed by Western blot analysis using crude *E. ruminantium* proteins as antigen.

Immunization of Mice with GroEL and GroES Constructs

Balb/c and C57BL/6 mice were used in this experiment. For genetic immunization, 10 mice per group were inoculated with a total of 1 μg DNA each: 0.5 μg delivered by intramuscular injection as well as 0.25 μg delivered by gene gun inoculations in both ears. The mice were inoculated three times at three-week intervals and were challenged with a lethal dose of *E. ruminantium* (Welgevonden) five weeks after the final boost.

Twenty mice were inoculated by intraperitoneal injection of 10^5 CFUs (colony-forming units) three times at three-week intervals with *Salmonella* expressing groEL, groES, or the empty vector. Ten mice from each group were challenged with a lethal dose of *E. ruminantium* (Welgevonden) five weeks after the final boost, and the remaining mice from each group were not challenged and were retained for lymphocyte proliferation assays.

Lymphocyte Proliferation Assay

Splenocytes were isolated and seeded in complete RPMI medium (2.5×10^5 cells per well). Crude *E. ruminantium* (Welgevonden) antigens, bovine endothelial antigen, and IL-2 (interleukin 2) were used as stimulators (1 μg per well). After an incubation period of 96 h, tritiated thymidine was added (0.5 μCi per well). Cells were harvested after 16 hours, and tritium incorporation was determined.

RESULTS AND DISCUSSION

Western blot analysis using sera from mice immunized by genetic immunization indicated that both the GroEL and ES proteins were expressed (data not shown). However, none of the mice inoculated with the GroEL genetic vaccine survived a lethal *E. ruminantium* challenge. When the GroES gene was used as an immunogen, 10% of the C57Bl/6J mice survived lethal challenge (TABLE 1).

TABLE 1. Survival of mice immunized with pCMVi UB vector

		Vector	GroEL	GroES
Balb/c	% Survival	0	0	0
	LD_{50}	2–6	2–6	2–6
C57BL/6J	% Survival	0	0	10
	LD_{50}	2–6	2–6	2–6

TABLE 2. Survival of mice immunized with *Salmonella* expressing GroEL/ES

		Trial 1			Trial 2		
		Vector	GroEL	GroES	Vector	GroEL	GroES
Balb/c	% Survival	0	0	0	0	10	30
	LD_{50}	2–6	2–6	2–6	15	15	15
	Lymphocyte proliferation	–	–	–	0/5	1/10	0/10
C57BL/6J	% Survival	0	30	20	0	30	10
	LD_{50}	6–8	6–8	6–8	3.1	3.1	3.1
	Lymphocyte proliferation	–	–	–	0/5	2/10	1/10

Western blot analysis using sera from mice immunized by bivalent *Salmonella* inoculation indicated that both the GroEL and ES proteins were expressed (data not shown). The *Salmonella* immunization experiment was repeated two times. In both trials, 30% of the C57BL/6J mice inoculated with *Salmonella* expressing GroEL survived (TABLE 2). None of the Balb/c mice survived in the first trial, but 30% survival for GroES and 10% survival for GroEL were observed in the second trial. C57BL/6J mice inoculated with the *Salmonella* expressing GroES had 20% survival in the first and 10% survival in the second trial (TABLE 2).

To determine if the mice inoculated with GroEL/ES *Salmonella* had a memory response to GroEL/ES, lymphocyte proliferation assays were done on the splenocytes of immunized, nonchallenged mice. The results obtained correlate with the survival rates in the challenged group, except for Balb/c mice inoculated with GroES (TABLE 2). The fact that anti-GroEL/ES antibodies could be detected in all mice suggests that there should be memory T cells present. The virtual absence of positive proliferation in the mice splenocytes might be attributed to the fact that crude antigen was used to stimulate the splenocytes. A better indication of immunological memory might be obtained using expressed GroEL and ES proteins instead of crude antigen. The memory lymphocytes might also reside in other lymph nodes that were not tested in this experiment.

In conclusion, the *E. ruminantium* GroES homologue seems to confer low levels of protection to a lethal *E. ruminantium* challenge in a murine model. We plan to test these constructs in sheep, as other DNA constructs tested in our laboratory that have shown no or little protection in mice, were found to be protective in sheep (Collins *et al.*, unpublished results).

REFERENCES

1. WANG, J.D. *et al.* 1998. GroEL-GroES mediated protein folding requires an intact central cavity. PNAS **95:** 12163–12168.
2. RETZLAFF, C. *et al.* 1994. Bacterial heat shock proteins directly induce cytokine mRNA and interleukin-1 secretion in macrophage cultures. Infect. Immun. **62:** 5689–5693.
3. VANET, A. & A. LABIGNE. 1998. Evidence for specific secretion rather than autolysis in the release of some *Heliobacter pylori* proteins. Infect. Immun. **66:** 1023–1027.

4. LALLY, N.C. *et al.* 1995. The *Cowdria ruminantium* groE operon. Microbiology **141:** 2091–2100
5. LAI, W.C. *et al.* 1995. Protection against *Mycoplasma pulmonis* infection by genetic vaccination. DNA Cell Biol. **14:** 643–651.
6. NAKAYAMA K., S.M. KELLY & R. CURTISS. 1988. Construction of an ASD+ expression cloning vector: stable maintenance and high level expression of cloned genes in a *Salmonella* vaccine strain. Biotechnology **6:** 693–697.
7. BRAYTON, K.A. *et al.* 1997. Development of the OPgun™ for bombardment of animal tissues. Onderstepoort J. Vet. Res. **64:** 153–156.

Sequence Analysis of Three *Ehrlichia ruminantium* LambdaGEM-11 Clones

ALRI PRETORIUS, N.E. COLLINS, H.C. STEYN, AND B.A. ALLSOPP

Molecular Biology Section, Onderstepoort Veterinary Institute, Pretoria, South Africa

ABSTRACT: Three Lambda GEM11 clones were isolated from a large-insert *Ehrlichia ruminantium* Welgevonden library. The inserts were amplified, sequenced, and analyzed. A total of 39 827 bp was obtained, and 18 different open reading frames (ORFs) were identified. Long repeats (100–200 kbp) were found in all three sequences. These repeats may play a role in the induction of antigenic variation. Along with a 20-kbp sequence of a clone from the *E. ruminantium* cosmid library, these sequences are the first large sequences to be yielded by the *E. ruminantium* genome sequencing project.

KEYWORDS: *Ehrlichia ruminantium*; genome sequencing of *E. ruminantium*; LambdaGEM-11 clones

In the past few years the number of available bacterial genome sequences has increased markedly. Molecular analyses of *Ehrlichia ruminantium*, an obligate intracellular parasite, have been hampered in the past because the organism is difficult to culture *in vitro*. The genome sequencing of *E. ruminantium* could provide the molecular basis for determining virulence factors, growth requirements, and ultimately tools for the design of genetic vaccines.[1] As part of the *E. ruminantium* genome sequencing project, clones from a large insert LambdaGEM-11 library were selected and sequenced. Identification of open reading frames (ORFs) will be targeted towards the development of vaccines.

METHODS

Three LambdaGEM-11 clones were isolated from a large insert *E. ruminantium* (Welgevonden) library. Two of the clones were identified by screening the library with a ~100-kbp *Ksp*I *E. ruminantium* (Welgevonden) fragment. The third clone was identified by screening a number of randomly picked clones with *E. ruminantium* (Welgevonden) genomic DNA. Phage DNA was isolated, and the ~15-kbp insert was amplified using long-template PCR. The amplified insert DNA was nebulized, size selected, and subcloned into the pMOS*Blue* blunt-ended cloning vector for sequenc-

Address for correspondence: Alri Pretorius, Molecular Biology Section, Onderstepoort Veterinary Institute, Pretoria, South Africa. Voice: +27 12-5299214; fax: +27 12-5299431.
Alri@moon.ovi.ac.za

Ann. N.Y. Acad. Sci. 969: 155–158 (2002). © 2002 New York Academy of Sciences.

TABLE 1. Open reading frames (ORFs) longer than 300 bases in length were translated and used in a PSI-BLAST[6] search for homologies with existing proteins

Clone	ORFs	ORF length	Closest homologies
WL2AP1	ORF 1	1230 bp (410 aa)	putative transport protein (*Legionella pneumophila* and others)
	ORF 2	609 bp (203 aa)	thymidylate kinase (DTMP kinase) (*Aquifex aeolicus* and others)
	ORF 3	963 bp (321 aa)	malonyl CoA-acyl carrier protein transacylase (*Sinorhizobium melioti* and others)
	ORF 4	792 bp (264 aa)	hypothetical protein RP 440 (*Rickettsia prowazekii* and others)
	ORF 5	927 bp (309 aa)	Inosine-5′-monophosphate dehydrogenase (*Aquifex aeolicus*)
	ORF 6	846 bp (282 aa)	hypothetical protein RP 444 (*Rickettsia prowazekii* and others)
	ORF 7	990 bp (330 aa)	pyruvate dehydrogenase E1 component (*Rickettsia prowazekii* and others)
	ORF 8 (partial)	~358 bp (~119 aa)	probable conjugal transfer protein (*Rickettsia prowazekii*)
WL2NEC1	ORF 1	3000 bp (1000 aa)	unknown protein (*Mesorhizobium loti*) and hypothetical RP780 (*Rickettsia prowazekii*)
	ORF 2	441 bp (167 aa)	ribonuclease H (*Caulobacter cresentus* and others)
	ORF 3	546 bp (182 aa)	none
	ORF 4	1248 bp (416 aa)	Mfd protein (*Rickettsia rickettsii* and others) and transcription repair coupling factor (*Caulobacter cresentus* and others)
WL2HCS1	ORF 1	435 bp (145 aa)	none
	ORF 2	525 bp (175 aa)	2-amino-4-hydroxy-6-hydroxymethyl-dihydropteridine pyrophosphokinase (*Aquifex aeolicus* and others)
	ORF 3	3033 bp (1011 aa)	phosphoribosylformlglycinamidine synthase–related protein (*Thermoplasma acidophilum* and others)
	ORF 4	969 bp (323 aa)	biotin synthase (*Pseudomonas aeruginosa* and others)
	ORF 5	456 bp (152 aa)	none
	ORF 6	588 bp (196 aa)	lipoprotein N1pD (*Neisseria meninggitidis* and others)

ing with the ABI 377 automated sequencer. The sequences were assembled and analyzed using gap4 and nip4.[2]

RESULTS AND DISCUSSION

The first clone, WL2AP1, is 13,470 bp in length and has a GC content of 32.5%. ORFs larger than 300 bp were identified. Four of the ORFs showed homology with housekeeping genes (TABLE 1). Two of the ORFs showed homology to transport proteins, and the remaining ORFs are homologous to hypothetical proteins of other bacteria. WL2AP1 also contains the DNA 23S rRNA gene. The sequence of WL2NEC1 is 12,300 bp in length with a GC content of 25.3 %. Four ORFs (>300 bp) were identified, three of which have homologies with existing genes (TABLE 1). One is similar to a hypothetical protein of *Rickettsia prowazekii*, the second has high homology with transcription-repair coupling factors of various bacteria, and the third is a ribonuclease H. WL2HCS1 has an insert size of approximately 14,057 bp and a GC content of 27.2%. A total of six ORFs (>300 bp) were identified; two have no homologies to known genes, while the remaining four are homologous to housekeeping genes (TABLE 1). The sequence of pcr9, a *E. ruminantium* sequence already published in Genbank, is also present in this contig. Long repeats (100–200 kbp) have been identified in all three sequences. Large repetitive sequences, at one time thought to be absent from compact genomes of prokaryotes, have recently been identified in a number of bacteria including *Mycoplasma*[3] and *Rickettsia*.[4] Repeated DNA sequences are located either within or just before the start of a gene, or may be located within the promoter region. The function of these repeats is unknown, but it is thought to play a role in the evolutionary mechanisms that allow bacteria to adapt to environmental changes. These mechanisms include the generation of antigenic diversity and the regulation of gene expression, where the length of the repeat dictates transcription of a particular gene.[1,3–5]

CONCLUSION

Along with a 20-kbp sequence of a clone from the *E. ruminantium* cosmid library, these sequences are the first large sequences to be yielded by the *E. ruminantium* genome sequencing project. The sequences of these clones have already been used to determine the codon usage of *E. ruminantium*. Selected ORFs from these clones will be subcloned into a genetic vaccine expression vector and tested in sheep for their ability to induce protective immunity to lethal *E. ruminantium* challenge.

REFERENCES

1. ROMERO, D. *et al.* 1999. Repeated sequences in bacterial chromosomes and plasmids: a glimpse from sequenced genomes. Res. Microbiol. **150:** 735–743.
2. STADEN, R. *et al.* 1998. The Staden Package. Computer Methods in Molecular Biology. S. Misener & S. Krawetz, Eds. Humana Press. Totowa, NJ.

3. GLEW, M.D. *et al.* 2000. Characterization of a multigene family undergoing high frequency DNA rearrangements and coding for abundant variable surface protein in *Mycoplasma agalactiae.* Infect. Immun. **68:** 4539–4548.
4. OGATA, H. *et al.* 2000. Selfish DNA in protein-coding genes of *Rickettsia.* Science **290:** 347–350.
5. ROCHA, E.P.C. *et al.* 1999. Functional and evolutionary roles of long repeats in prokaryotes. Res. Microbiol. **150:** 725–733.
6. ALTSCHUL, S.F. *et al.* 1997. Gapped BLAST and PSI-BLAST: a new generation of protein database search programs. Nucleic Acids Res. **25:** 3389–3402.

The Innate Resistance of Kenana Cattle to Tropical Theileriosis (*Theileria annulata* Infection) in the Sudan

M.A. BAKHEIT[a] AND A.A. LATIF[b]

[a]*Faculty of Veterinary Science, University of Khartoum, Sudan*

[b]*Faculty of Science, Midrand University, Halfway House 1685, South Africa*

ABSTRACT: A study was carried out to assess the innate resistance of the indigenous Kenana breed of cattle in the Sudan to tropical theileriosis, *Theileria annulata* infection of cattle. Nine susceptible Kenana calves were obtained from an area free from tropical theileriosis and the vector tick *Hyalomma anatolicum anatolicum* and were found negative to *T. annulata* antibodies in the indirect fluorescent antibody test. They were infected by inoculation of 1.0 mL *T. annulata* sporozoite stabilate. Three Friesian calves were also infected and served as susceptible controls. The percent of schizont parasitosis (Macroschizont Index, MSI) in the Kenana cattle was reduced by 70% compared to the Friesian calves. The percent of piroplasm parasitemia was also significantly lower in the Kenana calves. The rate of white blood cell reduction was significantly greater in the Friesian calves ($P < 0.05$). These differences were attributed to the high rate of schizont multiplication in the control cattle. Seventy-eight percent (7/9) of the Kenana cattle recovered spontaneously, and only 22% required treatment compared to 100% mortality in the Friesian controls. These differences were attributed to the high rate of schizont multiplication in the control cattle and, on the other hand, ability of the Kenana cattle to limit the MSI, resulting in less severe damage to the lymphoid tissue during the acute phase of the disease.

KEYWORDS: *Theileria annulata*; tick-borne disease; resistance to theileriosis; Kenana cattle in Sudan; *Hyalomma anatolicum anatolicum*

INTRODUCTION

Tick and tick-borne diseases are major health and management problems affecting the productivity of livestock in Sudan. Topical theileriosis (*Theileria annulata* infection of cattle, transmitted by *Hyalomma anatolicum anatolicum*) has emerged as a disease of economic importance with the introduction of exotic taurine breeds, mainly Holstein Friesian, to increase milk production. These imported breeds and their crosses proved to be highly susceptible when introduced onto endemic areas, and 40–60% mortalities have been reported.[1] The losses in 3000 imported pregnant

Address for correspondence: Dr. A.A. Latif, Faculty of Sciences, Midrand University, P.O. Box 2986, Halfway House, 1685, South Africa. Voice: +2711 315853; fax +2712 3436118. abdulal@edu.co.za

Ann. N.Y. Acad. Sci. 969: 159–163 (2002). © 2002 New York Academy of Sciences.

Friesian heifers introduced into Khartoum State were estimated at US$ 4.5–5.0 million.[2] The long-term approach for the control of tropical theileriosis would be to select cattle from the indigenous population for productivity while *Theileria* tolerance could be developed.[2,3] Among the local breeds of cattle in Sudan, the Kenana have high milk production potential, tolerate diverse environmental and nutritional conditions,[4] and are resistant to tick infestation.[5] The objective of this work was to investigate the innate resistance of the Kenana cattle to tropical theileriosis under laboratory conditions, to complement the previous studies on their tick resistance.

MATERIALS AND METHODS

Animals

Kenana calves (8 months old) were obtained from El Damazin, the Blue Nile province, 600 km south east of Khartoum, where tropical theileriosis and the vector *H. a. anatolicum* have not been known to occur.[6] They were transported by truck to University of Khartoum and kept at the animal house for 9 weeks before being used. They were sprayed with Amitraz, a short-acting acarcide, twice weekly. The sera of these animals were found negative to *T. annulata* schizont antigens in the indirect fluorescent antibody IFA test.[7] Three Friesian calves (4–5 months old) were also used as susceptible controls.

Infection of Cattle

The method of preparation of the *Theileria annulata* sporozoite stabilate has been previously described.[8] The ticks used had a 96.2% infection rate and 202.7 ± 155.0 infected acini per infected tick. Each animal received a subcutaneous inoculation of 1.0 mL of the stabilate (equivalent of 10 ticks) behind the right ear in front of the right parotid lymph node. Rectal temperature and blood smears were taken daily, while lymph node biopsy smears were taken when the glands were found swollen on palpation. The white blood cells (WBC) were counted, and the Macroschizont Index (MSI, percent of schizont parasitosis) was determined by counting the number of *Theileria* schizonts in 1000 mononuclear cells and multiplied by 0.1. The criteria used to record animal reactions to theileriosis have been described previously.[9] The two-sample Student's *t* test was used to compare the means of different parameters between the infected Kenana cattle versus the control Friesians. The differences were considered significant at $P < 0.05$.

RESULTS

TABLE 1 shows the performance of the Kenana and Friesian calves to *T. annulata* infection. All of the control Friesian calves developed severe and fatal theileriosis reactions; two died on day 11 and the third on day 13. The three calves did not respond to the treatment using butalex (buparvaquone, Coopers Pitman-Moore). Two of the nine Kenana cattle also developed severe reactions, were treated, and recovered. They were considered as susceptible as the controls and allocated a separate

TABLE 1. Clinical and parasitological reactions to *T. annulata* sporozoite stabilate infection in the Kenana cattle and the susceptible control Friesian calves

Cattle	No.	Fever		Schizonts			Piroplasm		Animal reactions
		Onset (d)	Duration (d)	Onset (d)	Duration (d)	Maximum MSI	Onset (d)	Maximum parisitemia	
KenanaR[a]	7	6.7 ± 1.4	7.7 ± 3.1	8.0 ± 1.7	9.3 ± 2.7	6.4 ± 7.0	11.1 ± 0.6	2.8 ± 3.9	1 mild 4 moderate 2 severe/ recovered
KenanaT[b]	2	7.5	9.0	6.5	9.5	57.0	11.0	7.0	2 severe/ treated
Friesian	3	6.2 ± 0.6	5.3 ± 1.5	7.0 ± 0.0	5.2 ± 1.2	57.0 ± 29.4	10.7 ± 0.6	12.6 ± 17.7	3 severe/fatal

[a]Kenana R: all recovered spontaneously.
[b]Kenana T: all treated and recovered.

group in TABLE 1. Of the seven Kenana calves one had mild reactions, four had moderate reactions, and two had severe reactions. However, all of them had recovered without treatment by day 14–19 after infection. The mean MSI was 6.4 ± 7.0 in the seven Kenana animals compared to 57.0 in the control Friesians and the two susceptible Kenana animals, and the difference was significant ($P < 0.05$). The MSI in the Friesian group increased to 45.8 and 80.5 by days 11 and 13, respectively, compared to 1.4 for the seven Kenana cattle. There was a significant reduction ($P < 0.05$) in the WBC counts in the two groups of cattle by day nine after infection. The counts were reduced by 48.7% and 58% in the Friesian calves by days 9 and 12, and the three animals died by day 13. The WBC counts dropped by 66% in the Kenana cattle by day 9, but there was a significant ($P < 0.05$) recovery by day 15 (58% reduction) and day 30 (46% reduction). The *Theileria* piroplasms parasitemia in the control Friesians was 4.5 times greater than in the Kenana cattle (12.6% and 2.8%, respectively), and the difference was significant ($P < 0.05$).

DISCUSSION

The artificial *T. annulata* challenge, which was used to infect the experimental cattle in the present study, was tremendous compared to the natural field challenge (25.7% and 30% tick infection rates in field ticks; unpublished data). The Kenana cattle showed different individual clinical and parasitological manifestations to the *T. annulata* infection. Thus, 78% (7/9) had recovered spontaneously, and only 22% required treatment compared to 100% mortality in the exotic Friesian cattle. Moreover, the two Kenana animals that were treated showed a faster response and recovered compared to the Friesians, which had transient improvement after treatment, resurgence of parasitemia, and eventually all died. Individual variations within cattle breeds to disease tolerance are reported in trypanotolerant cattle[10] and in host resistance to tick infestations.[11] A significant difference in the MSI was demonstrated between the Kenana and the Friesian calves. Since all animals were initially naïve to *T. annulata* infection as determined by the IFA test and had been maintained under the same experimental conditions, the differences in the body reactions between the two groups could be associated to a genetic factor(s). The Friesian control group had a maximum value of MSI three times greater than that of the Kenana in seven days. The Kenana cattle were also able to control the merozoite/piroplasm parasitemias and to tolerate low WBC counts. Therefore, the ability of the Kenana to control the enormous multiplication of the macroschizonts, resulting in less severe damage of the lymphoid tissues during the acute phase of the disease, is most probably the basis of their genetic resistance to tropical theileriosis. Similar findings were reported for Ankole cattle, a local breed in Rwanda.[12] These authors also found that the mean MSI level in the infected Ankole was three times less than that in the crossbred animals, and that there was a correlation between high mortality and a high MSI in the infected cattle. The innate resistance of the Kenana cattle to tropical theileriosis shown in this study and to tick infestations[5] would accentuate their suitability in breeding programs; this should be considered when planning long-term tick and tick-borne disease control policy, particularly in situations where farm management is judged to be poor and the resources for tissue culture immunization against theileriosis are not sustainable.

REFERENCES

1. BROWN, C.G.D. 1990. Control of tropical theileriosis (*Theileria annulata* infection of cattle). Parasitologia **32**: 23–31.
2. LATIF, A.A. 1994. Economic losses in exotic breeds of cattle due to tropical theileriosis in the Sudan. *In* Tropical Theileriosis in the Sudan. A.M. Atelmanan & S.M. Kheir, Eds.: 1–5. Central Veterinary Research Laboratories. Khartoum, Sudan.
3. YOUNG, A.S. 1981. The epidemiology of theileriosis in East Africa. *In* Advances in the Control of Theileriosis. A.D. Irvin, M.P. Cunningham & A.S. Young, Eds.: 38–55. Martinus Nijhoff Publishers. London.
4. SAEED, A.M., P.N. WARD, *et al.* 1987. Characterization of Kenana cattle at Um Banein, Sudan. ILCA Research Report 16. The International Livestock Centre for Africa. Addis Ababa, Ethiopia.
5. LATIF, A.A. 1984. Resistance to *Hyalomma anatolicum anatolicum* Koch (1844) and *Rhipicephalus evertsi evertsi* Neumann (1897) (Ixodoidea:Ixodidae) by cattle in the Sudan. Insect Sci. Appl. **5**: 509–511.
6. JONGEJAN, F., D. ZIVKOVIC, *et al.* 1987. Ticks (Acari: Ixodidae) of the Blue and White Nile ecosystems in the Sudan with particular reference to the *Rhipicephalus sanguinues* group. Exp. Appl. Acarol. **3**: 331–346.
7. BURRIDGE, M.J. & C.D. KIMBER. 1972. The indirect fluorescent antibody test for experimental East Coast fever (*Theileria parva* infection of cattle): evaluation of a cell culture schizont antigen. Res. Vet. Sci. **13**: 451–455.
8. FAO. 1993. Tick and tick-borne diseases control in eastern and southern Africa: Zimbabwe. Studies on theilerosis and economics of tick control. Manual of laboratory techniques. Field Document No. 3. Food and Agriculture Organization of the United Nations. Rome.
9. HOVE, T., F.L. MUSISI, *et al.* 1995. Challenge of *Theileria parva* (Boleni)-immunized cattle with selected East African *Theileria* stocks. Trop. Anim. Health Prod. **27**: 202–210.
10. ROELANTS, G.E., I. TAMBOURA, *et al* 1983. Trypanotolerance: an individual not a breed character. Acta Trop. **40**: 99–104.
11. LATIF, A.A., D.K. PUNYA, *et al.* 1991. Tick infestations on Zebu cattle in Western Kenya: individual host variation. J. Med. Entomol. **28**: 114–121.
12. PALING, R.W., C. MPANGALA, *et al.* 1991. Exposure of Ankole and crossbred cattle to theileriosis in Rwanda. Trop. Anim. Health Prod. **23**: 203–214.

Age-Related Innate Immune Response in Calves to *Babesia bovis* Involves IL-12 Induction and IL-10 Modulation

W.L. GOFF,[a] W.C. JOHNSON,[a] W. TUO,[a] R.A.VALDEZ,[a] S.M. PARISH,[b] G.M. BARRINGTON,[b] AND W.C. DAVIS[c]

[a]*Animal Diseases Research Unit, USDA-ARS, Pullman, Washington 99164, USA*

[b]*Department of Veterinary Clinical Sciences and* [c]*Department of Veterinary Microbiology and Pathology, College of Veterinary Medicine, Washington State University, Pullman, Washington 99164, USA*

ABSTRACT: There is a strong innate immunity in calves to infection with *Babesia bovis*. Interleukin (IL)-12 and IL-10 have been shown *in vitro* to be important immunoregulatory cytokines. Here we demonstrate *in vivo* that the protective innate response in young calves to infection with virulent *B. bovis* involves the early appearance of IL-12 and interferon-γ (IFN-γ) transcripts in the spleen. In contrast, IL-12 and IFN-γ mRNA expression in the spleens of adult cattle that succumbed to the infection was delayed and depressed and occurred within the context of IL-10 expression. Also in contrast with calves, there was no detectable antibody response before death in adults. A vigorous CD8[+] T-cell expansion occurred in the spleens of both calves and adults.

KEYWORDS: innate immune response; *Babesia bovis*; spleen; interleukin-12; interleukin-10

Humoral and cellular mechanisms are engaged in the bovine immune response against *Babesia bovis,* and a strong spleen-dependent innate immunity is manifested in young calves. In this study we compared the cytokine profile, antibody response, and, to some extent, cellular proliferation in the spleen between calves and adult cattle.

MATERIALS AND METHODS

Two groups of Holstein-Friesian castrated bull cattle (a group 4 months of age, and another group of adults) underwent a surgical procedure at 3 months of age to marsupialize the spleen in order to facilitate the sequential acquisition of spleen cells by percutaneous aspiration under local anesthesia during the course of infection.[1]

Address for correspondence: W.L. Goff, Ph.D., USDA-ARS-ADRU, P.O. Box 646630, 3003 ADBF, Washington State University, Pullman, Washington 99164-6630. Voice: 509-335-6003; fax: 509-335-8328.

wgoff@vetmed.wsu.edu

Ann. N.Y. Acad. Sci. 969: 164–168 (2002). © 2002 New York Academy of Sciences.

Each animal was experimentally infected with the virulent T_2Bo isolate of *B. bovis*.[2] Blood and spleen cells were collected on several occasions before and then daily for two weeks during acute infection. Differential blood leukocyte counts were made daily along with Giemsa-stained blood films for microscopic evidence of infection. In addition, hematocrit and rectal temperature were recorded daily. Plasma was assayed for the presence of interferon-γ (IFN-γ) using an ELISA.[3] Serum was assayed for specific antibody using indirect immunofluorescence.[4]

Spleen mononuclear cells (SMCs) were collected and processed for RT-PCR with cytokine-specific primers.[5] Also, SMCs were prepared for phenotype determination by flow cytometry.[6]

RESULTS AND DISCUSSION

As expected, the adult group experienced severe disease. There was no difference in hematocrit, with levels for both groups decreasing by approximately 50%. Each

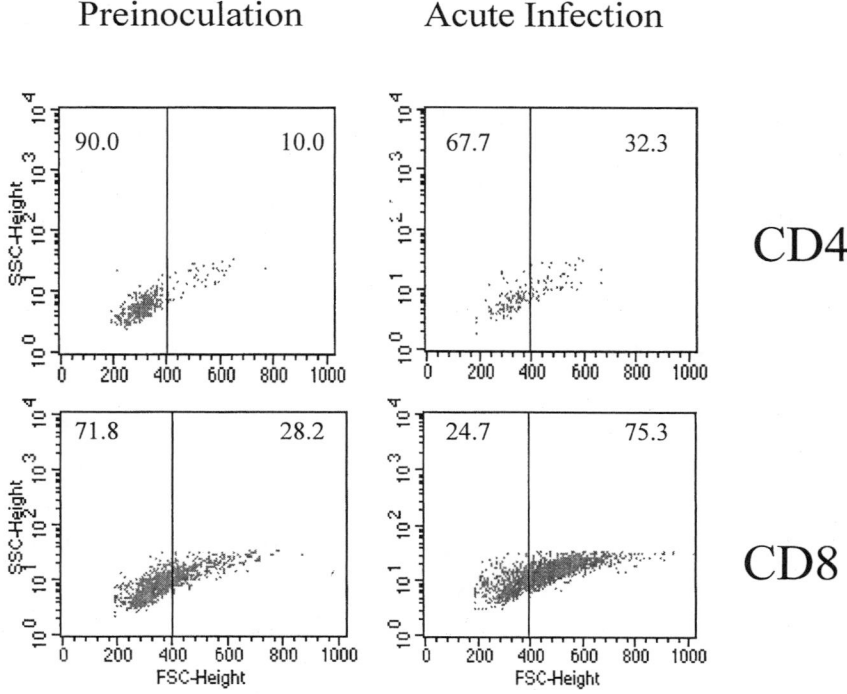

FIGURE 1. Flow cytometric evidence of lymphocyte proliferation in the spleen of a representative calf during *B. bovis* infection. SMCs were obtained before inoculation and at day 11 PI during the acute episode. SMCs were labeled with monoclonal antibodies (mAb) specific for leukocyte differentiation antigens. The data reflects the size shift (blast cells as a result of proliferation) resulting from gating on specifically labeled populations. The number in each quadrant is the percentage of the gated cells.

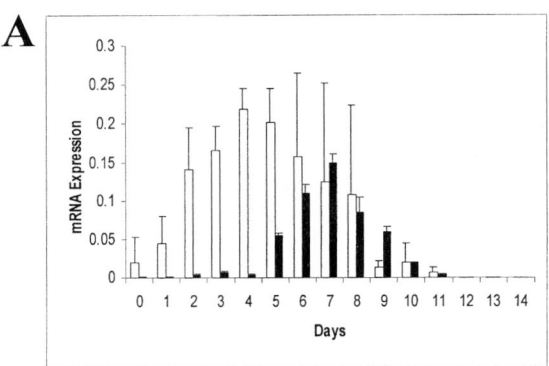

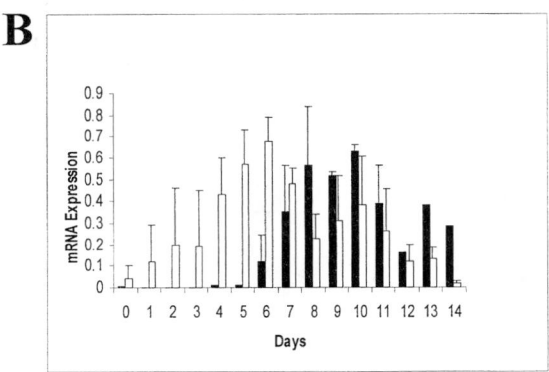

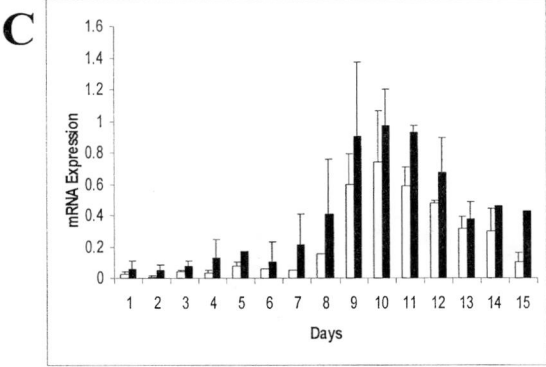

FIGURE 2. Kinetics of IL-12 **(A)**, IFN-γ **(B)**, and IL-10 **(C)** mRNA expression in SMC from calves (*white bars*) and adults (*black bars*) during *B. bovis* infection. The time to reach maximum expression from day zero was significantly different in calves and adults for IL-12 ($P < 0.01$) and IFN-γ ($P < 0.05$).

animal experienced a febrile response between 7 and 10 days post inoculation (PI), which lasted for 4–8 days in the calves and until immediately before death in the adults (between day 13 and 15 PI). There was microscopic evidence of parasitemia in each animal. As is characteristic with *B. bovis*, the level of parasitemia was low. However, robust parasites were detected in the peripheral blood from adults, whereas only crisis forms were noted from the calves.

Peripheral blood leukocyte numbers, primarily lymphocytes, decreased in both groups; but although the decrease continued until death in the adults, there was a return to normal in the calves, and by day 12 PI the difference between groups was significant ($P < 0.05$).

Specific antibody was detected in serum from the calves by day 11 PI but never detected in serum from adults. Isotype analysis was not done, but efforts are under way to determine whether there is a bias toward specific IgG_2, consistent with a type-1 response.

A vigorous $CD8^+$ proliferation occurred in the spleen of both groups (FIG. 1). We have shown that a $CD2^+$, $WC-1^-$, $\gamma\delta$ T-cell population exists in the spleen as a much larger proportion than in blood and that this population, when activated, expresses $CD8$.[6,7] This population has been shown to suppress proliferation of $CD4^+$ lymphocytes[7] and may well be playing this role in the splenic response during *B. bovis* infection.

Prominent among several parameters distinguishing the immune response of calves from adults was the early appearance of interleukin (IL)-12 and IFN-γ mRNA in the spleen (FIG. 2). Both molecules play a role in innate and acquired immunity, activating MP and providing a switch to synthesis of the opsonic immunoglobulin isotype IgG_2.[8,9]

IL-10 modulates type-1 responses, and this effect was apparent here. IL-10 modulation is necessary in order to prevent prolonged inflammatory responses that can result in pathologic conditions. IL-10 expression levels were greater and remained prominent longer in SMCs from adults. IL-12 and IFN-γ mRNA expression decreased following the induction of IL-10. IL-12 and IFN-γ induction in the spleen of calves occurred before the influence of IL-10, however, and the early induction of IL-12 and IFN-γ was associated with protection. This implies that, if IL-10 exerts its influence first, the type-1 response may be inhibited until too late to arrest the babesial disease process. Thus, the sequence of cytokine induction demonstrated here suggests that immune intervention strategies should consider means to incorporate or induce the timely production of IL-12.

REFERENCES

1. VARMA, S. & A.M. SHATRY. 1980. A technique for partial marsupialisation of the spleen in calves. Vet. Rec. **106:** 127–128.
2. GOFF, W.L., W.C. JOHNSON & C.W. CLUFF. 1998. *Babesia bovis* immunity: *in vivo* and *in vitro* evidence for IL-10 regulation of IFN-γ and iNOS. Ann. N.Y. Acad. Sci. **849:** 161–180.
3. AMETJI, B.N., D.C. BEITZ, T.A. REINHARDT & B.J. NONNECKE. 1996. 1,25-Dihydroxyvitamin D3 inhibits secretion of interferon-γ by mitogen- and antigen-stimulated bovine mononuclear leukocytes. Vet. Immunol. Immunopathol. **52:** 77–90.

4. GOFF, W.L., G.G. WAGNER, T.M. CRAIG & R.F. LONG. 1982. The bovine immune response to tick-derived *Babesia bovis* infection: serological studies of isolated immunoglobulins. Vet. Parasitol. **11:** 109–120.
5. GOFF, W.L., K.O. O'ROURKE, W.C. JOHNSON, *et al.* 1998. The role of IL-10 in iNOS and cytokine mRNA expression during in vitro differentiation of bovine mononuclear phagocytes. J. Interferon Cytokine Res. **18:** 139–149.
6. WYATT, C.R., C. MADRUGA, C.W. CLUFF, *et al.* 1994. Differential distribution of γδT-cell receptor lymphocyte subpopulations in blood and spleen of young and adult cattle. Vet. Immunol. Immunopathol. **40:** 187–199.
7. PARK, Y.H., L.K. FOX, M.J. HAMILTON & W.C. DAVIS. 1993. Suppression of proliferative response of BoCD4$^+$ T-lymphocytes by activated BoCD8$^+$ T-lymphocytes in the mammary gland of cows with *Staphylococcus aureus* mastitis. Vet. Immunol. Immunopathol. **36:** 137–151.
8. ESTES, D.M., N.M. CLOSSER & G.K. ALLEN. IFN-γ stimulates IgG$_2$ production from bovine B-cells costimulated with anti-μ and mitogen. Cell. Immunol. **154:** 287–295.
9. COLLINS, R.A., C.J. HOWARD, S.E. DUGGAN & D. WERLING. 1999. Bovine interleukin-12 and modulation of IFN-γ production. Vet. Immunol. Immunopathol. **68:** 193–207.

Residual Effect of Antibabesial Drugs on the Live Redwater Blood Vaccines

M.P. COMBRINK, P.C. TROSKIE, AND D.T. DE WAAL

Parasitology Division, Onderstepoort Veterinary Institute,
Onderstepoort, 0110, South Africa

ABSTRACT: It has been demonstrated that the attenuated organisms used in the unfrozen South African *Babesia bovis* and *B. bigemina* (redwater) vaccines are susceptible for longer periods to the residual effect of the anti-babesial drugs diminazene and imidocarb dipropionate than the virulent field strains. Reports of vaccine failures in some animals vaccinated with the frozen South African redwater vaccines after prophylactic treatment with imidocarb dipropionate have led us to reinvestigate the validity of the recommended prescribed waiting periods. Results indicated that waiting periods before administration of the frozen *B. bovis* and *B. bigemina* vaccines in animals that have been treated with diminazene at 3.5 mg/kg live weight, compare favorably with results initially obtained for the unfrozen vaccines at 4 and 8 weeks, respectively. However, the inhibitory effect of imidocarb dipropionate at 3.0 mg/kg live weight on the infectivity of both frozen *B. bovis* and *B. bigemina* vaccines is longer than previously anticipated and necessitated changing the minimum waiting periods before administration of these vaccines from 8 to 12 weeks and 16 to 24 weeks, respectively.

KEYWORDS: babesiosis; live redwater blood vaccines; diminazene; imidocarb; *Babesia bovis*; *Babesia bigemina*

The antibabesial drugs diminazene and imidocarb have long been used to successfully treat the Asiatic (*Babesia bovis*) and African (*Babesia bigemina*) forms of babesiosis in South Africa. It has been demonstrated, however, that the attenuated organisms used in the unfrozen South African *B. bovis* and *B. bigemina* (redwater) vaccines are susceptible for longer periods to the residual effects of diminazene and imidocarb dipropionate than the virulent field strains.[1]

The depletion kinetics of these drugs are therefore of great importance, especially where treatment may interfere with the efficacy of live *Babesia* vaccines that are often administered soon after treatment. The elimination half-life of diminazene has been estimated in cattle to be approximately 222 hours,[2] whereas imidocarb remains detectable in edible bovine tissues for up to 224 days.[3]

Address for correspondence: M.P. Combrink, Parasitology Division, Onderstepoort Veterinary Institute, Private Bag X05, Onderstepoort, 0110, South Africa. Voice: +27 12-5299204; fax: +27 12-5299434.

mike@moon.ovi.ac.za

Ann. N.Y. Acad. Sci. 969: 169–173 (2002). © 2002 New York Academy of Sciences.

Resent studies indicated that imidocarb had a longer than anticipated inhibitory effect on the infectivity of the frozen *B. bigemina* vaccine parasites compared to the unfrozen vaccine. On the basis of these findings, it was decided to reinvestigate the periods of residual effect of diminazene and imidocarb on the frozen *B. bovis* and *B. bigemina* vaccines.

MATERIALS AND METHODS

Animals

Nguni X Bonsmara cattle from Kaalplaas (an experimental farm adjacent to the Onderstepoort Veterinary Institute), ages ranging between 5 to 7 months old, were placed according to their susceptibility to *B. bovis* or *B. bigemina* into four experimental and four control groups of five animals each. Animals were dipped weekly with deltamethrin (Decatix 3, Hoechst Roussel Vet) and kept on pasture until they were vaccinated, after which they were housed in stables under tick-free conditions for the duration of the experiment. Notwithstanding these precautions, a number of the animals contracted redwater while on the veld and had to be excluded from the experiment.

Drug Administration and Vaccination

Commercially available antibabesial diminazene (Berenil, Intervet SA) and imidocarb dipropionate (Forray-65, Schering-Plough AH) were administered according to manufacturer's instructions (TABLE 1).

Thawing of the frozen *Babesia* vaccines was done by placing the vaccine directly from liquid nitrogen storage onto melting ice, where it was kept for 4 hours before intramuscular inoculation of an animal with 1 ml of the vaccine (TABLE 1).

Monitoring Redwater Reactions

Blood smears were prepared and monitored daily,[4] and antibodies against *Babesia* were determined in sera collected before and again 30 days after vaccination, using the indirect fluorescent antibody test technique.[5]

Evaluation of Infectivity

The criteria used to evaluate successful infectivity were either a positive blood smear diagnosis or positive seroconversion following vaccination. The unpaired *t*-test was used to determine whether results for the prepatent periods differed significantly.

RESULTS AND DISCUSSION

Diminazene-treated Animals

Results obtained for groups 1 and 2 (TABLE 1) showed no significant differences between the experimental and the respective control groups. Therefore, previously recommended waiting periods for the administration of the Asiatic and African red-

TABLE 1. Experimental animals treated with diminazene or imidocarb and inoculated using either frozen Asiatic (*Babesia bovis*) or African (*Babesia bigemina*) redwater vaccines

Drug treatment (day 0)	Vaccine	Group	Vaccine inoculation following treatment (weeks)	Number of animals	Number of animals positive on bloodsmear	Number of animals seroconverted	Prepatent period mean ± SD (days)*
Diminazene (3.5 mg/kg)	Asiatic[I]	1	4	5	5	4	13.4 ± 1.3^a
		control		5	4	5	8.5 ± 4.8^a
	African[II]	2	8	4	4	3	7.0 ± 1.2^a
		control		3	3	3	7.0 ± 1.0^a
		3	8	5	3	4	26.7 ± 4.7^a
Imidocarb (3.0 mg/kg)	Asiatic	control		2	2	2	15.0 ± 0.0^b
		3#	12	2	2	2	$15.0 \pm 5.7^{a,b,c}$
		control		2	2	2	$24.5 \pm 0.7^{a,c}$
	African	4	24	3	3	3	4.4 ± 1.5
		control		1	1	1	$5.0 \pm 0.0^{**}$

[I]*Babesia bovis* South African "S" strain.[6,7]
[II]*Babesia bigemina* Australian "G" strain.[8,9]
#Reinoculation of the two nonreactors of group 3.
*Means with different superscripts within a group and its control are significantly ($P < 0.05$) different.
**Insufficient data for statistical analysis.

TABLE 2. The inhibitory effect of diminazene and imidocarb on the live, frozen redwater vaccines

	Treatment (day 0)	
Babesia vaccine	Diminazene (3.5 mg/kg)	Imidocarb (3.0 mg/kg)
Asiatic form (B. bovis)	4 weeks[a]	12 weeks
African form (B. bigemina)	8 weeks	24 weeks

[a]Minimum period that prophylactic (residual) effect of drugs prevents effective vaccination/immunization.

water vaccines after diminazene treatment stay unchanged at 4 and 8 weeks, respectively (TABLE 2).

Imidocarb-Treated Animals

In group 3 (TABLE 1), *B. bovis* parasites could only be demonstrated in blood smears from three of the five animals and showed a significant difference in the mean prepatent period to that obtained for the control group. Reinoculation of the two non-reactors at 12 weeks after treatment with imidocarb proved to be successful because both animals became infected, indicating that imidocarb still has an inhibitory effect on the *B. bovis* vaccine parasite for at least 8 weeks after treatment.

Results from a previous study indicated the existence of an inhibitory effect of imidocarb on the infectivity of the frozen African redwater vaccine for up to 20 weeks. Inoculating animals in group 4 after a 24-week waiting period, however, proved to be successful (TABLE 1).

The infectivity of frozen vaccine is less predictable than that of unfrozen vaccine, mainly because of the dying off of parasites during freezing and thawing. Therefore, the inhibitory effect, especially of imidocarb, is more pronounced in the frozen *B. bovis* and *B. bigemina* vaccines, and the minimum waiting periods before administration of these vaccines should be adjusted accordingly to 12 and 24 weeks after treatment, respectively (TABLE 2).

It is important to remember that various factors, such as natural breed resistance to the organisms, methods of vaccine administration, and actual dose of the drug administered, can influence these waiting periods; and therefore only minimum waiting periods are recommended. In conclusion, it is evident that in those cases for which redwater (*Babesia*) vaccination is contemplated, the prophylactic use of either diminazene or imidocarb should be avoided.

REFERENCES

1. DE WAAL, D.T. 1996. Vaccination against babesiosis. Acta Parasitologica Turcica, **20**(Suppl. 1): 487–500.
2. GUMMOW, B., G.E. SWAN & J.L. DU PREEZ. 1994. A bioequivalence and pharmacokinetic evaluation of two commercial diminazene aceturate formulations administered intramuscularly to cattle. Onderstepoort J. Vet. Res. **61**: 317–326.
3. COLDHAM, N.G., A.S. MOORE., M. DAVE, et al. 1995. Imidocarb residues in edible bovine tissues and in vitro assessment of imidocarb metabolism and cytoxicity. Drug Metab. Dispos. **23**: 501–505.

4. DE WAAL, D.T. & F.T. POTGIETER. 1987. The transstadial transmission of *Babesia caballi* by *Rhipicephalus evertsi evertsi*. Onderstepoort J. Vet. Res. **54:** 655–656.
5. GRAY, S.J. & A.J. DE VOS. 1981. Studies on a bovine *Babesia* transmitted by *Hyalomma marginatum rufipes* Koch, 1844. Onderstepoort J. Vet. Res. **48:** 215–223.
6. DE VOS, A.J. 1978. Immunogenicity and pathogenicity of three South African strains of *Babesia bovis* in *Bos indicus* cattle. Onderstepoort J. Vet. Res. **45:** 19–124.
7. CALLOW, L.L., L.T. MELLORS & W. MCGREGGOR. 1979. Reduction in virulence of *Babesia bovis* due to rapid passage in splenectomized cattle. Int. J. Parasitol. **9:** 333–338.
8. DALGLIESH, R.J., L.L. CALLOW, L.T. MELLORS & W. MCGREGGOR. 1981. Development of a highly infective *Babesia bigemina* vaccine of reduced virulence. Aust. Vet. J. **57:** 8–11.
9. DE VOS, A.J., M.P. COMBRINK & R. BESSENGER. 1982. *Babesia bigemina* vaccine: comparison of the efficacy and safety of Australian and South African strains under experimental conditions in South Africa. Onderstepoort J. Vet. Res. **49:** 155–158.

Expression of RoTat 1.2 Cross-reactive Variable Antigen Type in *Trypanosoma evansi* and *T. equiperdum*

FILIP CLAES,[a,e] D. VERLOO,[a] D.T. DE WAAL,[b] T. URAKAWA,[c,d] P. MAJIWA,[c] B.M. GODDEERIS,[e] AND P. BÜSCHER[a]

[a]*Prince Leopold Institute of Tropical Medicine, Department of Parasitology, Antwerpen, Belgium*

[b]*Parasitology Division, Onderstepoort Veterinary Institute, Onderstepoort, South Africa*

[c]*International Livestock Research Institute (ILRI), Nairobi, Kenya*

[d]*London School of Hygiene & Tropical Medicine, London, United Kingdom*

[e]*Faculty of Agriculture and Applied Biological Sciences, Department of Animal Production, K.U. Leuven, Leuven, Belgium*

ABSTRACT: The variable antigen type (VAT) RoTat 1.2 has been cloned from a *T. evansi* strain, isolated in 1982 from a water buffalo in Indonesia. All *T. evansi* isolates hitherto tested express this VAT. In a study on the differential diagnosis of *T. equiperdum* and *T. evansi* in horses, we investigated serological evidence for the expression of RoTat 1.2 in 11 *T. evansi* and six *T. equiperdum* populations originating from Asia, Europe, Africa, and the Americas. Preinfection sera and sera of days 7, 14, 25, and 35 post-infection (p.i.) were analyzed for the presence of antibodies reactive with RoTat 1.2 in immune trypanolysis, ELISA/ *T. evansi* and CATT/*T. evansi*. Within the duration of the experiment, all rabbits infected with *T. evansi* became positive in the three serological tests. Five out of six rabbits infected with *T. equiperdum* also became positive in the three tests. Only one *T. equiperdum* strain (the OVI strain from South Africa) did not induce the production of antibodies reactive with RoTat 1.2 and thus might not contain or express a VSG that shares epitopes similar to those on the RoTat 1.2 VSG. The data lead to the conclusion that *T. equiperdum* can express VSGs containing epitopes serologically similar to those in the *T. evansi* RoTat 1.2 VAT. This explains, in part, why the antibody detection tests based on RoTat 1.2 VSG cannot reliably distinguish between the infections caused by *T. evansi* and those caused by *T. equiperdum*. There are no data that contradict the possibility that the putative *T. equiperdum* strains, which express VSGs with epitopes similar to those on RoTat 1.2, are actually *T. evansi*.

KEYWORDS: *Trypanosoma evansi*; *Trypanosoma equiperdum*; RoTat 1.2; surra; dourine; variable antigen type

Address for correspondence: Dr. Filip Claes, Prince Leopold Institute of Tropical Medicine, Department of Parasitology, Nationalestraat 155, B-2000 Antwerpen, Belgium. Voice: +32 3 247 63 69; fax: +32 3 247 63 73.

fclaes@itg.be

Ann. N.Y. Acad. Sci. 969: 174–179 (2002). © 2002 New York Academy of Sciences.

INTRODUCTION

The sexually transferred parasite *Trypanosoma equiperdum*, which causes the disease dourine in horses, is morphologically identical to *Trypanosoma evansi*, which causes surra in multiple species including horses. In many regions of the world, both parasites occur together, and current diagnostic tests are unable to distinguish between them.

Within the mammalian host, the cell membrane of a trypanosome is covered with a monolayer of variant surface glycoproteins (VSG).[1] This VSG, which determines the variable antigen type (VAT) of the individual trypanosome, is highly immunogenic and elicits VAT-specific antibodies with agglutinating and lytic activity.[2] Based on the RoTat 1.2 VAT, different diagnostic antibody detection tests for *T. evansi* have been developed, namely CATT/*T. evansi*,[3] LATEX/*T. evansi*, ELISA/ *T. evansi*,[4] and immune trypanolysis.[2] On the basis of anecdotal evidence, however, it appeared that *T. equiperdum*–infected laboratory animals and horses also reacted positively in the CATT/*T. evansi* test based on the RoTat 1.2 VSG. In order to define whether or not the RoTat 1.2 VSG is restricted to *T. evansi*, we studied the appearance of RoTat 1.2–specific antibodies in rabbits experimentally infected with 11 *T. evansi* and six *T. equiperdum* strains.

MATERIALS AND METHODS

Trypanosome Populations

A collection of 11 *T. evansi* and six *T. equiperdum* populations derived from strains isolated all over the world was used in this experiment (TABLE 1).

Rabbit Infections

Cryostabilates, stored in liquid nitrogen, were inoculated intraperitoneally in OF1 mice. Three days after infection, the mice were anesthetized and exsanguinated by cardiac puncture with a heparinized syringe. From this blood, a suspension in phosphate-buffered saline glucose (PSG) was prepared containing five trypanosomes per microscopic field (400× magnification) according to the matching method.[5] One milliliter of this suspension was injected intravenously into the ear vein of adult New Zealand white rabbits; parasitemia was monitored weekly by the mini-hematocrit centrifugation technique (MHCT) according to Woo.[6] Five milliliters of blood were taken from an ear vein at days 0, 7, 14, 25, and 35 post-infection for the preparation of serum. All sera were stored at −20°C.

Immune Trypanolysis with T. evansi RoTat 1.2

Immune trypanolysis was performed with *T. evansi* VAT RoTat 1.2 according to Van Meirvenne and others.[2] Rabbit sera were tested at a 1:4 dilution in phosphate-buffered saline (PBS). In the absence of lysis of the negative control, samples were considered positive when 50% or more of the trypanosomes were lysed.

TABLE 1. Data on the *T. evansi* and *T. equiperdum* populations used in this study

ITMAS cryo-stabilate code		Origin	Host	Year of isolation
Stock Philippines	060297	The Philippines	Water buffalo	1996
Stock Colombia	100297	Colombia	Horse	1973
Stock Kenya	110297	Kenya	Camel	1980
Stock Kazakhstan	060297	Kazakhstan	Camel	1995
Stock Br E18	020297	Brazil	Capybara	1986
Stock CAN 86K	170297	Brazil	Dog	1986
Stock STIB 816	020297	P.R. China	Camel	1978
RoTat 1.2	060297	Indonesia	Buffalo	1982
AnTat 3.1	270274C	South America	Capybara	1969
Stock Vietnam WH	101298	Vietnam	Water buffalo	1998
AnTat 3.2	190874A	South America	Capybara	1969
Alfort	241199A	Unknown	Unknown	Unknown
SVP	241199B	Unknown	Unknown	Unknown
OVI	241199C	South Africa	Horse	1977
Hamburg	251199A	Unknown	Unknown	Unknown
AnTat 4.1	210983A	Unknown	Unknown	Unknown
STIB 818	010999	P.R. China	Horse	1979

CATT/T. evansi

The direct agglutination test CATT/*T. evansi* is a direct card agglutination test that uses formaldehyde-fixed, freeze-dried trypanosomes of *T. evansi* VAT RoTat 1.2 stained with Coomassie blue.[3] The test was conducted on rabbit sera, diluted 1:8 in PBS.

ELISA/T. evansi

The antibody detection ELISA using RoTat 1.2 VSG was used as described by Verloo and others.[4] Percent positivity was calculated relative to a monovalent polyclonal serum obtained from a rabbit infected for 7 days with *T. evansi* RoTat 1.2. The cutoff was set at 60% positivity.

RESULTS

An overview of the results is summarized in TABLE 2. All rabbits were detected parasitologically positive in MHCT from day 7 post-infection onwards. In all 11 rabbits infected with different *T. evansi*, antibodies cross-reacting with the RoTat 1.2 VSG were detected in all tests used, within 30 days post-infection. Furthermore, five out of six *T. equiperdum* strains also induced antibodies cross-reacting with the

TABLE 2. Results of CATT/*T. evansi*, ELISA/*T. evansi* and immune trypanolysis RoTat 1.2 tests on day 35 post-infection sera from rabbits infected with different trypanosome populations

Code	Species	CATT/*T. evansi*	ELISA/*T. evansi*	Immune trypanolysis RoTat 1.2
RoTat 1.2	*T. evansi*	+	+	+
AnTat 3.1	*T. evansi*	+	+	+
AnTat 3.2	*T. evansi*	+	+	+
Stock Philippines	*T. evansi*	+	+	+
Stock Colombia	*T. evansi*	+	+	+
Stock Kenya	*T. evansi*	+	+	+
Stock Kazakstan	*T. evansi*	+	+	+
Stock Br E18	*T. evansi*	+	+	+
Stock CAN 86K	*T. evansi*	+	+	+
Stock STIB 816	*T. evansi*	+	+	+
Stock Vietnam	*T. evansi*	+	+	+
Alfort	*T. equiperdum*	+	+	+
SVP	*T. equiperdum*	+	+	+
OVI	*T. equiperdum*	–	–	–
Hamburg	*T. equiperdum*	+	+	+
AnTat 4.1	*T. equiperdum*	+	+	+
STIB 818	*T. equiperdum*	+	+	+

T. evansi RoTat 1.2 VSG. Only the South African *T. equiperdum* strain (OVI) did not react in any of the RoTat 1.2–based tests. A perfect concordance among these three serological tests was observed.

DISCUSSION

All RoTat 1.2 VSG-based diagnostic tests seem to have a good analytical sensitivity since all *T. evansi* strains tested positive consistently in all tests. Diagnostic sensitivity from the tests mentioned above was evaluated for *T. evansi* infections in water buffaloes[7] and camels.[8,9] Judging from the data obtained and from practical use in the field, the RoTat 1.2 VSG seemed to be a useful antigen in screening tests. Because genetic losses of the VSG genes can occur (as observed in the loss of the LiTat 1.3 VSG of *T. brucei gambiense*[11]), we cannot exclude the possibility that some strains of *T. evansi* might not express the predominant RoTat 1.2 VSG. Consequently, it is still necessary to evaluate the serological tests based on RoTat 1.2 in newly isolated *T evansi* populations.

Within six *T. equiperdum* isolates tested here, only the OVI strain did not generate antibodies reacting with RoTat 1.2 VSG during the test period. On the basis of their serological reactivity with the RoTat 1.2 VSG, all other *T. equiperdum* strains are indistinguishable from *T. evansi*. Although the OVI strain might express the RoTat 1.2 VAT in infections longer than 30 days, the results obtained might be explained by the absence of the RoTat 1.2 gene in the OVI repertoire.

Hitherto, the Rotat 1.2 VSG was only proven to appear in *T. evansi* and not in other trypanosomes from the *Trypanozoon* subspecies, including *T. b. brucei, T. b. gambiense* and *T. b. rhodesiense*.[4] Given the data obtained in this study, we cannot exclude the possibility that RoTat 1.2 VSG is restricted to *T. evansi*, that positive *T. equiperdum* stocks are actually misclassified as *T. evansi*, and that the OVI strain is the only real *T. equiperdum* in the studied collection. As in the beginning of the previous century,[12] antigens derived from *T. evansi* populations have been used in the complement fixation test (CFT) to eradicate dourine in the United States and Western Europe, it is possible that later on some of these diagnostic *T. evansi* strains might have been mistaken for *T. equiperdum*.

ACKNOWLEDGMENTS

F. Claes is funded by the Institute for the Promotion of Innovation by Science and Technology in Flanders (IWT). We wish to thank the following persons for kindly providing *Trypanosoma* strains: Dr. Reto Brun of the Swiss Tropical Institute Basel in Switzerland; Dr. Peter-Henning Clausen of the Free University Berlin in Germany; Dr. Joyce Hagebock and Dr. David Kinker of the National Veterinary Services Laboratories, United States Department of Agriculture, in the United States; Dr. Lun of Zhongshan University in the Peoples Republic of China; and Dr. Zablotsky of the All-Russian Research Institute for Experimental Veterinary Medicine (VIEV) in Russia. This investigation also received financial support from ILRI, Nairobi.

REFERENCES

1. PAYS, E. 1999. Antigenic variation in African trypanosomes. *In* Progress in Human African Trypanosomiasis, Sleeping Sickness. M. Dumas, B. Bouteille & A. Buguet, Eds.: 235–252. Springer. Paris.
2. VAN MEIRVENNE, N., E. MAGNUS & P. BÜSCHER. 1995. Evaluation of variant specific trypanolysis tests for serodiagnosis of human infections with *Trypanosoma brucei gambiense*. Acta Trop. **60:** 189–199.
3. BAJYANA SONGA, E. & R. HAMERS. 1988. A card agglutination test (CATT) for veterinary use based on an early VAT RoTat 1/2 of *Trypanosoma evansi*. Ann. Soc. Belge Méd. Trop. **68:** 233–240.
4. VERLOO, D., E. MAGNUS & P. BÜSCHER. 2001. General expression of RoTat 1.2 variable antigen type in *Trypanosoma evansi* isolates from different origin. Vet. Parasitol. **97:** 183–189.
5. HERBERT, W.J. & W.H.R. LUMSDEN. 1976. *Trypanosoma brucei*: A rapid "matching" method for estimating the host's parasitaemia. Exp. Parasitol. **40:** 427–431.
6. WOO, P.T.K. 1969. The haematocrit centrifuge for the detection of trypanosomes in blood. Can. J. Zool. **47:** 921–923.
7. VERLOO, D. *et al.* 2000. Comparison of serological tests for *Trypanosoma evansi* natural infections in water buffaloes from north Vietnam. Vet. Parasitol. **92:** 87–96.
8. VERLOO, D. *et al.* 1998. Performance of serological tests for *Trypanosoma evansi* infections in camels from Niger. J. Protozool. Res. **8:** 190–193.

9. GUTIERREZ, C. *et al.* 2000. Camel trypanosomosis in the Canary Islands: assessment of seroprevalence and infection rates using the card agglutination test (CATT/*T. evansi*) and parasite detection tests. Vet. Parasitol. **90:** 155–159.
10. CROSS, M., M.C. TAYLOR & P. BORST. 1998. Frequent loss of the active site during variant surface glycoprotein expression site switching in vitro in *Trypanosoma brucei*. Mol. Cell. Biol. **18:** 198–205.
11. DUKES, P. *et al.* 1992. Absence of the LiTat 1.3 (CATT antigen) gene in *Trypanosoma brucei gambiense* stocks from Cameroon. Acta Trop. **51:** 123–134.
12. MOHLER, J.R., A. EICHHORN & J.M. BUCK. 1913. The diagnosis of dourine by complement fixation. J. Agric. Res. **2:** 99–107.

Development of Resistance to Nymphs of *Amblyomma cajennense* Ticks (Acari: Ixodidae) in Dogs

LUCIANA S. MUKAI, A. CASTRO NETTO, M.P.J. SZABÓ, AND G.H. BECHARA

Faculdade de Ciências Agrárias e Veterinárias, Universidade Estadual Paulista, 14.884-900 Jaboticabal, SP, Brasil

ABSTRACT: Ticks have long been regarded as constraints to humans and domestic animals, but hosts often develop resistance to ticks after repeated infestations. The purpose of this investigation was to study the possible acquisition of immunity in domestic dogs to nymphs of *A. cajennense* by determining the tick alimentary performance after successive controlled infestations. Mean engorged weight of nymphs was not significantly different among the three infestations; molting rate from nymph to adult ticks, and the percentage of nymph recovery were also very close in all infestations. These results are similar to those obtained in studies of the dog–adult *Rhipicephalus sanguineus* interface. It is concluded that domestic dogs do not develop resistance against nymphs of *A. cajennense* ticks.

KEYWORDS: *Amblyomma cajennense*; *Rickettsia rickettsii*; tick infestation

Ticks have long been regarded as constraints to humans and domestic animals. In general, hosts develop resistance to ticks after repeated infestations.[1,2] Nevertheless, several studies on naturally occurring host–tick interactions were unable to detect host resistance to ticks even after repeated infestations.[3,4] Results from our laboratory in the last decade showed that, unlike guinea pigs and hamsters, dogs do not develop resistance to *Rhipicephalus sanguineus* ticks even after repeated infestations or vaccination.[5,6] The *Amblyomma cajennense* tick is widely distributed in South America; its immature stages are not host specific and can parasitize dogs. It is described as the main vector of the spotted fever agent, *Rickettsia rickettsii*, in Latin America and is associated with horses and capybaras. The purpose of this investigation was to study the possible acquisition of immunity in domestic dogs to nymphs of *A. cajennense* by determining the tick alimentary performance after successive and controlled infestations.

Address for correspondence: Dr. G.H. Bechara, Faculdade de Ciências Agrárias e Veterinárias, Universidade Estadual Paulista, 14.884-900 Jaboticabal, SP, Brazil. Voice: 55-16-3209-2662; fax: 55-16-3202-4275.
bechara@fcav.unesp.br

Ann. N.Y. Acad. Sci. 969: 180–183 (2002). © 2002 New York Academy of Sciences.

MATERIALS AND METHODS

A group of five dogs was infested three times with 80 nymphs of *A. cajennense* with a 30-day interval between infestations. Ticks were released on the shaved backs of the hosts into a feeding chamber glued onto the dog's skin. Engorged nymphs were collected after detachment and weighed in each infestation. Results were expressed as mean ± standard deviation and statistically analyzed via ANOVA.

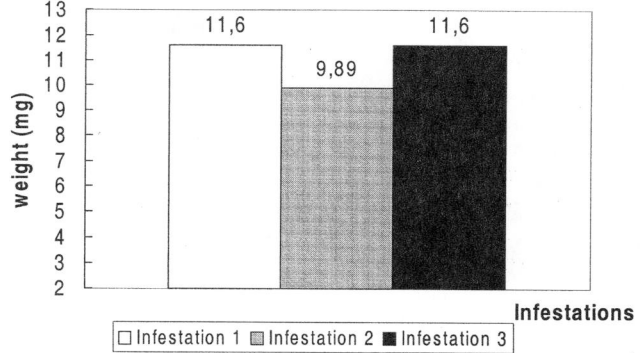

FIGURE 1. Weight (mg) of *A. cajennense* nymphs engorged and recovered in three succesive infestations of dogs. Results are expressed as means.

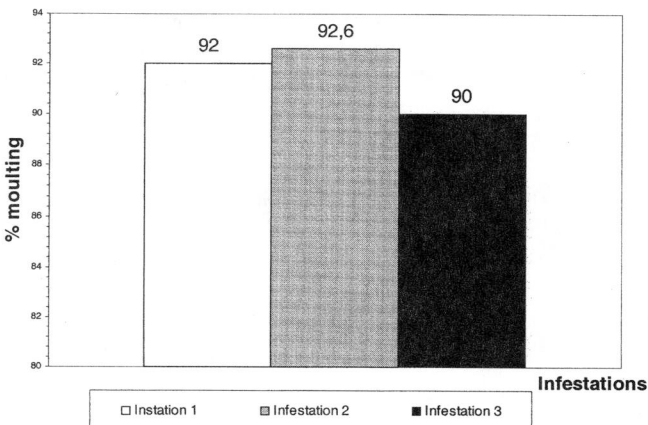

FIGURE 2. Molting (%) of *A. cajennense* nymphs engorged and recovered in three successive infestations of dogs. Results are expressed as means.

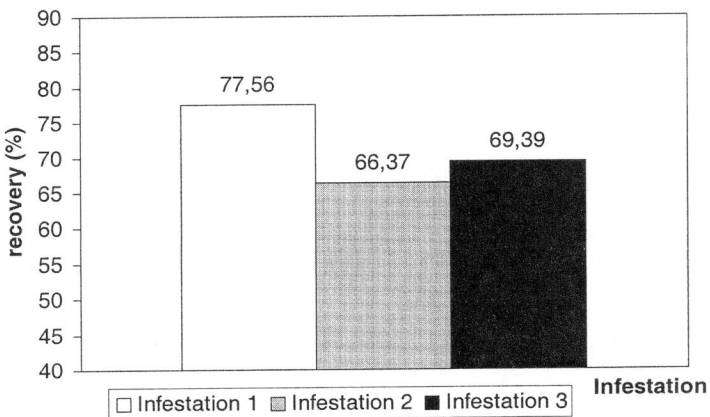

FIGURE 3. Recovering (%) of *A. cajennense* nymphs engorged and recovered in three successive infestations in dogs. Results are expressed as means.

RESULTS AND DISCUSSION

Under gross observation, dogs showed a light to moderate inflammatory reaction in the nymph feeding sites only. The mean engorged weight of nymphs was not significantly different among the three infestations, diminishing about 10% in the second infestation in relation to the first one (FIG. 1). The molting rate from nymph to adult ticks was about 90% in all infestations (FIG. 2), and the percentage of nymph recovery was also very close in all infestations, 77.6%, 66.4%, and 69.4% in the first, second, and third infestation, respectively (FIG. 3).

These results are similar to those obtained by Szabó *et al.*[5] and Bechara *et al.*,[6] who studied the dog–adult *Rhipicephalus sanguineus* interface, after repeated infestations and vaccinations, respectively. It is concluded that domestic dogs do not develop resistance against nymphs of *A. cajennense* ticks.

REFERENCES

1. RECHAV, Y. 1992. Naturally acquired resistance to ticks—a global view. Insect. Sci. Appl. **13:** 405–504.
2. WIKEL, S.K. 1996. Immunology of the tick–host interface. *In* The Immunology of Host–Ectoparasite Arthropod Relationships. S.K. Wikel, Ed.: 204–231. Cab International. London.
3. RANDOLPH, S.E. 1979. Population regulation in ticks: the role of acquired resistance in natural and unnatural hosts. Parasitology **79:** 141–156.

4. FIELDEN, L.J., Y. RECHAV & N.R. BRYSON. 1992. Acquired immunity to larvae of *Amblyomma marmoreum* and *A. hebraeum* by tortoises, guinea-pigs and guinea-fowl. Med. Vet. Entomol. **6:** 251–254.
5. SZABÓ, M.P.J., G.H. BECHARA, L.S. MUKAI & P.C.S. ROSA. 1995. Differences in acquired resistance in dogs, hamsters and guinea pigs infested with *R. sanguineus* tick. Braz. J. Vet. Res. Anim. Sci. **32:** 43–50.
6. BECHARA, G.H., M.P.J. SZABÓ, L.S. MUKAI & P.C.S. ROSA. 1994. Immunization of dogs, hamsters and guinea pigs against the tick *Rhipicephalus sanguineus* (Acarina:Ixodidae) using unfed adult tick extract. Vet. Parasitol. **52:** 79–90.

Hypersensitivity Induced in Dogs by Nymphal Extract of *Amblyomma cajennense* Ticks (Acari:Ixodidae)

LUCIANA S. MUKAI, A. CASTRO NETTO, M.P.J. SZABÓ, AND G.H. BECHARA

Faculdade de Ciências Agrárias e Veterinárias, Universidade Estadual Paulista, 14.884-900 Jaboticabal, SP, Brasil

ABSTRACT: In general, hosts develop resistance to ticks after repeated infestations; nevertheless, several studies on naturally occurring host–tick interactions were unable to detect resistance of hosts to ticks even after repeated infestations. The purpose of this investigation was to study the type of cutaneous hypersensitivity to unfed nymphal extract of *A. cajennense* in dogs, which, unlike guinea pigs, do not develop resistance. A first, but no second, peak in skin reaction was observed, suggesting that cellular immunity is an important mechanism of resistance to ticks. This may partially explain why guinea pigs, but not dogs, develop resistance against ticks.

KEYWORDS: *Amblyomma cajennense*; tick infestations; *Rickettsia rickettsii*

In general, hosts develop resistance to ticks after repeated infestations.[1,2] Nevertheless, several studies on naturally occurring host–tick interactions were unable to detect resistance of hosts to ticks even after repeated infestations.[3,4] In fact, results from our laboratory over the last decade showed that, unlike guinea pigs and hamsters, dogs do not develop resistance to *R. sanguineus* ticks even after repeated infestations.[5] In addition, an unfed adult extract of this tick species induced immediate-type hypersensitivity in both dogs and guinea pigs and a strong delayed-type reaction in guinea pigs only.[6] The *Amblyomma cajennense* tick is widely distributed in South America; its immature stages are not host specific and can parasitize dogs. It is described as the main vector of the spotted fever agent *Rickettsia rickettsii* in Latin America. The purpose of this investigation was to study the type of cutaneous hypersensitivity to unfed nymphal extract (UNE) of *A. cajennense* in dogs.

Address for correspondence: Dr. G.H. Bechara, Faculdade de Ciências Agrárias e Veterinárias, Universidade Estadual Paulista, 14.884-900 Jaboticabal, SP, Brasil. Voice: 55-16-3209-2662; fax: 55-16-3202-4275.

bechara@fcav.unesp.br

Ann. N.Y. Acad. Sci. 969: 184–186 (2002). © 2002 New York Academy of Sciences.

MATERIALS AND METHODS

Controlled Infestations

A group of four dogs was infested three times with 80 nymphs of *A. cajennense* ticks with a 30-day interval between infestations. Ticks were released on the shaved back of each host inside a feeding chamber fixed onto the host skin with atoxic glue.

Skin Test

A skin test was performed 15 days after the last infestation in the preinfested dogs. A group of four noninfested dogs was used as the control. UNE was injected intradermally in the left ear of the dogs (25 µg in 0.1 mL of PBS) and PBS only into the right ear. Reactions were evaluated by measuring the skin thickness at several times (10 min, 1, 2, 6, 18, 24, 48, and 96 h) post-UNE inoculation. The thickness of ears was measured three times at each interval with a Mitutoyo® device. The results were expressed as the mean percentage change in ear thickness in relation to prein-oculation values, and they were statistically analyzed by ANOVA.

RESULTS AND DISCUSSION

Dogs developed a strong immediate reaction whereby a 50% increase in ear thickness was observed 2 hours post-UNE inoculation (FIG. 1). A second and de-layed peak in skin reaction was not observed. The control animals did not develop

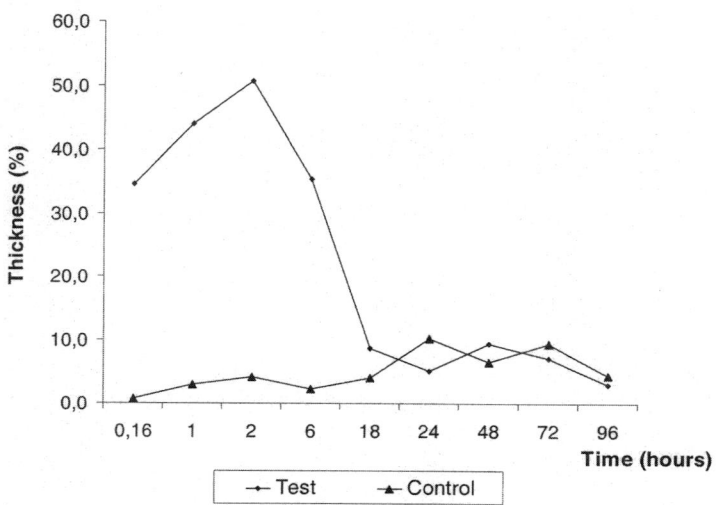

FIGURE 1. Skin test to show reactivity to unfed nymphs extract in a group of naïve dogs (control) and a group of dogs after three successive infestations (test). Results are ex-pressed as means.

any significant reaction to the extract, and PBS induced only mild reactions in the right ear of most the animals.

Intradermal inoculation of whole, unfed adult *Rhipicephalus sanguineus* extract in tick-sensitized hosts induced an immediate and a delayed-type hypersensitivity reaction in guinea pigs, but only a strong immediate reaction in dogs,[5] as observed here with the *A. cajennense* extract. A second peak in skin reaction was not observed, suggesting that cellular immunity is an important mechanism of resistance to ticks. This may partially explain why guinea pigs, but not dogs, develop resistance against ticks.

REFERENCES

1. RECHAV, Y. 1992. Naturally acquired resistance to ticks—a global view. Insect. Sci. Appl. **13:** 405–504.
2. WIKEL, S.K. 1996. Immunology of the tick–host interface. *In* The Immunology of Host–Ectoparasite Arthropod Relationships. S.K. Wikel, Ed.: 204–231. Cab International. London.
3. RANDOLPH, S.E. 1979. Population regulation in ticks: the role of acquired resistance in natural and unnatural hosts. Parasitology **79:** 141–156.
4. FIELDEN, L.J., Y. RECHAV & N.R. BRYSON. 1992. Acquired immunity to larvae of *Amblyomma marmoreum* and *A. hebraeum* by tortoises, guinea-pigs and guinea-fowl. Med. Vet. Entomol. **6:** 251–254.
5. SZABÓ, M.P.J., G.H. BECHARA, L.S. MUKAI & P.C.S. ROSA. 1995. Differences in acquired resistance in dogs, hamsters and guinea pigs infested with *R. sanguineus* tick. Braz. J. Vet. Res. Anim. Sci. **32:** 43–50.
6. SZABÓ, M.P.J., J. MORELLI, JR. & G.H. BECHARA. 1995. Cutaneous hypersensitivity induced in dogs and guinea-pigs by extracts of the tick *Rhipicephalus sanguineus* (Acari: Ixodidae). Exp. Appl. Acarol. **19:** 723–730.

The Possible Role That Buffalo Played in the Recent Outbreaks of Foot-and-Mouth Disease in South Africa

WILNA VOSLOO,[a] KARIN BOSHOFF,[a] RAHANA DWARKA,[a] AND
ARMANDA BASTOS[b]

[a]Onderstepoort Veterinary Institute, Onderstepoort 0110, South Africa

[b]Department of Zoology and Entomology, University of Pretoria, Pretoria, South Africa

ABSTRACT: African buffalo (*Syncerus caffer*) act as maintenance hosts for foot-and-mouth disease (FMD) in southern Africa. A single buffalo can become infected with all three of the endemic serotypes of FMD virus (SAT-1, SAT-2, and SAT-3) and pose a threat of infection to other susceptible cloven-hoofed animals. The floods of 2000 in southern Africa damaged the Kruger National Park (KNP) game fence extensively, and there were several accounts of buffalo that had escaped from the park. The VP1 gene, which codes for the major antigenic determinant of the FMD virus, was used to determine phylogenetic relationships between virus isolates obtained from the outbreaks and those previously obtained from buffalo in the KNP. These results demonstrate that buffalo were most probably the source of the outbreaks, indicating that disease control using fencing as well as vaccination is extremely important to ensure that FMD does not become established in domestic livestock.

KEYWORDS: African buffalo; foot-and-mouth disease; cattle; southern Africa; VP1 gene

INTRODUCTION

Foot-and-mouth disease (FMD) is an acute vesicular viral disease of cloven-hoofed animals. Although mortality is usually low in adult animals, morbidity can be very high, and the disease can cause severe production losses. The causative virus is an *Aphthovirus* of the family Picornaviridae and contains a single-stranded, positive sense RNA genome.

Free-living African buffalo (*Syncerus caffer*) act as maintenance hosts of the three SAT types of FMD in southern Africa. Most buffalo in the Kruger National Park (KNP) are infected with all three SAT types by the age of two years,[1] and the resultant carrier status is probably lifelong.[2] Transmission between carrier buffalo and susceptible cattle has been erratic under experimental conditions,[3–8] but these data,

Address for correspondence: Dr. Wilna Vosloo, Exotic Diseases Division, Onderstepoort Veterinary Institute, Private Bag X05, Onderstepoort 0110, South Africa. Voice: 27-12-5299592; fax: 27-12-5299543.

wilna@saturn.ovi.ac.za

Ann. N.Y. Acad. Sci. 969: 187–190 (2002). © 2002 New York Academy of Sciences.

together with circumstantial evidence, have indicated that carrier buffalo are the source of infection for other susceptible species. For this reason livestock surrounding the KNP are vaccinated twice annually to protect against FMD virus infection.

This study demonstrates the use of partial nucleotide sequencing of the main antigenic determinant of the FMD virus, VP1, in providing evidence that buffalo were the source of infection in the recent SAT-1 and SAT-2 outbreaks in South Africa.

MATERIALS AND METHODS

Study Area

Clinical material was submitted from affected cattle at a feedlot close to Middelburg and from the Nkomaas district, Mpumalanga, between November 29 and December 15, 2000. Clinical cases were also found in cattle in the Mhala district of the Northern Province between February 1 and May 30, 2001.

Virus Isolation and Typing

Virus was isolated from clinical material on primary pig kidney cells using standard techniques. The isolated virus was typed using the sandwich ELISA.[9]

Ribonucleic Acid Extraction, Gene Amplification, Nucleotide Sequencing, and Phylogenetic Analysis

The RNA extraction method, amplification of the carboxy-terminal part of the VP1 gene, and nucleotide sequencing were performed as previously described.[10] For the phylogenetic analysis of the SAT-1 and SAT-2 trees, 381 nucleotides of the VP1 gene were used. Gene trees were constructed using the neighbor-joining method included in the MEGA version 2.0 program.[11] Node reliability was established by 1000 bootstrap replications.

RESULTS

Serotype Determination of Isolates

All viruses isolated from clinical material in Mpumalanga were found to be SAT-1, whereas all viruses isolated from the Mhala district were typed as SAT-2 using the sandwich ELISA (results not shown).

Phylogenetic Analysis of Both Outbreaks

The first SAT-1 virus isolated from the feedlot had close homology to isolates obtained from buffalo in the south of the KNP (FIG. 1). SAR/32/00, the isolate from the feedlot, differs by 13% from KNP/22/96, a buffalo virus isolated near Lower Sabie during 1996 and by 16% from KNP/20/89, which originated from the Numbi Gate area in 1989. The first grouping is supported by a significant bootstrap value of 99% (FIG. 1).

The SAT-2 virus isolated at the start of the outbreak in Mhala, SAR01/01, differed by approximately 15% from buffalo isolates made in the Orpen area of the KNP dur-

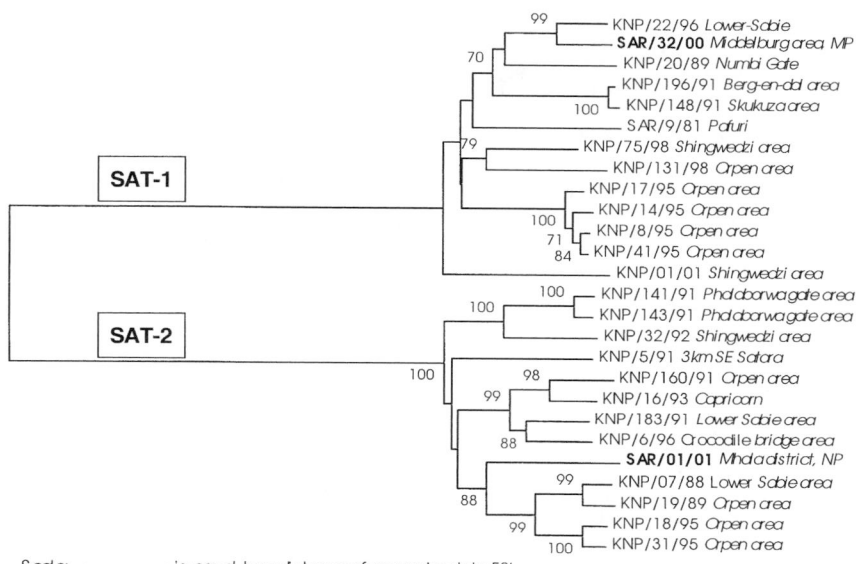

Scale: ⊢————⊣ is equal to a distance of approximately 5%

FIGURE 1. Neighbor-joining tree (Jukes and Cantor) based on partial VP1 gene nucleotide sequence data, depicting genetic relationships of SAT-1 and SAT-2 foot-and-mouth disease viruses from buffalo in the Kruger National Park and the recent outbreaks in South Africa. Bootstrap values based on 1000 replications and ≥70 and the origin of each buffalo isolate are indicated in the figure. SAR/32/00 is the SAT-1 isolate made from cattle in the feedlot close to Middelburg, and SAR/01/01 is the SAT-2 cattle isolate made in the Mhala district of the Northern Province.

ing 1988–1995 (FIG. 1; KNP19/89, KNP18/95, KNP31/95). This grouping is also supported by a high bootstrap value of 88%.

DISCUSSION

The VP1 gene, which codes for the major antigenic determinant of the FMD virus, has previously been used to determine phylogenetic relationships between different virus isolates and to trace possible origins of outbreaks.[12,13] It has also been shown unequivocally that buffalo were the source of outbreaks in impala in the KNP.[14] These sequence databases were used to determine the possible origins of the recent outbreaks of FMD outside the boundaries of the KNP.

The source of infection for the SAT-1 outbreak in the feedlot in Middelburg was traced to the Nkomaas region, south of the KNP, using serological evidence (results not shown). Phylogenetic relationships indicated that the virus that caused the outbreak was related to buffalo isolates obtained previously from the south of the KNP. This relationship was supported by a significant bootstrap value. Likewise, the SAT-2 virus isolated from cattle in the Mhala district was related to buffalo strains obtained from the neighboring Orpen area (FIG. 1).

During February 2000 severe flooding in southern Africa damaged the KNP game fence extensively, and there were several accounts of buffalo that had escaped from the park. Outbreaks of theileriosis in cattle were also recorded, indicating that buffalo had been in contact with cattle (Ben du Plessis and Edwin Dyasen, personal communication, 2000). Some of these stray buffalo were found in the FMD control areas where disease control relies on inspection only and animals are not vaccinated.

The sequencing results together with other epidemiological information demonstrate that buffalo were most probably the cause of the recent outbreaks of FMD in the areas surrounding the KNP, indicating that disease control using fencing as well as vaccination is extremely important to ensure that FMD does not become established in domestic livestock.

REFERENCES

1. THOMSON, G.R., W. VOSLOO, J.J. ESTERHUYSEN & R.G. BENGIS. 1992. Maintenance of foot-and-mouth disease virus in buffalo (*Syncerus caffer* Sparrman 1779) in southern Africa. Rev. Sci. Off. Int. Epiz. **11:** 1097–1107.
2. CONDY, J.B., R.S. HEDGER, C. HAMBLIN & I.T.R. BARNETT. 1985. The duration of foot-and-mouth disease virus carrier state in the African buffalo: (i) in the individual animals and (ii) in a free-living herd. Comp. Immunol. Micro. Infect. Dis. **8:** 259–265.
3. CONDY, J.B. & R.S. HEDGER. 1974. The survival of foot-and-mouth disease virus in African buffalo with non-transference of infection to domestic cattle. Res. Vet. Sci. **16:** 182–185.
4. ANDERSON, E.C., W.J. DOUGHTY & R. PALING. 1979. The pathogenesis of foot-and-mouth disease in the African buffalo (*Syncerus caffer*) and the role of this species in the epidemiology of the disease in Kenya. J. Comp. Pathol. **89:** 541–549.
5. BENGIS, R.G., G.R. THOMSON, R.S. HEDGER, *et al.* 1986. Foot-and-mouth disease and the African buffalo (*Syncerus caffer*). I. Carriers as a source of infection for cattle. Onderstepoort J. Vet. Res. **53:** 69–73.
6. GAINARU, M.D., G.R. THOMSON, R.G. BENGIS, *et al.* 1986. Foot and mouth disease and the African buffalo (*Syncerus caffer*). II. Virus excretion and transmission during acute infection. Onderstepoort J. Vet. Res. **53:** 78–85.
7. DAWE, P.S., F.O. FLANAGAN, R.L. MADEKUROZWA, *et al.* 1994. Experimental transmission of foot-and-mouth disease from carrier African buffalo (*Syncerus caffer*) to cattle in Zimbabwe. Vet. Rec. **134:** 211–215.
8. VOSLOO, W., A.D. BASTOS, E. KIRKBRIDE, *et al.* 1996. Persistent infection of African buffalo (*Syncerus caffer*) with SAT-type foot-and-mouth disease viruses: rate of fixation of mutations, antigenic change and interspecies transmission. J. Gen. Virol. **77:** 1457–1467.
9. ROEDER, P.L. & P.M. LE BLANC SMITH. 1987. Detection and typing of foot-and-mouth disease virus enzyme-linked immunosorbent assay: a sensitive, rapid and reliable technique for primary diagnosis. Res. Vet. Sci. **43:** 225–232.
10. BASTOS, A.D.S. 1998. Detection and characterization of foot-and-mouth disease virus in sub-Saharan Africa. Onderstepoort J. Vet. Res. **65:** 37–47.
11. KUMAR, S., K. TAMURA, I.B. JAKOBSEN & M. NEI. 2001. MEGA2: molecular evolutionary genetics analysis software. Bioinformatics, submitted.
12. BECK, E. & K. STROHMAIER. 1987. Subtyping of European foot-and-mouth disease strains by nucleotide sequence determination. J. Virol. **61:** 1621–1629.
13. VOSLOO, W., N.J. KNOWLES & G.R THOMSON. 1992. Genetic relationships between southern African SAT-2 isolates of foot-and-mouth-disease virus. Epidemiol. Infect. **109:** 547–558.
14. BASTOS, A.D., C.I. BOSHOFF, D.F. KEET, *et al.* 2000. Natural transmission of foot-and-mouth disease virus between African buffalo (*Syncerus caffer*) and impala (*Aepyceros melampus*) in the Kruger National Park, South Africa. Epidemiol. Infect. **124:** 591–598.

The Fencing Issue Relative to the Control of Foot-and-Mouth Disease

PAUL SUTMOLLER

Animal Health Consultant, Richmond, Virginia 23233, USA

ABSTRACT: Certain livestock diseases in sub-Saharan Africa, such as foot-and-mouth disease are difficult to control because of the large numbers of infected wildlife hosts. These wildlife disease reservoirs form a continuous hazard of transmittal of the diseases to domestic livestock, which limits the access of livestock products from southern Africa to international markets. The disease reservoirs are often found in border areas between countries with susceptible species and infected reservoir animals continuously crossing the border. A regional approach to disease control is probably the only way to achieve any real progress. Here we review the positive and negative attributes of fencing as a control mechanism for disease transmission.

KEYWORDS: foot-and-mouth disease (FMD); Cape buffalo; wildlife in southern Africa; livestock in southern Africa

INTRODUCTION

Certain livestock diseases in sub-Saharan Africa—such as foot-and-mouth disease (FMD)—are difficult to control because of the large numbers of infected wildlife hosts. For instance, a large percentage of Cape buffalo (*Syncerus caffer*) are long-term carriers of FMD virus, meaning that the animal is persistently infected without showing any signs of infection.[1] Apparently the Cape buffalo and the South African types (SAT) of FMD have found the ideal host/parasite equilibrium.

Buffalo calves lose their maternal antibodies at 2–6 months of age and thereafter show seroconversion for one or more of the three types of SAT virus. Apparently during that period they acquire the infection from their dams. It has been quite difficult to show that the infection can pass from buffalo to domestic livestock species, but studies of Thomson *et al.*[2] in 1992 indicated that young buffalo in the acute stage of infection are likely to be the most infectious animals in the herd. Those contagious calves are responsible for maintaining FMD virus in the herd and the spread of FMD to other wildlife or domestic livestock species.[3]

Address for correspondence: Dr. Paul Sutmoller, Animal Health Consultant, 1502 Largo Road, Richmond, Virginia 23233.
PaulSutmoller@compuserve.com

THE ISSUES

(1) Wildlife areas, and thus disease reservoirs, are often found in border areas between countries with susceptible and infected animals continuously crossing the border. A regional approach to disease control is probably the only way to achieve any real progress.

(2) Ecotourism based on wildlife is becoming increasingly profitable, and some large wildlife conservancies are being developed that can be more-effectively managed for optimal sustainable profitability. Containing the infectious agents within those wildlife conservancies becomes a major management effort in protecting adjacent domestic livestock populations.

(3) In several countries the policies of FMD control are dominated by the wish to export livestock products, particularly meat, to the more developed parts of the world. The control policy has been to prevent direct contact between buffalo and cattle through the erection of fences between National Parks and areas for safari, forestry hunting on the one side and farming on the other. Additional measures are the maintenance of vaccination buffer zones adjacent to the fences, disease surveillance, and livestock movement controls.

In these three issues, the separation of Cape buffalo and livestock by fences becomes the main topic. Fencing has been used in southern Africa to control movements of wildlife and domestic livestock for many years, but the policy has sparked heated debates about its efficacy and its deleterious effects on wildlife.

Fences for disease control must be designed and constructed with specific objectives in mind:

- What diseases must be controlled and in what species? The pathogenesis and the means by which the disease spreads or is transmitted must be considered. Is it by aerosol or direct contact; are insects or ticks involved in the transmission; are there intermediate hosts?

- Will the fence do the intended job? Is the fence high enough to stop the species concerned from jumping the fence? Is it likely to be damaged by the larger species such as elephant and giraffe?

- Will animal movement control give the expected results? Does it need to be complemented with other control measures such as vaccination of livestock and disease surveillance?

- Will the fence solve one problem, but cause a host of other (disease) problems? These problems may vary from cutting off wildlife from grazing grounds or water supplies to the use of the fence wires for snares by poachers.

- What is the impact on the environment? What is the impact on genetic exchange and on annual grazing movements?

Only lately have fencing policies been subjected to more formal risk analysis, environmental impact studies or cost/benefit analysis prior to being implemented.[4–6]

Risk assessments can indicate the best options for containing the disease in question. Environmental impact studies can determine which of the options have the least detrimental effect on wildlife and landscape and consequently on ecotourism (tourists don't like the sight of fences!). Finally, cost/benefit studies can show what the financial consequences will be of the selected options.

WILDLIFE CONSERVANCIES IN ZIMBABWE

The term "conservancy" is used for wildlife-management schemes in southern Africa and is usually applied to a group of adjacent properties managed as an ecological unit to enable more-efficient use and protection of the natural resources of the area.[7] A wide diversity of species and large populations that are easily visible are required by these enterprises. This results in large-scale translocation of wildlife and may be accompanied by the reintroduction of species that were previously eradicated such as the Cape buffalo in the traditional cattle ranching areas of south-eastern Zimbabwe.

The establishment of wildlife conservancies has created a problem with regard to FMD because the Office International des Epizooties (OIE) presently considers any territory on which buffalo infected with FMD viruses occur as "infected." Zones recognized as free of FMD by the OIE need to be separated from infected zones by a defined surveillance zone at least 10km deep (International Animal Health Code, 1992). According to the OIE recommendations this means that landowners acquiring even one infected buffalo "cause" their land to be in an infected zone and, by implication, their neighbors in a surveillance zone. However, in May 1997 it was accepted by the OIE that infected and free zones may be separated by a "barrier" instead of a surveillance zone.[8]

For wildlife conservancies in Zimbabwe, a relatively expensive, but practical solution to this problem was implemented. A double electrified fence barrier was constructed.[7] A defoliated strip of about 7.5m in width separates the two fences. The land one-meter on either side of each fence-line is also cleared of vegetation. The outer fence is a 1.9m high and "game proof" and the inner fence is 1.2m high and "buffalo proof."

Domestic stock are excluded from conservancies, but are present on adjacent land. In some places, the cattle immediately outside the conservancy were not vaccinated at the time the risk assessment was undertaken. The rationale for the double electrified fence was that FMD transmission by carrier buffalo to cattle would require close contact over a prolonged period[10] and that local circumstances would not favor airborne transmission.[11,12] The reasons for the apparent absence of airborne transmission of FMD in southern Africa are essentially the warm dry climate, the very small numbers of domestic pigs in the FMD-endemic areas, and the low stocking rates.[1,3]

There are three wildlife conservancies in the "Lowveld" area of Zimbabwe; the Save Valley Conservancy (SVC) is the largest and covers over 300,000 ha, comprising some 20 individual properties. The perimeter fence of SVC is about 350km long, and about 84% of this boundary is shared with communal land and resettlement areas. All of these areas have cattle, sheep and goats. In the SVC all cattle and other domestic livestock were removed upon their formation, but various wildlife species were introduced subsequently (including buffalo from other wildlife areas in Zimbabwe). The construction of the electrified double perimeter fence was completed in 1994. The other two conservancies have similar fencing arrangements.

TABLE 1. Buffalo-escape scenario: transmission of FMD by buffalo to cattle as a result of breaks in wildlife-conservancy fencing

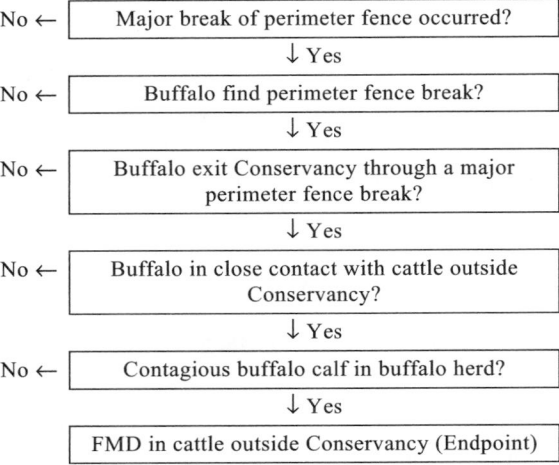

No ← | Major break of perimeter fence occurred?

↓ Yes

No ← | Buffalo find perimeter fence break?

↓ Yes

No ← | Buffalo exit Conservancy through a major perimeter fence break?

↓ Yes

No ← | Buffalo in close contact with cattle outside Conservancy?

↓ Yes

No ← | Contagious buffalo calf in buffalo herd?

↓ Yes

FMD in cattle outside Conservancy (Endpoint)

ASSESSMENT OF THE RISK OF FMD ESCAPE FROM THE SAVE VALLEY CONSERVANCY

Dr. Gavin Thomson and I were asked to make an estimate of the risk that FMD would be transmitted from buffalo in the SVC to unvaccinated cattle grazing in the vicinity of the Conservancy.[4] Quantitative risk assessments had never been used before to study these types of situations. Our method of choice was scenario-pathway analysis.[13,14]

We considered five different scenario pathways by which FMD virus could possibly be transmitted from infectious buffalo within the conservancies to livestock: Buffalo transmit FMD to cattle:

- following escape of buffalo from a conservancy through a fence break;
- entering and leaving a conservancy through a fence break;
- indirectly by infecting sheep and goats entering and leaving a conservancy;
- indirectly by infecting antelope that jump over the outer game fence of the conservancy; and/or
- by aerosol transported across the perimeter fence by air currents.

TABLE 1 is an example of the scenario pathways that we used.

For each of the questions in the scenario, a "Yes" or "No" answer was required. If the answer was "No" there would be no risk, but if the answer was "Yes" then the hazard would remain in the chain of events. In reality, the problem is more complicated because instead of a straightforward "Yes" or "No" answer there is a *probability* of the adverse event occurring. Moreover, if an attempt is made to estimate this probability, uncertainty needs to be allowed for both because of inherent variability of biological processes (variance) and because of lack of knowledge.[14] The final risk is an accumulation of the risk in each of the steps or events in the scenario pathway.

TABLE 2. Transmission of FMD by buffalo to cattle resulting from antelopes jumping over perimeter fences of a wildlife-conservancy

No ←	Buffalo infect antelope?

↓ Yes

No ←	Antelope contagious?

↓ Yes

No ←	Antelope exit the Conservancy by jumping the perimeter fence?

↓ Yes

No ←	Infected antelope/cattle contact outside Conservancy?

↓ Yes

No ←	Transmission of FMD to cattle outside Conservancy?

↓ Yes

FMD in cattle outside Conservancy (Endpoint)

Our analysis of the frequency of occurrence of adverse events (the risk) in the scenarios was based on technical, scientific, or circumstantial supporting evidence. The result of the analysis demonstrated an extremely low risk of this buffalo-escape scenario (somewhere of the order of 1:100,000 per 350 km peripheral fence per year), due to the small probability of occurrence of each of the steps in the scenario pathway.

In the past it was intuitively assumed that major fence breaks would be the highest risk for the escape of FMD from the conservancies. However, that proved to be a wrong perception. An analysis of the next scenario pathway will show that the transmission of FMD by buffalo to cattle resulting from antelopes jumping over perimeter fences of a wildlife-conservancy is a much greater risk.

Antelope often graze in the proximity of buffalo, and it is evident that antelope occasionally become infected (as shown by the presence of FMD antibody). Although the outer game fence stops most antelopes, there are some that jump over the fence (particularly the larger species). If such antelope develop FMD while in the proximity of cattle outside the conservancy they would probably be able to transmit the disease (TABLE 2).

Data from the Kruger National Park in South Africa showed that 18.4% of antelope had serum antibodies to SAT2 (Records of the Onderstepoort Veterinary Institute—surveillance data from the Kruger National Park). A serological survey of small game in Zimbabwean wildlife zones indicated that 2.4 to 7.8% of antelope had antibodies to FMD.[15] Following infection, antelope are likely to be contagious for 3 days, but not less than one or more than 5 days. The estimated life span of antelope was 1–8 years with a probable average of 4 years. From these values it follows that approximately 1:10,000 antelope may be contagious on any given day. However, these values could change owing to culling or to a lack of predators.

The number of antelope that are able to leave the conservancy annually by jumping the outer game fence was developed from the following information:

TABLE 3. Scenarios ranked by the annual risk of FMD posed to the cattle industry by buffalo within the Save Valley Conservancy in Zimbabwe

Scenario	Mean risk (350 km fence/year)	95th percentile
Buffalo infect cattle indirectly by infecting antelope that jump over the game fence of the conservancy	1:5000	1:1500
Buffalo infect cattle following escape of buffalo from the conservancy through a major fence break	1:200,000	1:60,000
Buffalo infect cattle by aerosol transported across the perimeter fence by air currents	10^{-5}	$10^{-4.7}$
Buffalo infect cattle entering and leaving the conservancy though a major fence break	10^{-7}	10^{-6}
Buffalo infect cattle indirectly by infecting sheep and goats entering and exiting the conservancy	Less than 10^{-10}	

Although no major break have been reported in the perimeter fence of the SVC, minor breaks of the top two strands of the game fence were found occasionally. Fence-patrol personnel reported up to a maximum of 10 minor fence breaks a year along their 10-km patrol. In some of those cases, antelope may have succeeded in jumping over the fence. Also, fence patrols regularly report observing game between the buffalo fence and the outer game fence, and, occasionally impala and kudu were found tangled in the fence wires.

Through interviews of fence-patrol personnel, it was estimated that the likelihood is that a total of some 300 antelope negotiate the outer game fence annually—but that number is unlikely to be less than 60 or more than 600. The interviews also indicated that number of antelope jumping the fence might be considerably higher when lions are present in the area. Based on expert opinion, we assumed that once contagious antelope get out of a conservancy, there is a fair chance of contact with cattle and likelihood of transmission to cattle. From these and other data it was estimated that the probability (risk) of an FMD outbreak in livestock outside the SVC from buffalo with antelope as intermediate hosts would likely be as high as 1:5000 per year.

The results of the risk assessments for the five scenarios are summarized in TABLE 3 in order of decreasing FMD risk posed to livestock in Zimbabwe.

It can be observed that the highest risk is of the antelope scenario. The combined risk of all scenarios would be very close to that risk since the risk of the other scenarios are several magnitudes smaller. Thus, the greatest risk (1:5000/350 km fence/year) posed by the double-fencing system in operation around conservancies in Zimbabwe is that contagious antelope (either in the incubation period or acute phase of infection) jump across the perimeter fence and cause FMD in cattle outside conservancies.

As mentioned before, it had been assumed that the greatest FMD risk posed to livestock outside conservancies would arise from a buffalo herd escaping through major breaks in the perimeter fence. However, this risk is about 40 times smaller than the risk that antelope act as intermediary host. The remaining scenarios all posed a negligible risk.

People or large animals, such as elephants could cause fence breaks. For the period for which data were available for the Zimbabwean conservancies, no such break had occurred—but the experience in South Africa has been less favorable. However, the fences in South Africa are constructed differently and stocking densities are usually higher—particularly for elephants, which cause most breaks. It is therefore likely that as the number of elephants in Zimbabwean conservancies increases the rate of fence breaks will increase.

Because the risk also increases proportionately with the length of the fencing, the antelope risk might rise with an increase of the number of conservancies. This could be accentuated by factors such as drought, which is likely to result in closer buffalo-antelope contact around water holes.

South Africa has suffered clinical outbreaks of FMD in impala in the Kruger National Park nearly every year over the last 20 years. Consequently, there has been concern that antelope might cross the single perimeter fence-line of the Kruger National Park. For that reason, the new perimeter fence is 2.4 m high; experience has shown that antelope are unable to clear such fences (S. Winterbach, personal communication). Based on this experience, raising the height of conservancy fences in Zimbabwe was considered in order to limit the risk of infected antelope getting out of conservancies.

It should also be remembered that risk assessments such as this one are based on simplified models and that unforeseen scenarios may occur. For instance, one can speculate that lion or other scavengers may possibly act as mechanical carriers of the virus after the kill of a viremic buffalo calf.

ASSESSMENT OF THE RISK OF LOW-MAINTENANCE BUFFALO FENCES IN ZIMBABWE

Dr. Euan Anderson and I carried out a more general risk assessment on the policy of FMD control in Zimbabwe particularly with regards to low maintenance buffalo fences.[5] These fences are 1.2 m high and have three cables. The top cable consists of 7-strand wire. The lower two cables are of 5-strand wire and are equally spaced below. In between and below these cables are two strands of high strain steel fencing wire. In places where there has been a high buffalo challenge 4 cables have been used, one of 7 strands and three of 5 strands.

The fence is not electrified. It is intended to be "buffalo proof" but allows the passage of other wildlife, while not being damaged by the larger species such as elephants.

We considered two scenarios "buffalo transmit FMD to cattle by direct buffalo-cattle contact and "buffalo transmit FMD to cattle indirectly by infecting antelope."

As with the SVC study, the first scenario proved to be of a very low risk because it required contagious buffalo and susceptible cattle to be both within a reasonably close distance at the same portion of the buffalo-control fence at same time. Secondly, climatic conditions had to be favorable for airborne transmission. Finally, FMD virus had to reach the cattle in sufficient amounts at the right receptor site to initiate infection.

It proved more difficult to make a quantitative estimation of the annual risk for the antelope scenario, because of the difficulty in estimating the number of antelope that might leave the area as they can freely move across the buffalo control fence. However, considering all risk factors it was concluded that the risk of FMD transmission from contagious buffalo herds to cattle separated by low-maintenance buffalo fences would be very low when the fencing was combined with additional measures such as the establishment of a buffer zone with low livestock density and/or vaccination zones.

During our fieldwork for this project we found that there have also been problems with the maintenance of low-maintenance fences. We observed stretches where wire was removed or where National Parks personnel had lowered the fence to allow their vehicles to pass. Often gates were not been maintained properly either.

One of our recommendations was that the fence should comprise three, and where necessary four, strands of thick (7-strand) cable, instead of one thick top cable and two thinner ones. No steel fencing wire should be employed. The thin wires and the steel wire are often stolen and can be used as snares.

Therefore the main recommendations for a low maintenance buffalo fence are that it must:

- be effective in mostly preventing the passage of buffalo;
- allow the passage of elephant or other large species without being damaged;
- not interfere with the normal migration of other species and allow the free passage of other wildlife;
- require minimal maintenance i.e. materials should not be attractive to poachers.

As with all other types of fences there are problems when crossing riverbeds etc. with some solutions having more success than others.

Our risk assessments were supposed to be followed by environmental impact study and cost/benefit studies of the various fencing options that we suggested, but unfortunately, political developments in Zimbabwe, so far have made these follow-up studies difficult.

WHAT MAKES SENSE?

Fences are supposed to prevent close contact between infected animals and non-infected animals from the same species or from different species. However, other transmission mechanisms, such as intermediate hosts, must be accounted for. How game fences will influence the ecology of a disease depends on the epidemiology and pathology of the disease in question.

In principle, wildlife fences should be constructed only *between* wildlife zones and the farming areas. They should not run through the middle of any wildlife zones, but between them and any commercial farms or communal lands. Also from a FMD control point of view there is no need to fence through communal lands or along international borders.

It appears that a modified low-maintenance buffalo control fence complemented with buffer zones or vaccination zones may be a cost-effective solution to the containment of FMD in wildlife zones. However, such fences might not be effective in preventing the risk of introducing other diseases such as tuberculosis from endemic wildlife populations. Such a situation would require a barrier that stops all buffalo and antelope movements. This could be a double fence as described for the wildlife conservancies in Zimbabwe or alternatively a single 2.4 meters-high buffalo-proof and that is electrified to prevent elephant damage. The local people should be involved in its maintenance to minimize theft.

The construction of a game fence along international borders if there are no wildlife areas in the neighboring countries would serve no purpose as far as FMD control is concerned. It would probably only serve as a source of fencing material! In these areas it would be preferable to implement a system of increased disease surveillance instead of fencing. The aim would be regular observation of the cattle population in the area and rapid response in the event of any clinical disease being observed.

Fencing policy planning involves teamwork of several scientific and technical disciplines: veterinarians, epidemiologists, biologists, environmentalists and engineers.

A risk analysis team can do useful work by assessing various scenarios showing ways by which the disease might spread and by evaluating levels of risks. Other teams should study cost/benefit aspects and environmental impacts of different fencing options. Of course, all stakeholders must be included from early on in the planning stage and community participation in planning and implementation is essential for its success.

Finally, I would like to emphasize our responsibilities as veterinary professionals when suggesting or recommending the erection or removal of fences for the purpose of disease control. Our recommendations may have far reaching consequences for the environment and wildlife and may impact severely (often negatively!) on the social and economic situation of the local population.

REFERENCES

1. THOMSON, G.R. 1994. Foot and mouth disease. *In* Infectious Diseases of Livestock with Special Reference to Southern Africa. J.A.W. Coetzer, G.R. Thomson & R.C. Tustin, Eds.: 825–852. Oxford University Press. Cape Town, London, New York.
2. THOMSON, G.R., W. VOSLOO, J.J. ESTERHUYSEN & R.G. BENGIS. 1992. Maintenance of foot and mouth disease virus in buffalo (*Syncerus caffer* Sparrman, 1979) in Southern Africa. Rev. Sci. Tech. Off. Int. Epizoot. **11:** 1097–1107.
3. THOMSON, G.R. 1995. Overview of FMD in Southern Africa. Rev. Sci. Tech. Off. Int. Epizoot. **14:** 503–520.
4. SUTMOLLER, P., G.R. THOMSON, S. HARGREAVES, *et al.* 1999. The foot-and-mouth disease risk posed by African buffalo within wildlife conservancies to the cattle industry of Zimbabwe. Prev. Vet. Med. **44** (2000): 43–60.
5. SUTMOLLER, P. & E. ANDERSON. 1999. Risk assessment of foot and mouth disease policies in Zimbabwe. Consultant Report. Veterinary Services, Ministry of Land, Agriculture and Rural Settlements, P.O. Box 8012, Causeway, Harare, Zimbabwe, pp. 35
6. SCOTT WILSON RESOURCE CONSULTANTS. 2000. Environmental Impact Assessment of the Veterinary Fences in Ngamiland, Summary Report for the Government of Botswana, September 2000, 105 pp.
7. ANONYMOUS. 1994. The lowveld conservancies: new opportunities for productive and sustainable land use. Save Valley, Bubiana and Chiredzi River Conservancies, Prive Waterhouse Wildlife, Tourism and Environmental Consulting (publishers). P.O. Box 453, Harare, Zimbabwe, 140 pp. plus appendices.

 8. OIE. 1992. International Animal Health Code. Mammals, birds and bees, 1993, 1994 and 1995 up-dates.
 9. OIE. 1997. Proceedings of the 65th General Session of the OIE.
10. THOMSON, G.R. 1996. The role of carrier animals in the transmission of foot and mouth disease. Comprehensive reports on technical items presented to the international committee or to regional commissions, pp. 87–103.
11. FOGEDBY, E.G., W.A. MALINQUIST, O.L. OSTEEN & M.L. JOHNSON. 1960. Airborne transmission of foot-and-mouth disease virus. Nord. Veterinaemed. **12:** 490–498.
12. DONALDSON, A.I. 1979. Airborne foot and mouth disease. Vet. Bull. **49:** 653–659.
13. AHL, A. 1991. Standardization of nomenclature for risk analysis studies. *In* Proceedings of the International Seminar on Animal Import Risk Analysis, August 1991. J.A. Acree & A.Ahl, Eds. Carlton University, Ottawa, Canada.
14. VOSE, D.J. 1997. Risk analysis in relation to the importation and exportation of animal products. Rev. Sci. Tech. Off. Int. Epizoot. **16**(1).
15. ANDERSON, E.C., C. FOGGIN, M. ATKINSON, *et al.* 1993. The role of wild animals other than buffalo in the current epidemiology of foot and mouth disease in Zimbabwe. Epidemiol. Infect. **11:** 559–563.

The Evolving Transmission Pattern of Rift Valley Fever in the Arabian Peninsula

SHAMSUDEEN F. FAGBO

M. Isa Mustafa, Jeddah 21332, Saudi Arabia

ABSTRACT: Vector-borne viruses are no respecters of international boundaries. The recent outbreak of Rift Valley fever (RVF) in the Kingdom of Saudi Arabia (KSA) and Yemen in September 2000 clearly sends a message that once pathogens cross their known geographic limits, they tend to adapt to the local ecology in order to survive and maintain transmission. This paper examines the various factors that may contribute to the establishment of RVF in the Arabian Peninsula (AP) and its possible spread to other countries. The annual influx of over 2 million pilgrims for the Hajj (annual pilgrimage for Muslims) in the KSA, as well as the large migrant population in this region, generates high human and animal traffic that presents a challenging agenda for public health. The potential risks within this period as well as other peculiar ecological factors are discussed.

KEYWORDS: Rift Valley fever; arbovirus; transmission; Arabian peninsula

INTRODUCTION

Rift Valley fever (RVF) was first described in Kenya in 1930.[1] An acute infection, it primarily affects domestic ungulates, causing abortion in gravid animals and mortalities, especially in the young. It is caused by an RNA arthropod-borne virus of the family Bunyaviridae, genus *Phlebotomus*. It remains infective for 3 months at room temperature and viable for almost 3 years in serum kept at $-4°C$. Various aspects of its molecular biology have been studied.[2] Demonstrated genetic reassortment between different strains of Rift Valley fever virus (RVFV) may aid vaccine development and widen understanding of its epidemiology.[3] Its pathogenesis and epidemiology in animals, especially in Africa, have been described.[4,5] An important arboviral zoonosis of humans, it may manifest clinically as undifferentiated fever, hemorrhagic fever, encephalitis, or ocular lesions with partial or permanent blindness.

The Arabian Penninsula (AP) refers to the sovereign lands south of the borders of Iraq and Jordan: Kuwait, the Kingdom of Saudi Arabia (KSA), United Arab Emirates (UAE), Qatar, Oman, Bahrain, and Yemen. Epidemiologically, however, the contiguity of a large portion of the KSA's northeastern border with Iraq cannot be overlooked. The KSA occupies about 80% of the AP, with extensive coastlines on the Red Sea and Persian Gulf. Generally, the climate is harsh with great extremes of temper-

Address for correspondence: Dr. Shamsudeen F. Fagbo, M. Isa Mustafa, P.O. Box 122656, Jeddah 21332, Saudi Arabia. Voice: 966 54 388 476; fax: 966 2 674 8914.
oshamsudeen@hotmail.com

Ann. N.Y. Acad. Sci. 969: 201–204 (2002). © 2002 New York Academy of Sciences.

ature and very little precipitation. However, areas such as the Tihama plains and Asir regions experience some rainfall and support agriculture.

VECTORS

RVFV is spread mainly by mosquitoes. Vector competence studies and virus isolation has been successful in more than 30 mosquito species.[6] There is a paucity of similar research on local strains of proven and potential vectors of RVFV—these include the *Culex, Aedes*, and *Anopheles* spp.;[7,8] in 1979, the Sindbis virus, another arbovirus, was first isolated from *Culex univittatus* in Eastern KSA. *Aedes albopictus* is also found in the region. RVFV vector competence has been demonstrated in the laboratory for *Phlebotomus duboscqi, P. papatasi*, and *Sergentomyia schwetzi*;[9] the latter two species are found in the AP. Phlebotomine flies should be tested for RVFV transmission: the region hosts many sandfly species—25 in the KSA alone.[10] Owing to their abundance, especially in areas with low or no mosquito densities, these flies may evolve for themselves a unique local role in viral transmission and, perhaps, maintenance in interepizootic periods. They readily adapt to man-derived urban biotypes and also infest potential rodent hosts of RVFV; they are known vectors of zoonotic leishmaniasis in the region. Other hematophagous insects, suspected of biological and mechanical transmission of RVFV,[11] also occupy niches in the region.

WILDLIFE RESERVOIR

Virus maintenance in the wild is yet to be full understood. Susceptible mammals can be found in the AP: 96 are known, of which 78 are found in the KSA.[12] The native Artiodyctyles, some of which are threatened species such as the *Capra ibex nubia, Hemitragus jayakari* (Arabian Tahr*), Gazella gazella*, and *Oryx leucoryx,* are potential wildlife reservoirs. Rodents include *Rattus rattus, Bandigota bengalensis, Gerbillus nanus* and others spanning over five families. RVFV antibodies have been detected in wild/commensal rodents in parts of Africa.[11] Chiropterid bats—there are over 30 species in the region[12]—are also possible reservoirs.[13]

TRANSMISSION PATTERNS

The recent epidemics were centered in the malarious areas of the Yemen and the KSA. Kuwait and the UAE are described as malaria-free, albeit with imported cases. Parts of the malarious regions in KSA have been studied by landsat images, and potential vector biotypes determined.[14] These biotypes, which harbor some of the candidate hosts and reservoirs mentioned earlier, may thus support the maintenance of the RVFV in the wild. The roles of the plethora of resident foreign workers in the region in transmission should be ascertained. Asymptomatic viremic migrants and their families could export the RVFV to their homelands: India (with the largest migrant population in the region), Philippines, or the USA. RVFV vectors have been identified in some of these countries[15] While limited secondary human transmission may occur in some places, there is a strong likelihood that infection of native mosquitos may exist in mosquito-endemic countries like India. This may lead to the inoculation of local ruminants and local establishment of the RVFV. It is also noteworthy that foreign workers are the least likely to have access to health facilities adequate for prompt detection: such facilities are increasingly becoming limited to citizens only on a free basis. Most workers in the slaughterhouses and abattoirs, especially during Hajj, are foreigners.

Annually, the KSA receives about 4 million visitors for the Hajj and Umrah (lesser pilgrimage) rites. The huge traffic during the Hajj season, often over 2 million people, is a public health challenge. Documented meningitis transmission amongst pilgrims[16] is an indication of probable RVFV transmission via contagion. During this season, over 2 million sheep, cattle, and camels are slaughtered; and there have been calls[17] for increased, stricter control of livestock movement with serosurveillance in abattoirs. Some pilgrims take home meat from slaughtered animals. Unlike foot and mouth disease (FMD), studies on the spread of RVFV via this route are lacking. One group more likely to transmit RVFV in this way are pilgrims from neighboring Arab/Gulf countries that come by road and engage in personal slaughtering of animals for their needs. It is highly feasible that, with the volume of meat being processed, infective amounts of the RVFV may become aerosolized and/or transmitted. This possibility is substantiated by the detection of RVFV antibodies in non-African livestock and abattoir workers in Makka—the Hajj focal point—in 1999.[18] The possible roles of feral cats in virus amplification should not be ruled out: Makka and some other urban areas of Saudi Arabia are known to have substantial feral cat populations that may not occur in RVF-endemic Africa. Cats, and dogs too, develop viremia without overt clinical disease upon exposure to RVFV.[15] Crows, widely established avian pests in the region, interact, along with cats, with the hitherto described urban biotypes and abattoirs in a manner that supports mechanical transmission. Their consumption of dead cat carcasses and slaughter-house remains may lead to viral inoculation and *in vivo* replication. They also transmit the West Nile virus, another arbovirus.

Nosocomial transmission is possible where there is little awareness or preparedness to handle the RVFV in health facilities. Such transmission may be enhanced by relocating viremic migrant workers as well as by unscreened donated blood. Nosocomial transmission of other blood-borne pathogens in the region has been recorded.[20]

CONCLUSION

The roles that the local fauna may play in RVFV transmission require urgent attention. The surveillance programs advocated should have the multiple effects of detecting latent arboviral activity (such as Crimean Congo Hemorrhagic and West Nile viruses) and aid public health education of the residents as well as pilgrims. A strong control program should incorporate customs peculiar to Muslim and Arab cultures (such as the abhorrence of autopsies, slaughtering customs, etc.) as well as revamped animal disease control protocols that emphasize greater collaboration between the veterinary and public health authorities. The integration of GIS and remote sensing technologies into surveillance activities is highly desirable.

ACKNOWLEDGMENTS

I appreciate the assistance of Prof. J.A.W. Coetzer (Head, Department of Veterinary Tropical Diseases, Faculty of Veterinary Science, University of Pretoria, South Africa) and Dr. Amadou Sall (Institut Pasteur de Dakar, Senegal).

REFERENCES

1. DAUBNEY, R., J.R. HUDSON & P.C. GRAHAM. 1931. Enzootic hepatitis or Rift Valley fever. An undescribed disease of sheep, cattle and man in East Africa. J. Pathol. Bacteriol. **34:** 545–579.
2. SALL, A.A. *et al.* 1999. Variability of the NSs protein among Rift Valley fever virus isolates. J. Virol. **73:** 2853–2858.
3. TURREL, M.J. *et al.* 1990 Generation and transmission of Rift Valley fever viral reassortants by the mosquito *Culex pipiens.* J. Gen. Virol **78:** 2307–2312.
4. SWANEPOEL, R. & J.A.W. COETZER. 1994. Rift Valley fever. *In* Infectious Diseases of Livestock with Special Reference to Southern Africa. J.A.W. Coetzer, G.R. Thompson & R.C. Tustin, Eds.: 688–717. Oxford University Press. Capetown, South Africa.
5. PETERS, C.J. 1997. Emergence of Rift Valley fever. *In* Factors in the Emergence of Arboviruses. J.F. Saluzzo & B. Dodet, Eds.: 253–264. Elsevier. Paris.
6. GAD, A.M. *et al.* 1987. Rift Valley fever virus transmission by different Egyptian mosquito species. Trans. R. Soc. Trop. Med. Hyg. **81:** 694–698.
7. WILLS, W.M. *et al.* 1985. Sindbis virus isolations from Saudi Arabian mosquitoes. Trans. R. Soc. Trop. Med. Hyg. **79:** 63–66.
8. CDC. 2000. Update: outbreak of Rift Valley fever—Saudi Arabia, August–November, 2000. MMWR **49:** 982–985.
9. DOHM, D.J. *et al.* 2000. Laboratory transmission of Rift Valley fever virus by *Phlebotomus dubosqi, Phlebotomus papatasi, Phlebotomus sergenti,* and *Sergentomyia schwetzi* (Diptera:Psychodidae). J. Med. Entomol. **37**(3): 435–438.
10. BUTTIKER, W. & D.J. LEWIS. 1983. Insects of Saudi Arabia: some ecological aspects of Saudi Arabian Phlebotomine sandflies (Diptera:Psychodidae). Fauna Saudi Arabia **5:** 479–527.
11. HOOGSTRAAL, H., J.M. MEEGAN & G.M. KHALIL. 1979. The Rift Valley fever epizootic in Egypt 1977–78. 2. Ecological and entomological studies. Trans. R. Soc. Trop. Med. Hyg. **73:** 624–629.
12. NADER, I.A. 1990. Checklist of the mammals of Arabia. Fauna Saudi Arabia **11:** 329–381.
13. FONTENILLE, D. *et al.* 1998. New vectors of Rift Valley fever in West Africa. Emerg. Inf. Dis. **4**(2): 289–293.
14. BUTTIKER, W. & K.P. FERGUSON. 1983. Fauna of Saudi Arabia: detection of faunal biotypes of medical importance in southwestern Saudi Arabia using landsat images. Fauna Saudi Arabia **3:** 10–27.
15. GARGAN, T.P. *et al.* 1988. Vector potential of selected North American mosquito species for Rift Valley fever virus. Am. J. Trop. Med. Hyg. **38**(2): 440–446.
16. AL-GAHTANI, Y.M. *et al.* 1995. Epidemiological investigation of an outbreak of meningococcal meningitis in Makka (Mecca), Saudi Arabia, 1992. Epidemiol. Infect. **115:** 399–409.
17. MEMISH, Z. 2001. Brucellosis control in Saudi Arabia: prospects and challenges. J. Chemother. **13**(S.1): 11–17.
18. TURKISTANI, A., A. GAD & N. AL-HAMDAN. 1999. Rift Valley fever among slaughter houses personnel in Makka during Hajj 1419H(1999). Eastern Med. J. Cited in: Alam, A.A. & A.G. Mohammed. 2000. Rift Valley fever: lessons to be learned. J. Fam. Comm. Med. **7**(3): 19–21.
19. KEEFER, G.V. *et al.* 1972. Susceptibility of dogs and cats to Rift Valley fever by inhalation or ingestion of virus. J. Infect. Dis. **125**(3): 307–309.
20. MEMISH, Z.A. & M.W. MAH. 2001. Brucellosis in laboratory workers at a Saudi Arabian hospital. Am. J. Infect. Control. **29**(1): 48–52.

Use of Sentinel Herds to Study the Epidemiology of Vesicular Stomatitis in the State of Colorado

BRIAN J. McCLUSKEY,[a] ELIZABETH L. MUMFORD,[b] MOWFAK D. SALMAN,[b] AND JOSIE J. TRAUB-DARGATZ[b]

[a]United States Department of Agriculture, Centers for Epidemiology and Animal Health, Ft. Collins, Colorado 80526, USA

[b]Department of Clinical Sciences, College of Veterinary Medicine and Biomedical Sciences, Colorado State University, Ft. Collins, Colorado 80526-8177, USA

ABSTRACT: Approximately 20 sentinel premises in Colorado were visited quarterly during a 3-year prospective study to investigate the persistence of VS viruses in horses. A survey to assess management practices, health events, animal movements and environmental data was completed at each visit. Collection of serum samples and oral swabs along with a clinical examination of sentinel horses were performed at each visit. Serum samples were tested by 2 or more of 4 available serological tests. The data collected for two years (August 1998 to August 2000) are reported here. During this period there was seroconversion in 1 and 8 horses based on capture IgM tests for seroytpes New Jersey and Indiana, respectively. Kaplan-Meier curves were generated for those premises with horses that seroconverted and the mean survival time was 4.17 quarters (range 1.85–7.0). The occurrence of seroconversions during periods when no clinical disease was observed suggests the persistence of vesicular stomatitis viruses in the environment of the sentinel premises.

KEYWORDS: sentinel herds; vesicular stomatitis; arthropod vectors

INTRODUCTION

Vesicular stomatitis (VS) in the United States is caused either by vesicular stomatitis virus New Jersey serotype (VSV-NJ) or vesicular stomatitis virus Indiana serotype (VSV-IN). These viruses are members of the family Rhabdoviridae, genus *Vesiculovirus*. Clinical VS has been seen in cattle, swine, llamas, and horses in the United States. However, serological evidence of virus exposure has been observed in many more species.[1,2] Reviews of the biological, pathological, and epidemiological aspects of this disease have been published.[3,4]

Address for correspondence: Dr. Brian J. McCluskey, United States Department of Agriculture, Centers for Epidemiology and Animal Health, 2150 Centre Ave., Building B, Mail Stop 2E7, Ft. Collins, CO 80526-8117.

brian.j.mccluskey@aphis.usda.gov

Ann. N.Y. Acad. Sci. 969: 205–209 (2002). © 2002 New York Academy of Sciences.

Outbreaks of VS in livestock in the southwestern United States occur sporadically. Most recently, outbreaks occurred in 1995, 1997, and 1998. Outbreaks typically begin in the late spring and end at the first frost. Also typical is a northward progression of disease over time, with the first positive premises in an outbreak typically identified in southern New Mexico, and with the last positive premises occurring in Colorado. The most recent outbreaks in the southwestern United States resulted in clinical disease in greater proportions in horses than cattle.[4] In VS endemic areas, including Central America and Ossabaw Island, Georgia, virus is transmitted by arthropod vectors.[5,6] Arthropods apparently also transmit VS viruses in the southwestern United States.[7,8] The objectives of this study were to investigate the persistence of VS viruses on equine premises previously identified as housing horses positive for VS and to identify potential factors associated with recurrence of VS on these premises.

MATERIALS AND METHODS

Sentinel equine premises were chosen from U.S. Department of Agriculture (USDA) databases developed during the 1995, 1997, and 1998 VS outbreaks in the United States. Selection criteria included one or more horses confirmed positive for VS in one or more of these three outbreaks in the 1990s, at least two horses on the premises at the time of the first study visit, and the willingness and ability to continue in the project for three years. Quarterly visits were made to each of the sentinel premises in which between 2 and 20 sentinel horses were given examinations of the mouth, nasal cavity, feet, and external genitalia. In addition, blood samples were drawn by jugular venipuncture, and swabs were collected from the oral cavity. Information about premises management practices, animal movement history, and other potential risk factors were collected by a standardized questionnaire at each visit.

All serum samples were tested by the competitive ELISA (cELISA) for antibody to both VSV serotypes. Samples positive by one or both cELISAs were tested by IgM capture ELISA, complement fixation tests, and serum neutralization tests for each serotype of the virus. Oral swab samples were frozen at $-70°C$ until the completion of serological testing.

Data were analyzed for two years (August 1998 to August 2000). Survival analysis was used to allow for inclusion of censored horses. A seroconversion was considered a "failure" in the survival analysis. Kaplan-Meir curves were generated for those premises with horses that seroconverted so that the mean survival time could be calculated. Mean survival time for each of the premises was used in a general linear model to evaluate management, environmental factors, and other factors associated with variations in survival times. Analyses were conducted using statistical software (SAS, v. 8, SAS Institute, Cary, NC).

RESULTS

Seroprevalences based on the cELISA for the New Jersey and Indiana serotypes for the first eight visits for all sentinel premises are presented in TABLES 1 and 2. The mean survival times and standard errors for those premises with seroconversions are

TABLE 1. Seroprevalence of VSV-NJ as determined by cELISA for sentinel premises in Colorado for quarterly visits (August 1998–August 2000)

Premises number	Visit 1 (%)	Visit 2 (%)	Visit 3 (%)	Visit 4 (%)	Visit 5 (%)	Visit 6 (%)	Visit 7 (%)	Visit 8 (%)
1	57	50	71	71	50	*	*	*
2	50	100	*	*	*	*	*	*
3	33	33	20	30	22	13	13	*
4	100	100	100	100	100	100	100	*
5	50	50	50	100	100	50	50	100
6	25	0	29	25	25	0	0	0
7	64	64	64	64	55	55	55	64
8	75	60	25	40	50	75	75	*
9	25	25	25	25	25	0	0	0
10	0	0	0	0	0	0	0	0
11	14	14	14	14	30	20	25	33
12	50	33	100	*	*	*	*	*
13	20	20	0	14	0	17	14	*
14	30	30	37.5	10	10	22	17	*
15	15	23	23	22	*	*	*	*
16	22	22	25	25	0	11	*	*
17	80	80	60	50	75	50	50	40
18	36	38	38	38	38	36	36	36
19	11	11	13	13	17	14	*	*
20	66	75	75	*	*	*	*	*

*Samples not obtained due to premises dropout or later entry into the study.

presented in TABLE 3. The final model included the total hours horses spent in a barn in a 24-hour period, the total hours horses spent on pasture in a day, the distance from where horses were housed to the nearest running water, the number of horses within a 1-mile radius of the premises, and premises owner's estimate of above-normal insect populations at the time of the initial visit. ($F = 4.16$, $P < 0.05$, $r^2 = 0.77$).

DISCUSSION

The occurrence of seroconversion in horses on the sentinel premises in this study during non–VS outbreak periods suggests that VS virus infections occur during non-outbreak periods. Existing virus-sequencing data suggest the viruses may survive in the southwestern United States through the winter months. Indeed, five virus isolates obtained in New Mexico in the spring of 1997 and in the summer of 1998 were identical to two virus isolates obtained in Colorado in 1997. This indicated that the same VS-IN virus caused outbreaks in the spring and summer of 1997 and 1998.[9] Vesicular stomatitis virus persistence on premises in the southwestern United States may

TABLE 2. Seroprevalence of VSV-IN as determined by cELISA for sentinel premises in Colorado for quarterly visits (August 1998–August 2000)

Premises number	Visit 1 (%)	Visit 2 (%)	Visit 3 (%)	Visit 4 (%)	Visit 5 (%)	Visit 6 (%)	Visit 7 (%)	Visit 8 (%)
1	57	50	57	57	50	*	*	*
2	0	0	*	*	*	*	*	*
3	0	0	0	0	0	0	0	*
4	100	100	100	100	100	100	100	*
5	100	100	100	100	100	100	100	100
6	63	29	29	25	25	0	0	0
7	64	64	64	64	64	55	64	64
8	25	20	0	20	25	50	25	*
9	75	50	50	50	50	50	50	50
10	44	50	22	44	30	30	50	40
11	100	86	71	71	83	40	75	100
12	50	66	100	*	*	*	*	*
13	60	60	20	43	43	50	43	*
14	20	30	13	20	10	11	0	*
15	31	23	23	33	*	*	*	*
16	57	50	57	57	50	*	*	*
17	0	0	*	*	*	*	*	*
18	0	0	0	0	0	0	0	*
19	100	100	100	100	100	100	100	*
20	100	100	100	100	100	100	100	100

*Samples not obtained due to premises dropout or later entry into the study.

TABLE 3. Mean survival times (in quarters of the year) and standard errors for VS (VSV-NJ or VSV-IN) sentinel premises in Colorado

Premises number	Mean survival time	Standard error
5	4.00	0.354
7	5.54	0.705
8	6.00	0.216
10	7.00	0.091
11	1.85	0.187
13	3.00	0.117
14	3.00	0.079
16	5.17	1.06
17	2.86	0.187
18	3.89	0.144
19	5.00	0.00
20	2.75	0.306

lead to alterations in the designation of VS as a disease foreign to the United States and in the establishment of control procedures.

A case-control study of VS previously conducted by this research group found the risk of having horses positive for VS was higher for premises where horses had access to pasture, where owners reported increased insect populations, and where horses were housed less than 0.25 miles from a source of running water.[10] This study also found that animals with access to a shelter or barn were at a reduced risk of developing VS. These factors also were found to make significant contributions to the final model developed in the study reported here.

REFERENCES

1. WEBB, P.A., T.P. MONATH & J.S. REIF. 1987. Epizootic vesicular stomatitis in Colorado, 1982: epidemiologic studies along the northern Colorado Front Range. Am. J. Trop. Med. Hyg. **36:** 183–188.
2. FLETCHER, W.O., D.E. STALLKNECHT & M.T. KEARNEY. 1991. Antibodies to vesicular stomatitis New Jersey type virus in white-tailed deer on Ossabaw Island, Georgia, 1985–1989. J. Wild. Dis. **27:** 675–680.
3. LETCHWORTH, G.J., L.L. RODRIGUEZ & J. DEL BARRERA. 1999. Vesicular stomatitis. Vet. J. **157:** 239–260.
4. McCLUSKEY, B.J., H.S. HURD & E.L. MUMFORD. 1999. Review of the 1997 outbreak of vesicular stomatitis in the western United States. J. Am. Vet. Med. Assoc. **215:** 1259–1262.
5. COMER, J.A., R.B. TESH, G.B. MODI, *et al.* 1990. Vesicular stomatitis virus, New Jersey serotype: replication in and transmission by *Lutzomyia shannoni* (Diptera: Psychodidae). Am. J. Trop. Med. Hyg. **42:** 483–490.
6. COMER, J.A., J.L. CORN, D.E. STALLKNECHT, *et al.* 1992. Titers of vesicular stomatitis virus, New Jersey serotype, in naturally infected male and female *Lutzomyia shannoni* (Diptera:Psychodidae) in Georgia. J. Med. Entomol. **29:** 368–370.
7. WALTON, T.E., P.A. WEBB, W.L. KRAMER, *et al.* 1987. Epizootic vesicular stomatitis in Colorado, 1982: epidemiologic and entomologic studies. Am. J. Trop. Med. Hyg. **36:** 166–176.
8. MEAD, D.G., C.J. MARE & F.B. RAMBERG. 1999. Bite transmission of vesicular stomatitis virus (New Jersey serotype) to laboratory mice by *Simulium vittatum* (Diptera: Simuliidae). J. Med. Entomol. **36:** 410–413.
9. RODRIGUEZ, L.L., T.A. BUNCH, M. FRAIRE & Z.N. LLEWELLYN. 2000. Re-emergence of vesicular stomatitis in the western United States is associated with distinct viral genetic lineages.Virology **271:** 171–181.
10. HURD, H.S., B.J. McCLUSKEY & E.L. MUMFORD. 1999. Management factors affecting the risk for vesicular stomatitis in livestock operations in the western United States. J. Am. Vet. Med. Assoc. **215:** 1263–1268.

Natural Aujeszky's Disease in a Spanish Wild Boar Population

C. GORTÁZAR,[a] J. VICENTE,[a] Y. FIERRO,[b] L. LEÓN,[c] M. J. CUBERO,[c] AND M. GONZÁLEZ[c]

[a]Instituto de Investigación en Recursos Cinegéticos (IREC, CSIC-UCLM), Ronda de Toledo, E-13005 Ciudad Real, Spain

[b]Yolfi Properties S.L., Abenójar, Ciudad Real, Spain

[c]Departamento de Patología Animal, Facultad de Veterinaria, Campus de Espinardo, 30.100 Murcia, Spain

ABSTRACT: We describe an outbreak of Aujeszky's disease (AD) in a wild boar (Sus scrofa) population from central Spain. Mortality was estimated to be at least 14% (14/100) in juveniles and 7.5% (3/40) in adults. Most of the affected animals (12/17) were between 4 and 8 months of age. Gross lesions mainly consisted of enlarged and congestive tonsils and lymph nodes, petechial hemorrhages on the small intestine, and engorged blood vessels in the brain and meninges. Histopathology revealed mild nonsuppurative meningoencephalitis. Positivity to the fluorescent antibody test was found in tissues from the affected animals. Seroprevalence of antibodies to AD virus (ADV) was 56% (9/16). To our knowledge, this is the first description of clinical cases in a wild suid population.

KEYWORDS: Aujeszky's disease; Spain; Sus scrofa; wild boar

INTRODUCTION

Aujeszky's disease (AD) is caused by an alpha-herpesvirus that mainly affects domestic swine.[1] Eradication programs are being implemented in several countries, including Spain, because of its economic importance in livestock. The wild boar is the most common wild ungulate in the Iberian peninsula and its population has increased in the last few decades.[2] In southcentral Spain, artificial feeding and watering may increase the risk of disease transmission. AD virus (ADV) can infect other domestic or wild species, and fatal cases in endangered carnivores have already been described.[3] This makes ADV of interest regarding conservation since endangered species such as the Iberian lynx (Lynx pardinus) share their habitat with the wild boar in southern Spain.

Address for correspondence: Dr. C. Gortázar, Instituto de Investigación en Recursos Cinegéticos (IREC, CSIC-UCLM), P. O. Box 535, E-13080 Ciudad Real, Spain.
gortazar@irec.uclm.es

Ann. N.Y. Acad. Sci. 969: 210–212 (2002). © 2002 New York Academy of Sciences.

To our knowledge, there have been no reports on clinical AD in free-living European wild boar populations. Thus, our aim was to describe the epidemiology and the pathological findings of a naturally occurring outbreak.

MATERIALS AND METHODS

The study area is located in a 900-ha hunting estate in southcentral Spain (38°55′ N; 0°36′ E; 600–850 m above sea level). Iberian red deer (*Cervus elaphus hispanicus*), introduced Barbary sheep (*Ammotragus lervia*), and mouflon (*Ovis ammon*) also inhabit the study area. The climate is Mediterranean and the habitat is characterized by scrubland and evergreen oak (*Quercus ilex*) woodlands with scattered pastures and small crops. The range is fenced in order to enclose the wild ruminants, but boars are able to cross under these fences. This wild boar population is kept inside the range by artificial feeding. The overall population of wild boar did not exceed 140 to 150 animals during the study period as estimated by the gamekeepers through repeated counts at the feeding places.

The first dead boar was found in March 2000. From then on, the gamekeepers were told to search actively for any sick boar or carcass. In total, 17 cases were registered, but only fresh carcasses (4) and sick found animals (2) were necropsied. Thus, all other dead boar are only suspected cases. Based on the tooth eruption patterns, boars less than 12 months of age were classified as juveniles and those above 1 year were classified as adults.

Unfixed samples of the brain (cerebrum and cerebellum) and tonsils as well as routine samples of other tissues were collected and stored at −20°C for immunofluorescence antibody test (IFAT) on tissues.[4] Sections of these tissues were fixed in 10% neutral buffered formalin and embedded in paraffin for histopathological examination by hematoxylin-eosin stain. Blood samples from 16 boars (6 affected; 10 shot) were collected, and sera were obtained and stored at −20°C until tested for antibodies against ADV-gII.[5] The threshold titer of optical densities was established based on the mean ± 3 SD of the negative control sera.

RESULTS

Dead or sick boars were found from March to October 2000, mainly at feeding (3/17) or watering places (7/17). The minimum mortality was estimated to be 7.5% (3/40) of the total adult population and 14% (14/100) of the juveniles. No sex-related differences were found. Apparently, no other wildlife species became affected. Eight of the 15 boar carcasses (53%) had been scavenged by other boar.

Clinical signs in the affected boars consisted of abnormal behavior. Individuals were unable to stand on their hind legs, showing tremor and incoordination. They were found inside the water holes, presumably due to a high body temperature. All affected animals were in good general condition. No exterior signs of pruritus or self-mutilations were seen in any animal. Postmortem examination showed frontal and temporal subcutaneous hematomas and edema of the chest and submandibular space. Common internal lesions in necropsied animals were inflammation of the tonsils and engorged blood vessels in the brain and meninges. Thoracic and abdominal lymph nodes also showed intense congestion. Two animals showed intestinal petechial hemorrhages and 1 had pulmonar edema and congestion. All animals had recently ingested food. Tuberculosis-like granulomas diagnosed as bovine TB were found in all (but 1) affected animals (manuscript in preparation). Mild diffuse non-suppurative meningoencephalitis with large amounts of leukocytes inside the blood vessels, but no perivascular cuffing, was present in the encephalon. No typical intranuclear herpesvirus inclusions were found.

All necropsied animals were positive to the IFAT in brain and tonsil sections, except for 1 autolyzed animal. Also, bronchial and mesenteric lymph nodes ($n = 3$), lung ($n = 1$), and intestine ($n = 4$) were positive. For the sera analyzed (including those of healthy, shot boar), seropositivity was 56.25% (9/16). Four out of 6 sera from affected animals were ELISA-positive.

DISCUSSION

A recent serosurvey indicates a seroprevalence to ADV of >35% in Spanish boar populations.[6] As in other countries,[7] the extent of clinical disease and the prevalence of latent infections in wild boars are unknown in Spain. The pathogenicity of the strains circulating among wild boars is unknown and other risk factors should also be taken into account. Mortality may be related to the susceptibility of the hosts. First, the affected animals were mainly juveniles. Second, their immune response could have been impaired by the concomitant bovine TB infection since humoral and cellular responses may be dichotomic.[8] Finally, cannibalism may contribute to the spread of the disease.[9] More research is ongoing in order to characterize any ADV isolates and to clarify the epidemiology of the disease in wild boars in Spain.

REFERENCES

1. METTENLEITER, T.C. 2000. Aujeszky's disease virus: the virus and molecular pathogenesis—state of the art, June 1999. Vet. Res. **31:** 99–115.
2. GORTÁZAR, C., J. HERRERO, et al. 2000. Historical examination of the status of large mammals in Aragon, Spain. Mammalia **64:** 411–422.
3. GLASS, C.M., R.G. MCLEAN, et al. 1994. Isolation of pseudorabies (Aujeszky's disease) virus from a Florida panther. J. Wildl. Dis. **30:** 180–184.
4. ALLAN, G.M., M.S. MCNULTY, et al. 1984. Rapid diagnosis of Aujeszky's disease in pigs by immunofluorescence. Res. Vet. Sci. **36:** 235–239.
5. QVIST, P., K.J. SORENSEN & A. MEYLING. 1989. Monoclonal blocking ELISA detecting serum antibodies to the glycoprotein gII of Aujeszky's disease virus. J. Virol. Methods **24:** 169–179.
6. VICENTE, J., L. LEÓN, et al. 2002. Antibodies to selected viral and bacterial pathogens in European wild boars from southcentral Spain. J. Wildl. Dis. **38**. In press.
7. MÜLLER, T., J. TEUFFERT, et al. 1998. Pseudorabies in the European wild boar from eastern Germany. J. Wildl. Dis. **34:** 251–258.
8. ZUCKERMANN, F.A. 2000. Aujeszky's disease virus: opportunities and challenges. Vet. Res. **31:** 121–131.
9. HAHN, E.C., G.R. PAGE, et al. 1997. Mechanisms of transmission of Aujeszky's disease virus originating from feral swine in the USA. Vet. Microbiol. **55:** 123–130.

Seroprevalence of Avian Paramyxovirus 1, 2, and 3 in Captive and Free-Living Birds of Prey in Spain (Preliminary Results)

Implications for Management of Wild and Captive Populations

URSULA HÖFLE,[a,b] J. M. BLANCO,[a] AND E. F. KALETA[b]

[a]Aquila Foundation and Centro de Estudios de Rapaces Ibéricas (JCCM), 45671 Sevilleja de la Jara, Toledo, Spain

[b]Institute for Avian and Reptile Diseases, Justus-Liebig-University, 35392 Giessen, Germany

ABSTRACT: Since December 1997, 700 blood plasma samples from 31 different species of captive and free-living birds of prey from Spain were analyzed by hemagglutination inhibition (HI) test for the presence of antibodies to avian paramyxovirus (aPMV) 1,2, and 3. Out of 700 birds, 120 tested positive for aPMV-1, 10 birds had antibodies to aPMV-2, and 4 birds tested positive against aPMV-3. Prevalence of antibodies against aPMV-1 was significantly higher in captive than in free-living birds of prey and in Falconiformes than in Strigidae and Accipitridae. Infection or exposure in captive birds may be due to the use of avian-derived food in rehabilitation and captive-breeding centers. This may be of concern at the time of reintroduction of these birds into free-living populations.

KEYWORDS: avian paramyxovirus 1, 2, and 3; Newcastle disease; birds of prey

INTRODUCTION

Wild birds, especially migratory waterfowl, birds of prey, and passerines, are frequently considered reservoirs or even vectors for avian pathogens of importance for commercial poultry.[1,2]

Recent experience in some captive breeding projects has shown that endangered species of birds of prey may be at risk of fatal infections by pathogens from avian-derived food.[3,4] In these cases, the pathogens were apathogenic for their original host, but had devastating effects on the infected kestrels and falcons. Also, serologic studies have shown that free-living birds can become exposed to galliform pathogens from the residues and runoff into ponds from farms,[5] as well as by ingestion of dumped chicken carcasses.[6]

Address for correspondence: Ursula Höfle, Aquila Foundation, Centro de Estudios de Rapaces Ibéricas, 45671 Sevilleja de la Jara, Toledo, Spain. Voice/fax: 0034-925-455004.
Uholfeh@nexo.es

Ann. N.Y. Acad. Sci. 969: 213–216 (2002). © 2002 New York Academy of Sciences.

Spain is one of the richest countries in western Europe in terms of birds of prey and is home to the Spanish imperial eagle (*Aquila adalberti*), one of the most endangered birds of prey in the world,[7] as well as many other endangered species of birds of prey. Captive breeding projects are under way for the Spanish imperial eagle, the Bonelli's eagle (*Hieraaetus fasciatus*), the peregrine falcon (*Falco peregrinus*), the lesser kestrel (*Falco naumanni*), and the Montagu's harrier (*Circus pygargus*) in different centers, in addition to the numerous rehabilitation centers distributed throughout the country where these same species may occur. Avian prey (especially galliform-derived, such as quail and red-legged partridges) or meat is used in most rehabilitation centers and in some captive breeding centers as a cheap food source.

In the present study, we report preliminary results on the seroprevalence of avian paramyxoviruses 1, 2, and 3 (aPMV-1, -2, and -3) in captive and free-living birds of prey in Spain. Avian paramyxovirus 1 is the causative agent of Newcastle disease, one of the most important diseases in domestic poultry, which can also be fatal for birds of prey.[1]

aPMV-2 and -3 occur mostly in turkeys, Passeriformes, and Psittaciformes and cause respiratory and central nervous system signs.[1]

MATERIALS AND METHODS

Blood samples from the superficial vena cutanea ulnares were obtained from 700 birds of prey of 31 species, in the field, upon admission to a rehabilitation center, during rechecks of birds that had spent considerable time at a rehabilitation center, or during routine health checks of birds of different breeding stocks (TABLE 1). Samples were maintained at 4°C until processing, and plasma was separated after centrifugation (12 min at $900 \times g$) and frozen at -20°C.

After thawing at 37°C and inactivation (30 min at 56°C) of the samples, they were tested against aPMV-1, -2, and -3 using the hemagglutination inhibition test.[8,9] The test strains used were as follows: for aPMV-1, the nonpathogenic strain F and the vaccine strain La Sota;[10] for aPMV-2, the Yucaipa strain (obtained from the Central Veterinary Laboratory, Weybridge, United Kingdom, 1984); for aPMV-3, the isolate 1571/83 (Institute for Avian and Reptile Diseases, JLU, Giessen, Germany, 1983). Results were compared by species/family of the birds, sex, age, captive or free-living status of the birds, and health status using the analysis of variance (ANOVA) test.

RESULTS

One hundred twenty out of 700 birds of prey and owls (17.1%) were found to have antibodies against aPMV-1. Seroprevalence was significantly higher in captive than in free-living birds of prey and owls ($P = 0.0023$), as well as in Falconidae as opposed to the other families ($P = 0.04$, TABLE 1). No significant differences were observed in seroprevalence among sex, different age classes, or health status of the investigated birds.

Antibodies against aPMV-2 were detected in 10 out of 700 birds (1.4%), all of these being diurnal, while only 4 of the 700 (0.6%) had antibodies against aPMV-3, all of them Accipitridae.

TABLE 1. Seroprevalence of antibodies against aPMV-1 in different families of captive and free-living birds of prey

Family	Total examined			Free-living			Captive		
	n	*n* Seropositive	%	*n*	*n* Seropositive	%	*n*	*n* Seropositive	%
Accipitridae	392	56	14.3	180	9	5	212	47	22.2
Pandionidae	2	0	0	1	0	0	1	0	0
Falconidae	141	46	32.6	23	3	13	118	43	36.4
Strigidae	122	17	13.9	69	8	11.6	53	9	17
Tytonidae	43	1	2.3	26	0	0	17	1	5.9
Total	700	120	17.1	299	20	6.7	401	100	24.9

DISCUSSION

The low seroprevalence of aPMV-1, -2, and -3 in free-living birds of prey is consistent with observations in birds of prey sampled in the field, principally in Germany.[11] Also, Falconidae are known to be more susceptible to infection by aPMV-1 than members of other families of birds of prey and owls.[12] This study is the first that compares seroprevalence of avian paramyxoviruses in captive and free-living birds of prey. The significantly higher seroprevalence of aPMV-1 in captive birds of prey is most probably due to the use of avian prey species (pigeons, quails, or partridges), 1-day-old chicks, or chicken meat in the rehabilitation and captive breeding centers. No direct evidence of the presence of aPMV-1 in these food items was sought, but the hypothesis is supported by the fact that, in previous cases, mortality of captive birds of prey due to other pathogens, for example, adenoviruses had been caused by contaminated avian-derived feed.[3,4]

Some endangered species are more susceptible to adenoviruses that are nonpathogenic in the chicken, a reason for which other investigators have previously recommended the use of different nonavian food items in captive birds of prey.[3] None of the seropositive birds showed clinical signs typical of an aPMV-1, -2, or -3 infection, which may, especially for aPMV-1, mean that the antibody production in these birds was due to exposure to a vaccine strain or to a mild abortive infection. Commercial vaccine strains against Newcastle disease have been used routinely in falcons in the Middle East with good success.[12] Nevertheless, the effect of these strains in different species is not yet known. Also, when ingesting avian prey, a bird may become exposed to a number of other potential pathogens in addition to aPMV-1.[3] For this reason, we recommend the use of different prey species, such as rodents, rabbits, or other small mammals, especially in captive breeding projects and in rehabilitation centers, for birds expected to be reintroduced into the wild.

REFERENCES

1. ALEXANDER, D.J. 1997. Newcastle disease and other avian paramyxoviruses. *In* Diseases of Poultry, 10th edit., pp. 541–569. Iowa State University Press. Ames, Iowa.
2. HLINAK, A. *et al.* 1998. Serological survey of viral pathogens in bean and white-fronted geese from Germany. J. Wildl. Dis. **34:** 479–486.
3. FORBES, N.A. *et al.* 1997. Adenovirus infection in Mauritius kestrels (*Falco punctatus*). J. Avian Med. Surg. **11:** 31–33.
4. RIDEOUT, B.R. *et al.* 1997. An adenovirus outbreak in captive Aplomado falcons (*Falco femoralis septentrionalis*) causing high morbidity and mortality. *In* Proceedings of the American Association of Zoo Veterinarians, pp. 45–46.
5. NAWATHE, D.R., O. ONUNKWO & I.M. SMITH. 1978. Serological evidence of bursal disease in wild and domestic birds in Nigeria. Vet. Rec. **102:** 444.
6. OÑA, A. *et al.* 2000. Epidemiological survey of infectious bursal disease virus in wild birds [abstract]. EWDA **4:** 39.
7. FERRER, M. 1993. El Águila Imperial Ibérica. Quercus. Madrid.
8. THAYER, S.G. & C.W. BEARD. 1998. Serologic procedures. *In* Isolation and Identification of Avian Pathogens, 4th edit., pp. 255–266. American Association of Avian Pathologists. Kennett Square, PA.
9. CEC. 1992. Richtlinie 92/66/EWG vom 14.07.1992 zur Einführung von Massnahmen zur Kontrolle der Newcastle Disease. Off. J. Eur. Community **L260:** 1–20.
10. WINTERFIELD, R.W., C.L. GOLDMAN & E.H. SEADALE. 1957. Newcastle disease immunization studies: 4. Vaccination of chicken with B1, F, and La Sota strains of NDV administered through the drinking water. Poult. Sci. **36:** 1076–1088.
11. SCHETTLER, E. *et al.* 2001. Seroepizootiology of selected infectious disease agents in free-living birds of prey in Germany. J. Wildl. Dis. **37:** 145–152.
12. HEIDENREICH, M. 1996. Greifvögel: Krankheiten, Haltung, Zucht. Blackwell Wissenschafts Verlag. Berlin/Vienna.

Serologic Survey of Selected Viral, Bacterial, and Protozoal Agents in Captive and Free-Ranging Ungulates from Central Kenya

KEVIN R. KIMBER,[a] JUAN LUBROTH,[b] EDWARD J. DUBOVI,[c] MARY LOU BERNINGER,[b] AND THOMAS W. DEMAAR[d]

[a]Wildlife Health Laboratory, Department of Population Medicine and Diagnostic Sciences, College of Veterinary Medicine, Cornell University, Ithaca, New York 14853, USA

[b]Plum Island Animal Disease Center, Greenport, New York 11944, USA

[c]New York State Veterinary Diagnostic Laboratory, College of Veterinary Medicine, Cornell University, Ithaca, New York 14853, USA

[d]Ol Jogi, Limited, Nanyuki, Kenya

ABSTRACT: Serologic evidence of exposure to various disease agents in free-ranging and captive ungulates at a private game ranch in Kenya is presented, and seroprevalence values inside a fenced-in area are compared with those found on the adjacent open savanna. Zebras outside the fence had a higher prevalence of equine rhinovirus-1 than zebras inside (Fisher's exact test, $P = 0.007$); for all other species and all other agents, there was no such difference ($P > 0.10$). Results highlight possible transmission of these agents from domestic species into wildlife or vice versa at our study site.

KEYWORDS: serology; zebra; antelope; giraffe; epidemiology; wildlife; survey; disease

INTRODUCTION

Serologic surveys influence wildlife management policies.[1,2] Translocation can introduce novel disease agents to unexposed populations of susceptible animals,[3] thus initiating epidemics in populations too small to sustain continuous infection.[4] Wildlife may act as reservoir hosts for disease in domestic species[5,6] and vice versa.[1] Serologic surveys of common wild species can reflect prevalence of disease within an ecological community, thereby assessing exposure risk among endangered taxonomically similar sympatric populations.[7] Artificial elevations of population density, as seen in game ranches and national parks,[8] can increase the significance of disease in limiting the carrying capacity of the environment.[9] Thus, comparison of the sero-

Address for correspondence: Dr. Kevin Kimber, Wildlife Health Laboratory, Department of Population Medicine and Diagnostic Sciences, College of Veterinary Medicine, Cornell University, Ithaca, NY 14853. Voice: 607-253-3572; fax: 607-253-3083.
krk2@cornell.edu

Ann. N.Y. Acad. Sci. 969: 217–223 (2002). © 2002 New York Academy of Sciences.

epidemiology of animals inside a game reserve with those outside the reserve may help predict and prevent epidemics.

MATERIALS AND METHODS

Ol Jogi ranch is a game sanctuary, with 13,000 acres fenced-in and 50,000 acres of open savanna ranch, located in the Laikipia district of central Kenya. In 1976, a single fence was erected to provide security for southern white rhinoceroses (*Ceratotherium simum simum*) and black rhinoceroses (*Diceros bicornis*) translocated that year. Burchell's zebra (*Equus burchelli*), buffalo (*Syncerus caffer*), Grant's gazelle (*Gazella grantii*), impala (*Aepyceros melampus*), reticulated giraffe (*Giraffa camelopardalis*), and other ungulates were enclosed when the fence was erected, and populations persist inside and outside the fence. Since 1976, southern white and black rhinoceroses and other ungulates have been introduced inside the fence. Cattle (*Bos indicus*), camels (*Camelus dromedarius*), horses (*Equus caballus*), and donkeys (*Equus asinus*) reside on the ranch, but do not enter the fenced-in area. Contact between herds of cattle and goats (*Capra* spp.) owned by pastoralists and animals in this study occurs.

Between 1995 and 1999, 222 serum samples were collected from Burchell's zebra, camels, buffalo, impala, Grant's gazelle, giraffe, and cattle during management culls and veterinary interventions, or from animals recently dead. No animals showed clinical signs or gross pathologic lesions consistent with infection for the agents tested. Camels and wildlife were unvaccinated; cattle were vaccinated for foot-and-mouth disease virus (FMDV) yearly and rinderpest virus (RPV) in 1995.

Samples were collected in plain glass clot tubes, placed on ice, and taken to the laboratory within 2 h; serum was aliquoted and frozen at −20°C until transport to the United States Department of Agriculture Foreign Animal Disease Diagnostic Laboratory (USDA/FADDL), where most ($n = 179$) were treated by 3 mrad of gamma irradiation prior to transshipment to the New York State Veterinary Diagnostic Laboratory (NYSVDL). Aliquots of zebra ($n = 46$) and nonequine ($n = 155$) sera were kept unirradiated by the USDA/FADDL and were analyzed for antibodies against African horse sickness virus (AHSV), bluetongue virus (BTV), FMDV, malignant catarrhal fever virus (MCFV), RPV, and trypanosomosis (TRYP). At the NYSVDL, samples were analyzed for antibodies against equine herpesvirus type-1 and type-4 (EHV-1 and -4), equine influenza virus (EIV), equine rhinovirus type-1 and type-2 (ERV-1 and -2), equine viral arteritis virus (EVAV), *Anaplasma* spp., bovine leukosis virus (BLV), bovine parainfluenza virus (PIV), bovine respiratory syncytial virus (BRSV), bovine viral diarrhea virus (BVDV), *Brucella abortus*, and infectious bovine rhinotracheitis virus (IBRV). Statistical comparisons used Fisher's exact test on SigmaStat (SPSS, Chicago, IL).

RESULTS

Results are listed in TABLES 1 and 2. Zebras outside the fence had a higher prevalence of ERV-1 ($P = 0.007$) than zebras inside. For all other species and all other

TABLE 1. Serological findings for equine viruses among Burchell's zebra (*Equus burchelli*) and dromedary camels (*Camelus dromedarius*) found near Ol Jogi ranch, Kenya

Disease agent	Test used (positive titer)	Number positive/n			
		IN[a]	OUT[b]	TOT[c]	Range[d]
African horse sickness virus	ELISA[e] (1:10)	22/23	23/23	45/46	1:10
Equine viral arteritis virus	SN[f] (≥1:8)	2/24	1/23	3/49	1:8–:16
Equine herpesvirus-1[g]	SN[f] (≥1:8)	21/24	22/23	45/49	1:8–1:96
Equine herpesvirus-4	SN[f] (≥1:8)	8/24	10/23	18/49	1:8–1:16
Equine influenza virus	HI[h] (≥1:8)	0/24	0/23	0/49	no positives
Equine rhinovirus-1[i]	SN (≥1:8)	2/24[j]	10/23[j]	12/49[f]	1:8–1:512
Equine rhinovirus-2	SN (≥1:8)	18/24	21/23	41/49	1:8–1:128

[a]IN = inside fence.
[b]OUT = outside fence.
[c]TOT = total.
[d]Range = range of positive titers.
[e]ELISA = enzyme-linked immunosorbent assay.
[f]SN = serum virus neutralization.
[g]50/50 camels were negative for equine herpesvirus-1. All resided outside fence.
[h]HI = hemagglutination inhibition.
[i]Four out of 49 camels were positive for equine influenza virus (titer range: 1:8–1:32). All resided outside the fence.
[j]Seroprevalence was significantly higher outside the fence than inside (Fisher's exact test, $P = 0.007$).

disease agents, the ratio of seropositive to seronegative animals outside the fence was not significantly different from the ratio inside the fence ($P > 0.10$).

DISCUSSION

Equine Viruses

In Laikipia, the seasonal population fluctuation of the vector for AHSV may be reduced compared to South Africa,[10] allowing for greater endemicity. The positive titers to EVAV in this study could be due to exposure to EVAV or a similar cross-reacting viral species. Titers to EHV-1 among zebra in our study were often higher than to EHV-4, suggesting the virus present was more closely related antigenically to EHV-1.[2,11] Serologic surveys for equine rhinoviruses have not been reported in wild or captive zebras. The rapid spread, high morbidity, duration of positive titers, and persistence of viral shedding in recovered horses make ERV-1 a possible indicator for exposure of wild equids to agents from domestic horses.[12] Our results suggest limited exposure to ERV-1 among zebra inside the fence when compared with zebra outside.

TABLE 2. Results of serology tests for nonequine diseases[a,b] among ungulates found near Ol Jogi Ranch, Kenya

Disease agent	Test used (positive titer)	Number positive/n			
		IN[c]	OUT[d]	TOT[e]	Range[f]
Anaplasma spp.[g]	CF (= 1:5)[h]				
Buffalo (*Syncerus caffer*)		0/1	1/7	1/10	1:5
Bluetongue virus	ELISA (= 1:8)[i]				
Camel (*Camelus dromedarius*)[j]		0/0	10/10	10/10	not applicable
Cattle (*Bos indicus*)		0/0	55/55	55/55	not applicable
Buffalo		0/0	4/4	4/4	not applicable
Grant's gazelle (*Gazella grantii*)		3/5	2/3	5/8	not applicable
Impala (*Aepyceros melampus*)		12/19	4/7	16/26	not applicable
Reticulated giraffe (*Giraffa camelopardalis*)		0/0	1/1	1/1	not applicable
Bovine parainfluenza-3 virus	SN ($\geq$1:8)[k]				
Cattle		0/0	55/55	55/55	1:16–$\geq$1:512
Buffalo		1/1	5/7	6/10	1:8–1:192
Grant's gazelle		4/5	2/3	6/8	1:8–1:64
Impala		3/27	2/8	5/36	1:8–1:24
Reticulated giraffe		1/11	0/3	1/14	1:8
Bovine respiratory syncytial virus	SN ($\geq$1:8)[k]				
Cattle		0/0	17/55	17/55	1:8–1:32
Buffalo		0/1	2/7	2/10	1:8–1:16
Grant's gazelle		1/5	3/3	4/8	1:8–1:24
Impala		5/27	2/8	7/36	1:8–1:128
Reticulated giraffe		2/11	1/3	3/14	1:8–1:12
Bovine virus diarrhea virus[l]	SN ($\geq$1:8)[k]				
Cattle		0/0	30/55	30/55	1:16–1:384
Brucella abortus[m]	CF ($\geq$1:10)[h]				
Dromedary camel		0/0	2/21	2/21	1:20–1:640
Cattle		0/0	7/55	7/55	1:10–1:40
Foot-and-mouth disease virus[l]	VIAA[n]				
Cattle[o]		0/0	40/55	40/55	not applicable

TABLE 2. Results of serology tests for nonequine diseases[a,b] among ungulates found near Ol Jogi Ranch, Kenya (*continued*)

Disease agent	Test used (positive titer)	IN[c]	OUT[d]	TOT[e]	Range[f]
Infectious bovine rhinotracheitis virus[p]	SN ($\geq$1:8)[k]				
Cattle		0/0	18/55	18/55	1:8–1:384
Buffalo		1/1	4/7	6/10	1:8–1:32
Grant's gazelle		0/5	1/3	1/8	1:8
Rinderpest virus[l]	TCVN ($\geq$ 1:12)[q]				
Cattle[o]		0/0	46/55	46/55	1:12–$\geq$1:110

[a]Camels, cattle, buffaloes, Grant's gazelles, impalas, and reticulated giraffes were negative for bovine leukosis virus (BLV) by ELISA at $\geq$1:8, for malignant catarrhal fever virus by immunoperoxidase at $\geq$1:20, and for trypanosomosis by immunofluorescent antibody at $\geq$1:150.

[b]There was no significant difference in seroprevalence inside vs. outside the fence for any agent in any species.

[c]IN = inside fence.

[d]OUT = outside fence.

[e]TOT = total.

[f]Range = range of positive titers.

[g]Camels, cattle, Grant's gazelles, impalas, and reticulated giraffes were negative for *Anaplasma* spp.

[h]CF = complement fixation test.

[i]ELISA = enzyme-linked immunosorbent assay.

[j]Camels were not tested for BLV, bovine parainfluenza-3 virus, or bovine respiratory syncytial virus.

[k]SN = serum virus neutralization test.

[l]Camels, buffaloes, Grant's gazelles, impalas, and reticulated giraffes were negative for bovine virus diarrhea virus, foot-and-mouth disease virus, and rinderpest virus.

[m]Buffaloes, Grant's gazelles, impalas, and reticulated giraffes were negative for *Brucella abortus*.

[n]VIAA = virus infection associated antigen test.

[o]Cattle were vaccinated.

[p]Camels, impalas, and reticulated giraffes were negative for infectious bovine rhinotracheitis virus.

[q]TCVN = tissue culture virus neutralization.

Nonequine Disease Agents

Cattle at Ol Jogi are regularly diagnosed with anaplasmosis by blood smear evaluation and concurrent clinical signs, but seropositive cattle were not observed in this study. Our data concur with other studies suggesting BTV is endemic in wildlife and domestic livestock in Laikipia.[13] African wildlife have not been tested for BLV to date.[14] Antibodies to PIV have not been reported previously in giraffe and Grant's gazelle. The low titer in the giraffe in this study may be due to exposure to a closely related virus or to the presence of antiviral factors in the serum. Strong titers and high prevalence of antibodies to PIV in all other species suggest the positive titer in the giraffe is genuine. Serologic testing for BRSV in African wildlife and camels has not been reported. The low titers found could be the result of antigenically related viruses or the presence of antiviral factors in the sera. Brucellosis (with associated abortions and seropositivity) has been reported in cattle near our study site,[15] and transmission from cattle to wildlife has been suggested.[16] The absence of titers to IBRV in giraffes and camels in our study suggests opportunity for interspecific transmission, as in Tanzania.[17] The absence of titers to FMDV and RPV in several cattle in this study suggests a lack of vaccination coverage. Transport of FMDV, MCFV, or RPV to our study site could occur from wildlife or livestock owned by pastoralists, whose vaccination practices are unknown. *Trypanosoma congolense* and *T. brucei* are probably not present at our study site because no animals were positive, and insect traps in riverine bush areas at our study site have not recovered the tsetse fly (*Glossina* spp.) vector (DeMaar, unpublished data).

REFERENCES

1. PALING, R.W., D.M. JESSETT & B.R. HEATH. 1979. The occurrence of infectious diseases in mixed farming of domesticated wild herbivores and domestic herbivores, including camels, in Kenya. I. Viral diseases: a serologic survey with special reference to foot-and-mouth disease. J. Wildl. Dis. **15:** 351–358.

2. BARNARD, B.J.H. & J.T. PAWESKA. 1993. Prevalence of antibodies against some equine viruses in zebra (*Zebra burchelli*) in the Kruger National Park (1991–1992). Onderstepoort J. Vet. Res. **60:** 175–179.

3. STANLEY-PRICE, M.R. 1991. A review of mammal re-introductions, and the role of the Re-introduction Specialist Group of IUCN/SSC. *In* Beyond Captive Breeding: Symposium of the Zoological Society of London. Volume 62: 9–25. Oxford Sci. Pub. New York/London.

4. LYLE, A.M. & A.P. DOBSON. 1993. Infectious disease and intensive management: population dynamics, threatened hosts, and their parasites. J. Zoo Wildl. Med. **24:** 315–326.

5. PLOWRIGHT, W. & B. MCCULLOCH. 1967. Investigations on the incidence of rinderpest virus infection in game animals of N. Tanganyika and S. Kenya, 1960/63. J. Hyg. **65:** 343–358.

6. NYAGA, P.N. *et al.* 1981. Prevalence of antibodies to parainfluenza-3 virus in various wildlife species and indigenous cattle sharing the same habitats in Kenya. J. Wildl. Dis. **17:** 605–608.

7. ALEXANDER, K.A. *et al.* 1994. Serologic survey of selected canine pathogens among free-ranging jackals in Kenya. J. Wildl. Dis. **30:** 486–491.

8. PRINS, H.H.T. & F.J. WEYERHAEUSER. 1987. Epidemics in populations of wild ruminants: anthrax and impala, rinderpest, and buffalo in Lake Manyara National Park, Tanzania. Oikos **49:** 28–38.

9. ANDERSON, R.M. 1981. Population ecology of infectious disease agents. *In* Theoretical Ecology, Principles, and Applications, 2nd edit., pp. 318–355. Blackwell. Oxford.

10. BARNARD, B.J.H. 1998. Epidemiology of African horse sickness and the role of the zebra in South Africa. *In* African Horse Sickness, pp. 12–19. Springer-Verlag. New York/Berlin.

11. MONTALI, R.J. *et al.* 1985. Equine herpesvirus type 1 abortion in an onager and suspected herpesvirus myelitis in a zebra. J. Am. Vet. Med. Assoc. **187:** 1248–1249.

12. MCCOLLUM, W.H. & P.J. TIMONEY. 1991. Studies on the seroprevalence and frequency of equine rhinovirus-1 and -2 infection in normal horse urine. *In* Equine Infectious Diseases VI: Proceeding of the Sixth International Conference, pp. 83–87. R&W Pub. Newmarket, UK.

13. DAVIES, F.G. & A.R. WALKER. 1974. The distribution in Kenya of bluetongue virus and antibody, and the *Culicoides* vector. J. Hyg. **72:** 265–272.

14. SCHOEPF, K.C. *et al.* 1997. Serological evidence of the occurrence of enzootic bovine leukosis (EBL) virus infection in cattle in Tanzania. Trop. Anim. Health Prod. **29:** 15–19.

15. KADOHIRA, M. *et al.* 1997. Variations in the prevalence of antibody to brucella infection in cattle by farm, area, and district in Kenya. Epidemiol. Infect. **118:** 35–41.
16. WAGHELA, S. & L. KARSTAD. 1986. Antibodies to *Brucella* spp. among blue wildebeest and African buffalo in Kenya. J. Wildl. Dis. **22:** 189–192.
17. RWEYEMAMU, M.M. 1974. The incidence of infectious bovine rhinotracheitis antibody in Tanzanian game animals and cattle. Bull. Epizoot. Dis. Afr. **22:** 19–22.

Avian Cholera on North Coast California

Distinctive Epizootiological Features

RICHARD G. BOTZLER

Department of Wildlife, Humboldt State University, Arcata, California 95521-8299, USA

ABSTRACT: Between 1945 and 2001, avian cholera (*Pasteurella multocida* infection) was confirmed at 27 epizootics in 18 different years on northcoastal California. Estimated mortality ranged from 1 to 6750 birds per site, with a median total mortality of about 1000 birds per year. Eight epizootics involved <150 birds; thus, minor epizootics were common. Annual total wildfowl mortality ranged from 0.4% to 7.0% of estimated live populations; median annual mortality for American coots (*Fulica americana*) (11.5%) surpassed that of tundra swans (*Cygnus columbianus*) (0.2%) and ducks (0.2%). Coots comprised >50% of total wildfowl mortality in 16 of 17 epizootics. Overall, coots comprised 82% of known avian cholera mortality, but only 34% of the live wildfowl present; ducks and swans died much less frequently. Wildfowl at one site consistently died in a sequential pattern; there was no sequential mortality at other sites.

KEYWORDS: avian cholera; epizootiology; California north coast; *Pasteurella multocida*; wildfowl

INTRODUCTION

Avian (fowl) cholera (*Pasteurella multocida* infection) is a serious disease of wildfowl in North America, including American coots (*Fulica americana*), tundra swans (*Cygnus columbianus*), ducks, geese, and other associated aquatic species.[1] First reported in the 1943–44 winter in both Texas[2] and northern California,[3] it was observed on the north coast of California (Humboldt and Del Norte Counties) the following year[4] and has since spread to all major waterfowl flyways of North America.[5] Because of an extended avian cholera history, relatively isolated setting, and consistent habitat and land use, the north coast of California has provided a unique opportunity to evaluate the epizootiology of this disease.

My objectives were to (a) summarize the history of avian cholera on California's north coast, (b) assess the impact of avian cholera on north coast wildfowl, (c) assess the evidence for differential host susceptibility, and (d) assess any sequence in species mortality at each site.

Address for correspondence: Dr. Richard G. Botzler, Department of Wildlife, Humboldt State University, Arcata, CA 95521-8299. Voice: 707-826-3724; fax: 707-826-4060.
rgb2@humboldt.edu

Ann. N.Y. Acad. Sci. 969: 224–228 (2002). © 2002 New York Academy of Sciences.

STUDY AREAS

Humboldt and Del Norte Counties are the two northernmost coastal counties in California. Avian cholera has occurred regularly on four sites of this region. Centerville (40°30′ N, 124°20′ W) is a 100-ha private pastureland used for cattle grazing on the Eel River Delta; two ponds on the site, 3.9 and 5.5 ha, respectively, are leased out to a private club each year for waterfowl hunting.[6] Humboldt Bay National Wildlife Refuge (40°40′ N, 124°15′ W) on South Humboldt Bay was established in 1971 and comprises 900 ha of pastureland and bay-shore wildlife habitat. North Humboldt Bay (40°52′ N, 124°05′ W) includes about 1000 ha of private and state-owned pasturelands and wetlands, as well as the City of Arcata Oxidation Ponds.[7] Lake Earl Wildlife Area (41°48′ N, 124°10′ W) includes 2000 ha of grasslands, wetlands, and dunes administered by the California Department of Fish and Game since 1977 for waterfowl management.

METHODS

Data on estimated avian cholera mortality at epizootic sites came from California Department of Fish and Game files. Since 1972, systematic daily mortality surveys to obtain complete carcass counts were conducted when possible at affected sites by trained students in conjunction with state and federal personnel. Site-specific live counts of each wildfowl species were based on annual United States Fish and Wildlife Service (USFWS) surveys of Humboldt and Del Norte Counties conducted in early January.

Avian cholera impact on wildfowl was estimated by comparing complete carcass counts for all species to the respective estimated live counts. This was done for all wildfowl collectively, as well as for the respective individual species.

Coots previously were reported at Centerville as comprising a far greater proportion of the dead birds observed than that of the respective live populations.[6,8] To determine whether such host selection was consistent here and at other sites, records were assessed for 12 epizootics involving ≥100 birds, which also had thorough carcass counts, and for which live bird estimates were available. Host selection for a species was considered to occur if that species' percent composition in the carcass collection of an epizootic was at least 5 percentage points higher than in its respective live population (e.g., if a species comprised an estimated 20% of the live population, it needed to comprise ≥25% of the recorded mortality to be considered as experiencing host selection).

A consistent sequence in species mortality was reported at Centerville in 1977 and 1978, with coots, swans, and wigeon dying early in these epizootics and with pintail and shovelers dying later.[6,8] The consistency of this sequence at Centerville and at the other sites was evaluated by ranking the mean day of death for each species in an epizootic; Friedman's test[9] was used to determine whether the species rankings were consistent between years for each site. An alpha equal to 0.05 was used to determine statistical significance for statistical tests.

RESULTS AND DISCUSSION

Avian Cholera History

Between 1945 and 2001, there were 27 confirmed occurrences of avian cholera in 18 different years and 4 unconfirmed, but probable, epizootics of avian cholera in 3 additional years. Three confirmed occurrences involved single mortality events for which no subsequent mortality was known to occur at these respective sites. These birds likely flew in from nearby epizootics.

The observed mortality patterns had a northerly shift during this period. Between 1945 and 1979, all known epizootics of avian cholera were reported first or only at Centerville; however, no mortality has been reported at this site since 1979. Between 1971 and 1991, mortality was observed irregularly on South Humboldt Bay, but with no reports since 1991. In contrast, mortality has been recorded on North Humboldt Bay and Lake Earl starting in 1976 and has occurred only at these sites since that time. One other site, Freshwater Lagoon (41°16′ N, 124°05′ W), 29 km north of North Humboldt Bay, had one known epizootic: 2800 birds died in 1994; it was the only known site affected that year.

Total swan mortality declined during this northerly shift. Based on Spearman's rank correlation test,[9] there was a significant ($P < 0.01$) decline in annual swan mortality from 1972 to 2001. In contrast, there was no significant change in the corresponding estimated live counts based on USFWS mid-winter live population surveys.

Impact of Avian Cholera

From 1945 to 2001, estimated avian cholera mortality ranged from 1 to 6750 birds per confirmed occurrence,[8] with a median of about 500 birds dying per site per year. The median total mortality was about 1000 total birds for all sites in avian cholera years. Eight of the 27 confirmed occurrences involved ≤150 birds and there were 3 cases of single bird mortality in which no further mortality was observed at the respective sites. Thus, minor mortality events appeared to be relatively common on the north coast.

There were 11 avian cholera years in which both thorough carcass counts were made and live counts were available. In these years, total coot, duck, and swan losses ranged from 0.4% to 7.0% (median: 2.1%) of the total estimated live population of these groups, collectively. Coot losses alone ranged from 4.6% to 30.2% (median: 11.5%), duck losses ranged from <0.1% to 2.1% (0.2%), and swan losses ranged from 0% to 20.6% (0.2%) of their respective live populations. Because of the difficulty in finding all carcasses during an epizootic, these are probably minimum mortality estimates.

Site-specific avian cholera impact also was assessed. For four epizootics at Centerville, total mortality ranged from 14% to 57% (median: 37%) of the respective total wildfowl population estimates. In contrast, with 6 epizootics at Lake Earl, total carcass counts ranged from 1% to 98% (median: 6%) of estimated live counts. For one epizootic at North Bay and two epizootics at South Bay, collectively, total carcass counts ranged from only 1% to 2% of the total wildfowl counts.

TABLE 1. Species comparison of mortality in dead population to estimated live population, California north coast, 1972 to 2001

Species	Percent mortality (%)[a]		Percent live population (%)[b]		Host selection[c]
	Median	Range	Median	Range	
American coot (*Fulica americana*)	82	4–97	34	11–65	11/12
Ruddy duck (*Oxyura jamaicensis*)	<1	0–62	3.5	<1–34	1/12
Shoveler (*Anas clypeata*)	1.2	0–17	2.2	<1–30	1/10
American wigeon (*Anas americana*)	<1	0–24	10	<1–33	0/12
Tundra swan (*Cygnus columbianus*)	1.1	0–10	3.5	<1–11	0/10
Northern pintail (*Anas acuta*)	1.5	0–5	9	<1–41	0/10
Other duck species	<1	0–7	1.9	<1–33	0/10

[a]Percent of collected carcasses comprising this species (n = 12 epizootics).
[b]Percent that this species comprises in estimated live count (n = 12 epizootics).
[c]Number of cases where percent of dead count is at least 5 percentage points greater than live count/number of epizootics where this species was present.

Host Selection

Coots were the most common species affected by avian cholera on the north coast. For 17 confirmed epizootics with thorough carcass composition counts, coots comprised >50% of total mortality in 16 cases and >70% of known mortality in 13 cases.

Coots consistently comprised a greater proportion of dead birds collected than of the live populations; all other species comprised smaller proportions of their dead populations than respective live populations (TABLE 1). Coots also had evidence for host selection in 11 of 12 epizootics, whereas other species rarely did (TABLE 1).

Sequential Mortality

The mean day of death was ranked for each species in 10 epizootics for which daily carcass totals were available: four epizootics at Centerville, four at Lake Earl, and two at South Bay. Using Friedman's test[9] on these rankings, the sequence of coots, swans, wigeon, pintail, and shovelers was consistent ($P < 0.05$) between all 4 years at Centerville. In contrast, there were no consistent ($P > 0.10$) mortality sequences between years for Lake Earl or for South Bay.

Summary

Avian cholera occurs at only a limited number of sites on California's north coast. Yet, despite the apparent similarity of habitats, climate, and land use, the history and epizootiology of avian cholera have been distinctive at each site.

ACKNOWLEDGMENTS

I greatly appreciate the assistance of countless Humboldt State University students, as well as J. G. Mensik, M. Kuehner, K. Kovacs, D. Yparraguirre, and C. Feldheim, in the fieldwork and preparation of this manuscript.

REFERENCES

1. BOTZLER, R.G. 1991. Epizootiology of avian cholera in wildfowl. J. Wildl. Dis. **27:** 367–395.
2. QUORTRUP, E.R., F.B. QUEEN & L.J. MEROVKA. 1946. An outbreak of pasteurellosis in wild ducks. J. Am. Vet. Med. Assoc. **108:** 94–100.
3. ROSEN, M.N. & A.I. BISCHOFF. 1949. The 1948–49 outbreak of fowl cholera in birds in the San Francisco Bay area and surrounding counties. Calif. Fish Game **35:** 185–192.
4. TITCHE, A. 1979. Avian cholera in California. Wildl. Mgmt. Branch Admin. Rep. 79-2. Calif. Dept. Fish and Game, Sacramento, CA.
5. FRIEND, M. 1999. Avian cholera. *In* Field Manual of Wildlife Diseases. Biol. Res. Div. Inform. Tech. Rep. 1999-001, pp. 75–92.
6. MENSIK, J.G. & R.G. BOTZLER. 1989. Epizootiological features of avian cholera at Centerville, Humboldt County, California. J. Wildl. Dis. **25:** 240–245.
7. HAZLEWOOD, R.M., A.F. ODDO, R.D. PAGAN & R.G. BOTZLER. 1978. The 1975–76 avian cholera outbreaks in Humboldt County, California. J. Wildl. Dis. **14:** 229–232.
8. ODDO, A.F., R.D. PAGAN, L. WORDEN & R.G. BOTZLER. 1978. The January 1977 avian cholera epornitic in northwest California. J. Wildl. Dis. **14:** 317–321.
9. LANGLEY, R. 1970. Practical Statistics. Dover. New York.

The Hook Lake Wood Bison Recovery Project

Can a Disease-Free Captive Wood Bison Herd Be Recovered from a Wild Population Infected with Bovine Tuberculosis and Brucellosis?

J. S. NISHI,[a] B. T. ELKIN,[b] AND T. R. ELLSWORTH[a]

[a]Resources, Wildlife, and Economic Development (RWED), Government of the Northwest Territories (GNWT), Fort Smith, Northwest Territories X0E 0P0, Canada

[b]Resources, Wildlife, and Economic Development (RWED), Government of the Northwest Territories (GNWT), Yellowknife, Northwest Territories X1A 3S8, Canada

ABSTRACT: The Hook Lake Wood Bison Recovery Project (HLWBRP) is a wildlife conservation project aimed at recovering a captive, disease-free herd of wood bison (*Bison bison athabascae*) from a wild herd infected with bovine tuberculosis (*Mycobacterium bovis*) and brucellosis (*Brucella abortus*). The disease eradication protocol that we have used involves a combination of techniques, including (1) orphaning of newborn wild-caught calves to minimize exposure to *B. abortus* and *M. bovis*, (2) testing calves for maternal antibodies to brucellosis in the field prior to inclusion in the project, (3) isolating calves in pairs to prevent potential spread of disease, (4) prophylactic treatment using antimycobacterial and anti-*Brucella* drugs, and (5) an intensive whole-herd testing program for both diseases and removal of reactors. From 1996 to 1998, we captured a total of 62 calves; presently, 58 individuals comprise the founder herd. The captive-born cohorts consist of 7 two-year-olds, 21 yearlings, and 22 calves. To date, there have been no cases of bovine tuberculosis or brucellosis in the captive herd.

KEYWORDS: wood bison; wildlife conservation; disease eradication; bovine tuberculosis; bovine brucellosis; *Bison bison athabascae*; *Mycobacterium bovis*; *Brucella abortus*

INTRODUCTION

An overabundance of plains bison (*Bison bison bison*) in National Buffalo Park (NBP) at Wainwright, Alberta, resulted in the Canadian government's decision to ship 6673 bison from NBP to the newly created Wood Buffalo National Park (WBNP) between 1925 and 1928.[1] In addition to being a separate subspecies, the plains bison also introduced two exotic cattle diseases, bovine tuberculosis (*Mycobacterium bovis*) and brucellosis (*Brucella abortus*). Tuberculosis was first recognized in a single

Address for correspondence: J.S. Nishi, Resources, Wildlife, and Economic Development, Government of the Northwest Territories, P.O. Box 390, Fort Smith, Northwest Territories X0E 0P0, Canada. Voice: 867-872-6446; fax: 867-872-4628.
John_Nishi@gov.nt.ca

Ann. N.Y. Acad. Sci. 969: 229–235 (2002). © 2002 New York Academy of Sciences.

WBNP bison in 1937 and brucellosis was first noted in 1956.[1] Both diseases have maintained enzootic proportions in WBNP bison.[2]

Concern over the diseases and their implications to the health status of the Canadian cattle herd led to a federally appointed Northern Diseased Bison Environmental Assessment Process from 1988 to 1990, which culminated in a recommendation to eradicate all existing free-ranging diseased bison in and around WBNP and to replace those herds with healthy wood bison (*Bison bison athabascae*).[1] This proposed action was met with conflicting mandates and perceptions, and opposing fundamental values of the interest groups involved, with strong public opposition mostly from First Nations' communities and environmental organizations. Two major concerns expressed during this process were the possible impairment of ecosystem integrity and the loss of genetic diversity represented by infected herds.

One of the herds that was considered in the environmental assessment process was the Hook Lake herd, a wood bison population infected with bovine brucellosis and tuberculosis located northeast of WBNP and east of the Slave River. In 1971, there were approximately 1700 bison in the herd, but the population declined through the 1970s and, since 1980, the population has persisted at low density and fluctuated between 200 and 500 animals[3] (RWED, unpublished data). Key factors that have been implicated for the decline and continuous low density of bison in the Hook Lake area are brucellosis and tuberculosis, wolf predation, habitat succession, and hunting.[3]

In 1996, the Deninu Kue' First Nation, the Fort Resolution Aboriginal Wildlife Harvesters' Committee (AWHC), and the Government of the Northwest Territories implemented a pilot project—the Hook Lake Wood Bison Recovery Project (HLWBRP)—to determine the feasibility of genetic salvage of diseased bison.[4,5] Specific objectives were (1) to conserve genetic integrity of the wild herd by capturing an adequate number of bison calves, (2) to provide veterinary care and preventative drug treatment to eliminate tuberculosis and brucellosis from the captive calves, and (3) to raise a disease-free herd of captive wood bison from the salvaged calves.

METHODS

Capture, Care, and Prophylaxis of Wild-Caught Calves

We captured HL wood bison calves (estimated age from 1 to 10 days old) in May of 3 consecutive years (1996, 1997, and 1998) by netting them from a helicopter.[4,5] In May 1996, we captured 20 calves and brought them back to an isolation facility at Fort Resolution, Northwest Territories. During the subsequent two capture sessions in 1997 and 1998, we used the Brewer's Card Test (BCT) to test calves in the field for antibodies to *B. abortus*. All BCT-positive reactors were returned to their site of capture and released within ca. 30 minutes of capture, whereas test-negative calves (20 in 1997 and 22 in 1998) were transported to the isolation facility for prophylaxis and hand-rearing.

We housed each cohort of calves as isolated pairs in 1.3-m × 2.5-m wooden sheds during their first 2 weeks of captivity. During this period, calves were habituated to people, trained to feed from a bottle, and treated with antibiotics via intramuscular injection (see TABLE 1). After the initial 2-week period, we released calves as isolated pairs into larger 13-m × 23-m isolation paddocks. These paddocks were double-fenced to prevent direct contact between adjacent calf pairs. The double fences were also lined by plastic tarps (in 1999, tarps were replaced by plywood) to act as a solid visual barrier and to reduce direct airflow between adjacent paddocks. Additional disease-control measures put in place included the use of protective clothing by handlers, disinfectant boot baths, and restrictions on movement into and between isolation pens.

During the first 4 to 5 months of captivity, we followed a feeding regimen of colostrum replacer[6] for 2 days, then a combination of colostrum and milk replacer (powdered milk composition of 24% protein and 22% fat by weight) for 2 weeks, and finally a milk replacer alone that served as the medium for administering oral antibiotics. Antibiotic protocol and prescribed dosages[4] and duration of treatment are summarized in TABLE 1. We also offered calves a high-quality alfalfa-timothy hay and, after ca. 4 weeks of age, a medication-free 18% protein calf starter *ad libitum* throughout the isolation period. When calves were about 5 months of age, we replaced the calf starter with rolled barley at a rate of ca. 1 kg/calf/day.

Disease-Testing Protocol

Our disease-testing regime comprises a whole-herd test conducted twice annually in the months of February and November. To test for exposure to bovine tuberculosis, we employ the intradermal caudal fold test using *M. bovis* PPD (tuberculin).[7] In the event of positive or suspicious reactors, the comparative cervical test is used to discriminate between reactors to *M. bovis* versus *M. avium*. We have also used the Fluorescence Polarization Assay (FPA)[8] as an ancillary serological test[2] for tuberculosis in the two most recent whole-herd tests. For bovine brucellosis, Agriculture and Agri-Food Canada's Animal Disease Research Institute (ADRI) in Lethbridge, Alberta, conducts the following assays on blood serum: Buffered Plate Antigen Test (BPAT),[9] Standard Tube Agglutination Test (STAT),[10] Compliment Fixation Test (CFT),[10] Competitive Enzyme-Linked Immunosorbent Assay (C-ELISA),[11] and FPA.[12] All whole-herd tests are conducted with a veterinarian accredited by the Canadian Food Inspection Agency (CFIA), and all FPA tests are conducted at ADRI, Nepean, Ontario.

Another important part of the disease-testing protocol is detection of latent infections of *B. abortus*.[13] Our approach for detecting latent infection has been to test for seroconversion and bacterial shedding following first calving of all wild-caught dams. To reduce potential risks of disease exposure from latently infected females, we place each pregnant cow into an isolation pen following a negative brucellosis test conducted early in the third trimester. We closely monitor these cows until parturition or abortion resolves the pregnancy. Placentas (and fetuses in the event of abortion) are collected immediately after calving and are submitted for brucellosis culture at the United States Department of Agriculture's National Veterinary Services Laboratory in Ames, Iowa. Serum is collected from each cow/calf pair at 3 days, 30 days, and 6 months postcalving to look for evidence of seroconversion of latent infections.

TABLE 1. Capture dates and durations for bottle-raising and antibiotic treatment of wild-caught wood bison calves potentially exposed to bovine brucellosis and tuberculosis (Hook Lake Wood Bison Recovery Project, Fort Resolution, NT, 1996–98)

Capture year (median date)	1996 (12 May)	1997 (11 May)	1998 (5 May)
Capture period	5 days	3 days	2 days
Colostrum replacer	13 days	12 days	8 days
Milk replacer	5.3 months	5.5 months	4.1 months
Dihydrostreptomycin (25 mg/kg IM[a], EOD[b])	11 days	14 days	15 days
Oxytetracycline[c] (25 mg/kg IM, EOD)	11 days	14 days	7 days
Enrofloxacin (10 mg/kg PO[d], daily)	1.3 months	1.5 months	3.2 months
Isoniazid (10 mg/kg PO, daily)	4.9 months	5.3 months	3.7 months
Rifampin[e] (10 mg/kg PO, daily)	—	1.5 months	2.8 months

[a]IM: intramuscular injection.
[b]EOD: every other day.
[c]In 1998, oxytetracycline was administered *per os* every day for 7 days.
[d]PO: *per os*, oral administration with milk.
[e]Administered in 1997 and 1998, but not in 1996.

RESULTS

Throughout the course of preventative treatment with antibiotics, we maintained all calves in pairs under strict isolation during their first 10 months. Our criterion for release of calf pairs into a larger cohort herd was that each individual calf should test negative on two successive disease tests conducted at least 60 days apart. We conducted the first whole-herd test on the 1996 calf cohort in November 1996; all tests conducted were negative. However, during the second whole-herd test of that cohort, in February 1997, 1 female calf reacted to the caudal fold test for tuberculosis and, as a precautionary measure, the calf and its pen mate were slaughtered in March 1997 (TABLE 2). A subsequent postmortem on both calves found no gross visible lesions suggestive of infectious diseases. Histopathological observations determined that acid fast bacteria were present in a single minute granulomatous lesion in a mediastinal lymph node of the reactor calf, but laboratory culture by CFIA did not isolate any mycobacterial species.[4] In April 1997 during a follow-up disease test, 1 male produced a suspicious reaction on the Brewer's card test and STAT (3-3-1) for brucellosis, but tested negative on both the BPAT and CFT.[4] That calf and its pen mate were kept in isolation and retested on 25 June 1997 with negative results on all 4 tests. The remaining 16 bison remained test-negative and were released to a common pasture in April 1997. In subsequent years, we completed the disease-testing process for the 1997 and 1998 cohorts with all bison cohorts testing negative. Presently, the 1996, 1997, and 1998 wild-caught cohorts have undergone 11, 8, and 6 whole-herd tests respectively. Aside from the 2 cases described above, there have been no subsequent serological reactors to brucellosis and no reactors to the caudal fold test nor the recently employed FPA test for tuberculosis.

TABLE 2. Current number of bison, Hook Lake Wood Bison Recovery Project, Fort Resolution, NT, July 2001 (numbers in parentheses represent mortalities)

Cohort	Male	Female
Wild-caught		
1996	5 (1)	13 (1)[a]
1997	4 (0)	16 (0)
1998	6 (0)	14 (2)[b]
Captive-born		
1999[c]	3 (0)	4 (2)
2000[d]	10 (2)	11 (2)
2001[e]	11 (2)	11 (2)
Total	39 (1)	69 (3)

[a]Female bison reacted on caudal fold test. She and male pen mate were killed on 5 March 1997 for postmortem examination (see text).

[b]Female calf euthanized on 15 August 1998 due to severe ataxia after 3.5 months of unsuccessful treatment (culture-negative for tuberculosis and brucellosis). Female short yearling died on 12 April 1999 from accidental neck injury.

[c]The 1999 cohort mortalities: nutritional myopathy, unknown.

[d]The 2000 cohort mortalities: late-term abortion (nondisease-related), stillborn (hypoxia resulting from dystocia), trauma (kicked in head), unknown.

[e]The 2001 cohort mortalities: trauma (exposure), shock, suspected nutritional myopathy (2 calves).

At the time of writing, 40 of 43 wild-caught cows have calved and been tested at 3 days and 4 weeks postcalving. Of those 40 cow/calf pairs, there have been no reactors for brucellosis. We also collected 15 placentas from 29 cows in the 1996 and 1997 cohorts, and all placental tissues were culture-negative for *B. abortus*.

With the final capture of 22 wild bison calves in May 1998 and 4 mortalities since the beginning of the project, the captive herd now consists of 58 founders in 3 separate cohorts (TABLE 2). The captive-born cohorts comprise another 50 bison, including 7 two-year-olds (1999 cohort), 21 yearlings (2000 cohort), and 22 calves (2001 cohort) (TABLE 2).

DISCUSSION

Despite rigorous disease testing, there have been no confirmed cases of either bovine tuberculosis or bovine brucellosis in the HLWBRP. This strongly suggests that the diseases are not present in this captive bison herd. However, we realize that sole reliance on an absence of caudal fold or serological reactors to conclude that tuberculosis and brucellosis are absent from the captive Hook Lake herd may be too simplistic and emphasizes an unrealistic assumption that the disease tests employed have perfect sensitivity and specificity. Additional issues such as incomplete validation of diagnostic tests for bison, dependence among diagnostic tests, efficacy of prophylaxis, and uncertainty in the epidemiological characteristics and frequency of latent infections in bison need to be considered. To account for these uncertainties, determination of health status of the captive Hook Lake bison herd will require a science-based risk-assessment approach.[14] The task of defining and recognizing this herd as disease-free remains a critical step that must be resolved before further plans can be made to use captive-born progeny in a reintroduction program within the Northwest Territories or elsewhere in Canada.

ACKNOWLEDGMENTS

A long-term project of this scope requires commitment and collaboration of many individuals, too numerous to name individually. Nevertheless, we are particularly grateful to program staff, K. Delorme and S. Cuthbert, and the many volunteers whose hard work has been critical to the program success thus far. We also recognize D. Balsillie, D. Beaulieu, R. Boucher, C. Gates, and T. Unka for the early vision and inception of this program. We thank the Deninu Kue' First Nation, the Aboriginal Wildlife Harvesters' Committee, and the community of Fort Resolution for their ongoing support. ADRI Lethbridge and ADRI Nepean have provided in-kind support by conducting all diagnostic serology. The Government of the Northwest Territories (RWED) has provided base funding.

REFERENCES

1. CONNELLY, R.G. et al. 1990. Northern diseased bison: report of the Environmental Assessment Panel. Minister of Supply and Services Canada, Ottawa, Ontario.
2. JOLY, D.O. & F. MESSIER. 2001. Limiting effects of bovine brucellosis and tuberculosis on wood bison within Wood Buffalo National Park. University of Saskatchewan, Saskatoon, Saskatchewan.
3. REYNOLDS, H.W. & A.W.L. HAWLEY. 1987. Bison ecology in relation to agricultural development in the Slave River Lowlands, NWT. Canadian Wildlife Service Occasional Paper 63. Ottawa, Ontario.
4. GATES, C.C., B.T. ELKIN & D.C. BEAULIEU. 1998. Initial results of an attempt to eradicate bovine tuberculosis and brucellosis from a wood bison herd in northern Canada. In International Symposium on Bison Ecology and Management in North America, pp. 221–228. Montana State University, Bozeman, Montana.
5. NISHI, J.S. et al. 2001. An overview of the Hook Lake Wood Bison Recovery Project: where have we come from, where are we now, and where we would like to go? In Proceedings of the Second International Bison Conference, pp. 215–233. Bison Center of Excellence, Edmonton, Alberta.
6. CHELACK, B.J., P.S. MORLEY & D.M. HAINES. 1993. Evaluation of methods for dehydration of bovine colostrum for total replacement of normal colostrum in calves. Can. Vet. J. 34: 407–412.
7. MONOGHAN, M.L. et al. 1994. The tuberculin test. Vet. Microbiol. 40: 111–124.
8. LIN, M. et al. 1996. Modification of the Mycobacterium bovis extracellular protein MPB70 with fluorescin for rapid detection of specific serum antibodies by fluorescence polarization. Clin. Diagn. Lab. Immun. 3: 438–443.
9. NIELSEN, K.H. et al. 1996. Comparison of enzyme immunoassays for the diagnosis of bovine brucellosis. Prev. Vet. Med. 26: 17–32.
10. STEMSHORN, B.W. et al. 1985. A comparison of standard serological tests for the diagnosis of bovine brucellosis in Canada. Can. J. Comp. Med. 49: 391–394.
11. GALL, D. & K. NIELSEN. 1994. Improvements to the competitive ELISA for detection of antibodies to Brucella abortus in cattle sera. J. Immunol. 15: 277–291.

12. GALL, D. *et al.* 2000. Validation of the fluorescence polarization assay and comparison to other serological assays for the detection of serum antibodies to *Brucella abortus* in bison. J. Wildl. Dis. **36:** 469–476.
13. SUTHERLAND, S.S. & J. SEARSON. 1990. The immune response to *Brucella abortus*: the humoral response. *In* Animal Brucellosis, pp. 65–81. CRC Press. Boca Raton, Florida.
14. NISHI, J.S., C. STEPHEN & B.T. ELKIN. 2002. Implications of agricultural and wildlife policy on management and eradication of bovine tuberculosis and brucellosis in free-ranging wood bison of northern Canada. This volume.

Implications of Agricultural and Wildlife Policy on Management and Eradication of Bovine Tuberculosis and Brucellosis in Free-Ranging Wood Bison of Northern Canada

J. S. NISHI,[a] C. STEPHEN,[b] AND B. T. ELKIN[c]

[a]Resources, Wildlife, and Economic Development (RWED), Government of the Northwest Territories (GNWT), Fort Smith, Northwest Territories X0E 0P0, Canada

[b]Center for Coastal Health, Nanaimo, British Columbia V9R 5S5, Canada

[c]Resources, Wildlife, and Economic Development (RWED), Government of the Northwest Territories (GNWT), Yellowknife, Northwest Territories X1A 3S8, Canada

ABSTRACT: Although disease is often an important factor in the population dynamics of wild ungulates, it is largely the threat—both real and perceived—that sylvatic disease reservoirs pose to the health status of commercial livestock or game farm industry that has led governments to establish policy and legislation for disease management, trade, and movement. With respect to bovine tuberculosis and brucellosis in wildlife, policies are largely borrowed from the existing regulatory framework for domestic livestock. In this paper, we review how general policy goals for managing these reportable diseases in domestic livestock have also affected conservation and management of bison in Canada. We argue that there is a need to better integrate conservation biology with agricultural livestock policy to develop management options and better address the unique conservation challenges that diseased free-ranging bison populations present.

KEYWORDS: bison; *Bison bison*; conservation; agricultural policy; disease eradication; herd health status; bovine tuberculosis; *Mycobacterium bovis*; bovine brucellosis; *Brucella abortus*

INTRODUCTION

Zoonotic diseases that exist within a host-parasite continuum between wildlife, domestic animal, and human populations represent important threats to conservation of biological diversity, economic sustainability of livestock industries, and human health.[1] In fact, implications for production and trade, and the zoonotic potential of infectious diseases, have been an important force behind a common approach to dis-

Address for correspondence: J.S. Nishi, Resources, Wildlife, and Economic Development, Government of the Northwest Territories, P.O. Box 390, Fort Smith, Northwest Territories X0E 0P0, Canada. Voice: 867-872-6446; fax: 867-872-4628.

John_Nishi@gov.nt.ca

Ann. N.Y. Acad. Sci. 969: 236–244 (2002). © 2002 New York Academy of Sciences.

ease eradication used by government agencies charged with the regulation of trade and husbandry practices of domestic livestock.

In general, the "agriculturalist" approach involves classifying diseases according to several criteria including zoonotic risk. Combined with specific knowledge on the diseases' epidemiology in livestock, regulations are applied that work towards minimizing prevalence and/or eradicating the pathogens. In most cases, livestock diseases that pose threats to international trade or have serious socioeconomic and human health consequences are defined as "reportable". A person diagnosing or suspecting a "reportable disease" in a farm animal is required by law to notify government authorities within a specific time frame so that disease-control measures can be implemented.[2] For reportable zoonotic diseases in livestock such as bovine tuberculosis (*Mycobacterium bovis*) and brucellosis (*Brucella abortus*), agricultural agencies conduct regular market surveillance and, in the event of reactors, they may implement epidemiological trace-backs, test and slaughter, or whole-herd eradication programs.[3–6]

On the other hand, the approach used by "wildlife conservationists" in addressing the implications of reportable diseases to conservation and translocation programs of wild ungulates has been less well defined and is relatively new.[7–9] Compared to the extensive scientific literature of reportable diseases in livestock, knowledge of basic epidemiology, pathogenesis, and natural history of those same diseases in wildlife is incomplete. A result is an associated lack of well-designed policy on managing health of wildlife populations—both free-ranging and captive. This is particularly relevant to conservation and captive-breeding programs of wild ungulates that are enzootic with reportable diseases because a principal objective is to salvage genetic diversity by establishing "disease-free" herds. In the absence of policies or accepted protocols for defining health status of captive wildlife, uncertainty on health status of a salvaged herd may reduce conservation options such as translocation and reintroduction.[8,9]

THE NORTHERN DISEASED BISON ISSUE IN CANADA

In northern Canada, bovine tuberculosis and brucellosis are endemic in wood bison (*Bison bison athabascae*) herds in and around Wood Buffalo National Park (WBNP). Those diseases were introduced with the translocation of 6673 plains bison (*B. b. bison*) from National Buffalo Park (NBP) at Wainwright, Alberta, to WBNP in the 1920s.[10] Original exposure and infection of the NBP plains bison with the bovine diseases was likely a result of "spill over" from contact with diseased cattle. The continued presence of those bovine diseases in free-ranging WBNP bison[11] presents a pathogen reservoir for potential "spill back" from diseased wild herds to nearby healthy bison populations and commercial bison and cattle ranches, and potentially to humans who may hunt and consume disease-exposed bison.[10]

IMPLICATIONS OF AGRICULTURAL POLICIES

Canada initiated national programs to eradicate tuberculosis and brucellosis from domestic livestock in 1923.[5,6] Canada's national cattle herd was declared free of brucellosis in 1985,[6] although it continues to have cases of tuberculosis in farmed cervids and sporadic cases in cattle.[5] Upon achieving brucellosis-free status in 1985, attention was centered on WBNP because its bison were the primary nidus of brucellosis in Canada.[12] In 1990, following two years of public consultation, the federally appointed "Northern Diseased Bison Assessment Panel" recommended depopulation of all infected free-ranging bison in and around WBNP followed by replacement with disease-free wood bison.[10] The recommendation was not undertaken because of strong opposition from First Nations' communities and environmental organizations and concerns with possible impairment of ecosystem integrity and loss of genetic diversity represented by infected bison herds. In the absence of management action, there has been continued deliberation, research, and surveillance programs to contain the diseases.

IMPLICATIONS OF CONSERVATION PRINCIPLES

Wood bison are listed under Appendix II of the Convention for International Trade in Endangered Species and are considered an endangered subspecies under the United States Endangered Species Act. The Committee on the Status of Endangered Wildlife in Canada considers wood bison a threatened species of American bison. Through a collaborative effort by jurisdictions in Canada and the United States under the umbrella of the Recovery of Nationally Endangered Wildlife Program, the Wood Bison Recovery Team (WBRT) has recently finalized a national recovery plan for wood bison. Three conservation principles have been endorsed by the WBRT and are identified in the plan: "(1) preserving intraspecific and biological diversity; (2) restoring and maintaining the interaction of wood bison with their natural environment to perpetuate evolution; and (3) promoting recovery efforts within original range."[13]

The WBRT considers that "eliminating the two bovine diseases from bison herds in the WBNP region would remove the greatest obstacle to the recovery of wood bison in Canada."[13] Despite being diseased, free-ranging bison in and around WBNP represent the greatest source of genetic diversity for wood bison.[14] Consequently, genetic conservation of those populations is a prerequisite to disease management and long-term conservation of the threatened subspecies.

ELK ISLAND NATIONAL PARK, ALBERTA, CANADA: BISON CONSERVATION AND DISEASE ERADICATION

Plains Bison

In 1906, the Canadian government purchased the Pablo holding of plains bison and translocated the first few shipments of bison to Elk Island National Park (EINP) as an interim location while fencing was being completed at the newly created Wainwright NBP. Between 1907 and 1912, a total of 716 bison were received. In 1909, all but 48 bison were moved from EINP to NBP.[15] By 1929, the EINP bison population had grown to 823, warranting the first slaughter of 225 animals to reduce population size. All carcasses were inspected and found free of tuberculosis and brucellosis. In 1935, a second slaughter resulted in veterinary inspection of 512 bison; no significant diseases were noted. Additional inspected slaughters of 800 and 600 bison in 1939 and 1944, respectively, led managers to consider that the herd was disease-free.[16]

However, in 1945, tests revealed that 6 (16%) of 37 park bison were positive for brucellosis; 5 (14%) were suspicious reactors.[16] To eliminate brucellosis, a separate isolation area was created and a strategy of only sending test-negative animals to the isolation area was adopted. This approach failed. By the mid-1950s, prevalence of brucellosis had increased to 32% (11% suspicious reactors), and the disease spilled over into elk and was found in bison within the isolation area.[15] In 1959, after 12 years of testing and slaughtering reactors and sending seronegative animals to the isolation area, the population still had a seroprevalence rate of 52%.[16]

A more intensive disease eradication program prescribed large-scale population reduction followed by vaccination (strain 19 *Brucella* vaccine) of young age classes and test and slaughter of seropositive and nonvaccinated bison.[16] Twice-yearly herd testing was also initiated. By 1964, prevalence was reduced to 21%. In 1965, the herd was further reduced to 493 head and most nonvaccinated and reactor animals had been slaughtered. By 1969, only 2 bison tested positive for brucellosis. Over the next two years, there were no serological reactors during disease tests. In 1972, EINP plains bison were officially declared free of brucellosis.[16]

Wood Bison

In 1965, 47 wood bison were captured in northern WBNP and 21 that tested negative for bovine brucellosis and tuberculosis were shipped to an isolation area at EINP.[13] Despite the initial screening of reactors, tuberculosis and brucellosis were detected in the translocated herd in 1968. In 1969, the herd was divided in two: original animals and captive-born calves (including 2 calves shipped after 1966).[16] After the pregnant females calved, all original animals were slaughtered and calves were hand-reared. Following removal of founders in 1970, remaining animals were test-negative for tuberculosis and brucellosis. The herd was declared free of the diseases in 1971.[13] By 1976, the population of 114 bison was providing source stock for zoos and other facilities. The EINP herd has been the cornerstone for wood bison recovery in Canada and has provided disease-free founding stock for 6 free-ranging populations, captive-breeding herds, zoo and park herds, and private commercial herds.[13] Wood and plains bison at EINP are subjected to the same testing requirements imposed on ranched bison in Canada. Both herds are tested annually and there have been no positive reactors since the 1970s.

NORTHWEST TERRITORIES, CANADA: BISON CONSERVATION AND MANAGEMENT

Mackenzie Bison Sanctuary: Establishing a Healthy Wild Herd

In late February 1963, 77 bison were driven by helicopter into a corral in the Needle Lake area of WBNP.[17] Those animals were considered to be part of an isolated herd of pure wood bison recently discovered in the northwest region of WBNP.[13] Fourteen animals were not handled further because they suffered from capture myopathy. Of the remaining 63 animals, 24 of 46 (52%) animals handled tested positive for brucellosis.[17] One 4-year-old bull tested positive for tuberculosis; a subsequent postmortem revealed an advanced infection.[17] In early March 1963, 19 of the 21 bison that tested negative for brucellosis and tuberculosis were transported to a holding corral near Fort Smith, Northwest Territories, to establish a captive-breeding herd.[18] Three calves were born the following spring, raising herd size to 22 bison. After an outbreak of anthrax in bison in the nearby Grand Detour area in summer 1963, it was decided to relocate the captive herd. In July 1963, calves were vaccinated for brucellosis and the rest of the herd were tested again for brucellosis and tuberculosis. All animals tested negative and, "since this was the second test, the Health of Animals Branch (Canada Department of Agriculture) declared the herd disease-free."[18] Of 21 bison declared fit for transport, 18 bison were barged to Fort Providence in the Northwest Territories, then transported by cattle liner, and released in an area 24 km northeast of the community and now known as the Mackenzie Bison Sanctuary.[13,18] The Mackenzie herd exhibited a classic pattern of eruptive oscillation, increasing sigmoidally since 1964 and reaching a peak at ca. 2400 bison in 1989 and subsequently stabilizing at ca. 2000 animals.[19]

A cursory check on herd health was conducted in 1982 when 9 adult bison were collected. There was no gross evidence of tuberculosis or brucellosis on postmortem inspection and all animals were seronegative for *B. abortus*.[20] The herd was considered free of bovine tuberculosis and brucellosis based on the absence of any gross histological or bacteriological evidence during postmortems on 51 bison collected between 1986 and 1988, and on the absence of antibody titers to *B. abortus* in those 51 animals or an additional 112 bison that were either chemically immobilized or shot by hunters between 1986 and 1990.[21] Blood sera collected from 153 hunter-killed bison between 1993 and 2001 were all seronegative for *B. abortus*. Since 1988 to early 2001, hunters have shot 419 bison and there have been no reports of tuberculosis-like lesions.

Hook Lake: Salvaging Healthy Wood Bison

In 1996, the Hook Lake Wood Bison Recovery Project (HLWBRP) was initiated cooperatively between the Government of the Northwest Territories, the Deninu Kue' First Nation, and the Aboriginal Wildlife Harvesters' Committee in Fort Resolution, Northwest Territories. The HLWBRP represents an attempt to conserve the genetic diversity of a diseased, free-ranging wood bison herd in the Slave River Lowlands through the capture, isolation, and prophylactic treatment of wild-caught newborn calves.[22] Over three years (1996, 1997, and 1998), a total of 62 wild newborn bison calves were captured by helicopter net-gunning. Each year, calves were paired and hand-raised at an isolation facility, treated for brucellosis and tuberculosis using a combination of antibiotics, and subjected to an intensive testing protocol that has included biannual whole-herd tests and postcalving testing for brucellosis. Currently, the captive-breeding herd consists of a total of 108 bison (58 founders and 50 captive-born offspring) and there have been no cases of either bovine tuberculosis or brucellosis after extensive disease testing.[22] A fundamental objective of this recovery project is to establish a "disease-free" captive-breeding herd that would provide healthy progeny for reintroduction back to their original range, but contingencies may also include translocation to other jurisdictions as part of the National Wood Bison Recovery Plan.

DISCUSSION

We reviewed three past examples of bison salvage and disease eradication programs in Canada—plains and wood bison at Elk Island National Park, and the Mackenzie wood bison herd. In the end, those programs achieved the desired objective of eliminating bovine tuberculosis and brucellosis, but at the cost of reduced genetic variability.[14] However, it is impossible to know exactly what combination of factors contributed to their eventual success. Consequently, it is difficult to prescribe specific recommendations for current or future bison salvage and conservation initiatives based only on those experiences.

The Hook Lake Wood Bison Recovery Project exemplifies a current approach to genetic salvage and disease eradication of free-ranging wood bison infected with bovine tuberculosis and brucellosis.[22] However, to progress beyond the phases of genetic salvage and captive breeding and into a full-scale recovery program involving translocation and reintroduction of captive-born animals, the health status of the founding herd must be defined and evaluated.

While the Canadian Health of Animals Regulations (Health of Animals Act)[2] establishes criteria for the eradication of tuberculosis and brucellosis in Canada, it is important to note that "bovines" are defined as "cattle or bison domestically raised or kept and ... does not include a bison that has ever been in contact with or part of a wild herd." As such, the federal agricultural regulations do not presently provide a policy framework that can be used to establish criteria to define a nationally recognized disease-free bison herd within the context of a species recovery program. Although wildlife conservation does not fall within the federal agricultural mandate, the far-reaching implications of the diseased bison issue require that a comprehensive policy framework be developed cooperatively so that it meets the needs and addresses the concerns of agriculturalists and conservationists alike. Over the longer term, such a policy framework would provide a better tool for both planning and evaluating conservation programs rather than an ad hoc review of projects on a case-by-case basis. From an international perspective, the two best examples of these comprehensive approaches include the protocols outlined by interdisciplinary and interagency working groups for Yellowstone bison[3,23] and sub-Saharan African buffalo.

In August 2000, the United States Department of the Interior published a final environmental impact statement (EIS) on bison management for the state of Montana and Yellowstone National Park.[23] The purpose of the EIS was "to maintain a wild, free-ranging population of bison and address the risk of brucellosis transmission to protect the economic interest and viability of the livestock industry in the state of Montana."[23] The interagency team agreed that elimination of brucellosis was not within the scope of the management plan, but that it was a long-term objective. A series of eight alternate options were evaluated in the EIS, with each containing a combination of methods to work towards eventual elimination of brucellosis in bison. Methods included (1) vaccination of bison once a safe and effective vaccine was developed, (2) capture and slaughter of seropositive bison and/or removal of sero-negative animals to a quarantine facility, and (3) control of bison population size and movement.[23] In considering the option of isolating seronegative animals under quarantine, the interagency team described a protocol that would allow brucellosis-exposed bison originating in Yellowstone or Grand Teton National Park to qualify as brucellosis-free under a rigorous testing regime.[3,23] Bison that qualify as brucellosis-free would be available to Native American tribes, parks, preserves, and other requesting organizations and could be moved intrastate or interstate following authorization by state animal health authorities.

In the greater Kruger National Park and the Natal Central Complex Reserves in South Africa, free-ranging African buffalo (*Syncerus caffer*) are endemically infected with a number of significant livestock diseases including foot-and-mouth disease (*Aphthovirus* spp.), corridor disease (*Theileria parva*), and bovine tuberculosis and brucellosis. Buffalo are highly prized because of their ecological and ecotourism value, but concerns about transmission of disease to livestock limit their movements by humans. The motivation for a disease-free buffalo-breeding program is to conserve the buffalo genotype in the affected areas and to translocate healthy buffalo to other national parks, game reserves, or game ranches outside the traditional buffalo range. A Specialist Veterinary Regulatory Panel recognizes a two-phase approach to establishing disease-free herds and outlines diagnostic testing requirements, breeding systems, and movement protocols.

Although the Yellowstone bison and African buffalo projects lay out a specific protocol that must be followed in order to qualify for "disease-free" status, the question remains of how confident that status is and what amount of risk, that is, the probability of false-negatives, is deemed acceptable. The HLWBRP faces a similar challenge. Resolution of this question may lie in part with the approach that has been recently adopted internationally by the World Health Organization and the Office International des Epizooties for resolving livestock health issues—the risk analysis.[24] The issue of "disease-free" status in captive wildlife revolves around epidemiological issues such as test sensitivity and specificity, lack of independence in diagnostic test data (arising from serial sampling of the same individuals and diagnostic tests that rely on the same physiological mechanisms, that is, cell-mediated versus humoral immune response), and uncertainty in the basic epidemiological characteristics of the disease in the host. In conservation projects where additional measures are taken to prevent or treat disease, i.e., use of antibiotic prophylaxis in the HLWBRP,[22] there is the added uncertainty in efficacy of those measures. These issues lend themselves well to risk assessment.[24] An additional benefit of the risk assessment is that model assumptions must be clearly acknowledged and, in so doing, the assessment identifies knowledge gaps and provides useful direction for future research.

Herd depopulation within a test and slaughter regime has provided a tried-and-true method for disease eradication in livestock industries at regional and national levels,[3–6] but the technique precludes genetic conservation when applied to diseased wildlife populations. There is an important need to develop a foundation of science-based research and policy to develop management options and tackle the unique conservation challenges that are posed by free-ranging diseased bison populations in northern Canada. At a minimum, this will require increased integration between the practitioners of conservation biology and veterinary epidemiology,[9] and increased collaboration among the respective agencies. Without this interaction and in the absence of progress towards developing feasible management options, agencies and stakeholders may tend to revert back to traditional agriculturalist approaches that may not be beneficial for conservation of wood bison. Evaluating and improving protocols for salvaging and establishing healthy captive herds from disease-exposed wild bison populations will be fundamental to the long-term interests of both the agriculturalist and wildlife conservationist.

ACKNOWLEDGMENTS

We thank R. Bengis, D. Grobler, and M. Hofmeyr for insight and unpublished information on the African buffalo breeding projects. A. Michel and M. Sutherland provided helpful comments on an earlier version of the manuscript.

REFERENCES

1. DASZAK, P., A.A. CUNNINGHAM & A.D. HYATT. 2000. Emerging infectious diseases of wildlife—threats to biodiversity and human health. Science **287:** 443–449.
2. GOVERNMENT OF CANADA. 1990. Health of Animals Act—1990, c. 21 [on-line—URL: http://laws.justice.gc.ca/en/H-3.3/index.html].
3. UNITED STATES DEPARTMENT OF AGRICULTURE (USDA). 1998. Brucellosis eradication: uniform methods and rules, effective February 1, 1998. APHIS 91-45-001. USDA. Washington, District of Columbia.
4. MARTIN, S.W. *et al.* 1994. Livestock Disease Eradication: Evaluation of the Cooperative State-Federal Bovine Tuberculosis Eradication Program. Nat. Acad. Press. Washington, District of Columbia.
5. ESSAY, M.A. & M.A. KOLLER. 1994. Status of bovine tuberculosis in North America. Vet. Microbiol. **40:** 15–22.
6. KELLAR, J.A. & A. DORE. 1998. Surveillance for bovine brucellosis (*B. abortus*) in Canada: a new direction. Animal Disease Surveillance Unpublished Report. Canadian Food Inspection Agency, Ottawa, Ontario.
7. CUNNINGHAM, A.A. 1996. Disease risks of wildlife translocations. Conserv. Biol. **10:** 349–353.
8. WOODFORD, M.H., Ed. 2000. Quarantine and Health Screening Protocols for Wildlife prior to Translocation and Release. IUCN Species Survival Commission—Veterinary Specialist Group and the OIE [online—URL: http://wildlife.usask.ca/RiskAnalysis/Quarantine.pdf].
9. DEEM, S.L., W.B. KARESH & W. WEISMAN. 2001. Putting theory into practice: wildlife health in conservation. Conserv. Biol. **15:** 1224–1233.
10. CONNELLY, R.G. *et al.* 1990. Northern diseased bison: report of the Environmental Assessment Panel. Minister of Supply and Services Canada, Ottawa, Ontario.
11. JOLY, D.O. & F. MESSIER. 2001. Limiting effects of bovine brucellosis and tuberculosis on wood bison within Wood Buffalo National Park. Final report submitted to Wood Buffalo National Park. University of Saskatchewan, Saskatoon, Saskatchewan.
12. TESSARO, S.V., L.B. FORBES & C. TURCOTTE. 1990. A survey of brucellosis and tuberculosis in bison in and around Wood Buffalo National Park, Canada. Can. Vet. J. **31:** 174–180.
13. GATES, C.C. *et al.* 2001. National recovery plan for the wood bison (*Bison bison athabascae*). National Recovery Plan No. 21. Recovery of Nationally Endangered Wildlife (RENEW), Ottawa, Ontario.
14. WILSON, G.A. & C. STROBECK. 1999. Genetic variation within and relatedness among wood and plains bison populations. Genome **42:** 483–496.

15. CORNER, A.H. & R. CONNELL. 1958. Brucellosis in bison, elk, and moose in Elk Island National Park, Alberta, Canada. Can. J. Comp. Med. **22:** 9–20.
16. BLYTH, C.B. 1995. Dynamics of ungulate populations in Elk Island National Park. M.Sc. thesis. University of Alberta, Edmonton, Alberta.
17. NOVAKOWSKI, N.S. 1963. Report on the transfer of wood bison, 1963. Unpublished Report CWS-37-63. Canadian Wildlife Service, Edmonton, Alberta.
18. NOVAKOWSKI, N.S. 1963. Wood Bison transfer—completion report. Unpublished Report CWS-357-63. Canadian Wildlife Service, Edmonton, Alberta.
19. LARTER, N.C. *et al.* 2000. Dynamics of reintroduction of an indigenous large ungulate: the wood bison of northern Canada. Anim. Conserv. **4:** 299–309.
20. HAWLEY, V.D. 1983. Fort Smith regional bison studies, 1979–1983. Northwest Territories Wildlife Service Unpublished Report. Fort Smith, Northwest Territories.
21. TESSARO, S.V., C.C. GATES & L.B. FORBES. 1993. The brucellosis and tuberculosis status of wood bison in the Mackenzie Bison Sanctuary, Northwest Territories, Canada. Can. J. Vet. Res. **57:** 231–235.
22. NISHI, J.S., B.T. ELKIN & T.R. ELLSWORTH. 2002. The Hook Lake Wood Bison Recovery Project: can a disease-free captive wood bison herd be recovered from a wild population infected with bovine tuberculosis and brucellosis? This volume.
23. ANONYMOUS. 2000 (August). Final Environmental Impact Statement of the Interagency Bison Management Plan for the State of Montana and Yellowstone National Park. Vol. 1. United States Department of the Interior, National Park Services. Washington, District of Columbia.
24. ZEPEDA, C., M. SALMAN & R. RUPPANNER. 2001. International trade, animal health, and veterinary epidemiology: challenges and opportunities. Prev. Vet. Med. **48:** 261–271.

Emergency Response Planning for Anthrax Outbreaks in Bison Herds of Northern Canada

A Balance between Policy and Science

J. S. NISHI,[a] D. C. DRAGON,[b] B. T. ELKIN,[b] J. MITCHELL,[c] T. R. ELLSWORTH,[a] AND M. E. HUGH-JONES[d]

[a]Resources, Wildlife, and Economic Development (RWED), Government of the Northwest Territories (GNWT), Fort Smith, Northwest Territories X0E 0P0, Canada

[b]Resources, Wildlife, and Economic Development (RWED), Government of the Northwest Territories (GNWT), Yellowknife, Northwest Territories X1A 3S8, Canada

[c]Wood Buffalo National Park (WBNP), Parks Canada, Fort Smith, Northwest Territories X0E 0P0, Canada

[d]Department of Epidemiology and Community Health, School of Veterinary Medicine, Louisiana State University, Baton Rouge, Louisiana 70803-8404, USA

ABSTRACT: Anthrax outbreaks in northern Canada have implications for on-going recovery efforts for the threatened wood bison and may pose a health risk to humans, other wildlife, and domestic livestock. RWED and WBNP maintain Anthrax Emergency Response Plans (AERPs) for their respective jurisdictions. An AERP is a preplanned logistical framework for responding effectively and rapidly to an outbreak so as to minimize spread of the disease, reduce environmental load of spores available for future outbreaks, and minimize risk to public health. In this paper, we describe the main components of an AERP and outline areas for future research.

KEYWORDS: anthrax; bison; northern Canada; AERP

ANTHRAX IN NORTHERN CANADA

Within the general area of northern Alberta and the adjacent Northwest Territories, Canada, there are several free-roaming wood bison (*Bison bison athabascae*) herds residing in the Mackenzie Bison Sanctuary, Slave River Lowlands, and Wood Buffalo National Park (WBNP). In 11 of the last 40 years, outbreaks of anthrax have been observed in at least one of these three regions that are now considered endemic for the disease.[1] During the outbreaks, surveillance and clean-up crews found 1585 bison carcasses (TABLE 1). This is an underestimate of actual losses as seroepidemio-

Address for correspondence: J.S. Nishi, Resources, Wildlife, and Economic Development, Government of the Northwest Territories, P. O. Box 390, Fort Smith, Northwest Territories X0E 0P0, Canada. Voice: 867-872-6446; fax: 867-872-4628.

John_Nishi@gov.nt.ca

Ann. N.Y. Acad. Sci. 969: 245–250 (2002). © 2002 New York Academy of Sciences.

TABLE 1. Number of bison carcasses found during anthrax outbreaks in northern Canada[1]

| | | Region affected | | | | | | | | | | |
| | | Slave River Lowlands | | Wood Buffalo National Park | | | | Mackenzie Bison Sanctuary | | | | |
Year	Carcass treatment/ disposal technique	Hook Lake	Grand Detour	Park Central	Lake One	Davidson Tower	Falaise Lake	Boulogne Lake	Slave Point	Calais Lake	Mink Lake	Total
1962	Lime/deep burial, m[a]	281[b]	NS[c]	NS	NS	NS	NS	NS	NS	NS	NS	281
1963[d]	Lime/deep burial, m	15	242	47	NS	NS	NS	NS	NS	NS	NS	304
1964[d]	Lime/deep burial, m	44	259	49	11	NS	NS	NS	NS	NS	NS	363
1967	Incineration/burial, m	0	0	0	120	NS	NS	NS	NS	NS	NS	120
1968	Incineration/burial, m	0	0	0	1	NS	NS	NS	NS	NS	NS	1
1971	Incineration/burial, m	33	0	0	0	NS	NS	NS	NS	NS	NS	33
1978	Incineration/burial, m	12	27	40	0	NS	NS	NS	NS	NS	NS	79
1991	Lime/deep burial	0	0	32	0	NS	NS	NS	NS	NS	NS	32
1993	3–5% formaldehyde/ incineration	0	0	0	0	NS	110[e]	26	7[f]	23	3	169
2000[g]	None	0	0	0	48	52	0	0	0	0	0	100
2001	Incineration None	12[h]	0	0	91[i]	0	0	0	0	0	0	103
Total		397	528	168	271	52	110	26	7	23	3	1585

[a]Mounded. [b]One black bear and a moose carcass were found in the affected region, but were inconclusive for *B. anthracis* because of advanced decomposition of specimens. [c]NS = no surveillance performed in the region. [d]Anthrax was also diagnosed in moose carcasses in the same general area. The number of moose mortalities was not specified. [e]One moose carcass was also found in the area and *B. anthracis* was successfully isolated from it. [f]Two moose carcasses were also found in the area and *B. anthracis* was successfully isolated from 1 carcass. [g]Three moose and 3 black bear carcasses were also found in the affected regions during the outbreak. *Bacillus anthracis* was isolated from the circulatory system of 1 moose carcass and from the digestive tract of 2 bear carcasses. [h]A 13th bison carcass was also found in the affected area, but was deemed a wolf kill. The bison cow carcass had been reduced to dismembered bones that were starting to bleach and there were no clumps of sloughed hair or edematous discharges typically observed around anthrax carcasses. [i]One moose carcass was also found in the affected area.

logical research suggests that additional anthrax mortalities in these herds have gone undetected[2] and carcasses under forest canopy may have been missed.[3]

HISTORICAL RESPONSES

Anthrax outbreaks in northern Canada have implications for ongoing recovery efforts for the threatened wood bison and may pose a health risk to humans, other wildlife, and domestic livestock. Federal and territorial agencies have historically initiated control measures aimed at breaking the cycle of infection (TABLE 1). These measures include large-scale carcass detection and disposal operations to minimize scavenging and release of anthrax spores into the environment.[1,3] During the 1960s and 1970s, additional preventative measures included depopulation by helicopter out of interherd regions to establish buffer zones and contain outbreaks. However, in all cases, buffer zones were repopulated within weeks. Between 1965 and 1977, large-scale vaccination roundups were also conducted, but were discontinued due to public concern over bison mortalities, increasing costs, and questions of effectiveness. A minimum of 1426 bison mortalities was associated with those depopulation and vaccination programs.[1]

CHALLENGES

In northern Canada, the challenges of responding to anthrax epizootics include remoteness of regions involved, unpredictable timing of outbreaks, and large requirements for monetary and human resources. Additional complications arise from a loss of experience through staff turnover during intervening years and difficulty in conducting field research due to the sporadic, abrupt nature of outbreaks.

ANTHRAX EMERGENCY RESPONSE PLANS

RWED and WBNP maintain Anthrax Emergency Response Plans (AERPs) for their respective jurisdictions. An AERP is a preplanned logistical framework for responding effectively and rapidly to an outbreak so as to minimize spread of the disease, reduce environmental load of spores available for future outbreaks, and minimize risk to public health. Below, we describe the main components of an AERP and also outline areas for future research.

Identification of Potential Outbreak Conditions

Outbreaks appear to be associated with a specific season and weather pattern and have generally occurred in late summer during prolonged hot, dry weather following periods of spring flooding.[1] Several climatic and environmental factors in years with and without outbreaks need to be evaluated to determine exactly which factors may trigger an outbreak or what environmental variables and associated thresholds may provide predictive capabilities.

Aerial Surveillance for Dead Animals

Aerial surveillance is conducted during typical outbreak periods and in traditional bison range. Current surveillance efforts should detect mid- to large-scale outbreaks. Once suspect carcasses are located, aerial surveillance is initiated in both immediate and surrounding areas. Daily aerial surveillance is conducted with fixed-wing and/or rotary-wing aircraft using a search pattern based on the dispersion of carcasses. After confirmation of anthrax in the index case(s), a helicopter-mounted infrared sensor can be used to find carcasses under heavy forest cover.[3] Owing to variable success, technicians should be trained and the technique validated.

Diagnostic Confirmation of Anthrax

Swabs of blood and other body fluids are preferred samples. Diagnostic success is increased if samples are air-dried to stimulate sporulation; the spore protects the bacterium from contaminants and temperature fluctuations during shipment. Once the index case has been confirmed as anthrax, further diagnostic submissions are limited to suspected cases in new species or new geographical regions. Additional samples may be archived for genotyping.

Disposal of Carcasses

In an intact carcass, anthrax bacilli are destroyed by natural putrefaction within a few days of death. However, scavengers often do not allow a carcass to remain intact long enough for putrefaction to occur. If vegetative cells of anthrax are released from a carcass due to scavenging and then encounter suitable conditions of humidity, temperature, and nutrient depletion, they can form resistant spores that will contaminate the soil. Consequently, various methods of carcass disposal and treatment have been used in an effort to destroy the vegetative anthrax bacilli before they can sporulate.

Used singly or in different combinations, methods have included putrefaction, treatment with lime or formaldehyde, burial, and incineration. Liming and burial are no longer considered useful. Lime is ineffective in deterring scavengers and provides an alkaline-rich environment that may prolong spore viability.[4] Carcass burial may maintain a reservoir of spores that can be spread by burrowing wildlife and can also contaminate groundwater. Treatment of carcasses with formaldehyde is considered a useful technique. It decontaminates sites containing high concentrations of spores and is an effective deterrent to scavengers. Long-term environmental effects of formaldehyde applied at carcass sites are negligible.[5,6] Complete carcass incineration is as effective because spores are destroyed and no remains are left for scavengers. Incomplete burning may not destroy all anthrax spores[7] and, in such cases, the sites should be reburned or treated with formaldehyde. There is a need to test effectiveness of carcass treatment and disposal techniques through appropriate sampling for anthrax spores (i.e., Before and After Control Impact design).

Protection of Public Health

Following confirmation of anthrax, access to affected areas may be restricted through media advisories, public announcements, highway signage, and blocked access at hiking trails. Community health centers are provided information on symptoms and treatment of anthrax.

Media Relations

A spokesperson should be designated to field media inquiries in a consistent manner and to provide regular updates.

Research Planning

Information gaps, potential research opportunities, research hypotheses, and sampling designs should be identified in advance of an outbreak. Collaborators, research team members, and responsibility for maintenance of sampling equipment should also be predetermined.

CONCLUSIONS

(1) The infrequency and unpredictability of anthrax outbreaks requires a pre-planned, organized, and adaptive approach to ensure a timely and effective response.

(2) An AERP provides a knowledge base and adaptive management framework that allows experience gained during one outbreak to be used to improve the response to future outbreaks. The framework outlined in an AERP allows for areas of improvement to be identified, and the research methodology incorporated into the plan allows for the evaluation of proposed improvements as well as testing of relevant epizootiology hypotheses during the next outbreak.

(3) Interagency cooperation and collaboration will further help to improve effectiveness and consistency of the response to anthrax outbreaks in northern Canada.

ACKNOWLEDGMENTS

We thank A. Moreland, P. Gale, B. Goldsteyn-Thomas, E. Tanaka, S. Tessaro, G. Tiffin, H. Epp, L. Jones, M. Pybus, B. Samuel, and G. Wobeser for participating in a joint WBNP-RWED anthrax research and management workshop on which this paper was based.

REFERENCES

1. DRAGON, D.C. & B.T. ELKIN. 2001. An overview of early anthrax outbreaks in northern Canada: field reports of the Health of Animals Branch, Agriculture Canada, 1962–71. Arctic **54:** 32–40.

2. RIJKS, J. 1999. A serological study of bison (*Bison bison*) in an area of northern Canada experiencing sporadic and epizootic anthrax. M.Sc. thesis. University of London, London, United Kingdom.

3. GATES, C.C., B.T. ELKIN & D.C. DRAGON. 1995. Investigation, control, and epizootiology of anthrax in a geographically isolated, free-roaming bison population in northern Canada. Can. J. Vet. Res. **59:** 256–264.

4. DRAGON, D.C. & R.P. RENNIE. 1995. The ecology of anthrax spores: tough but not invincible. Can. Vet. J. **36:** 295–301.

5. MILES, J., P.M. LATTER, I.R. SMITH & O.W. HEAL. 1988. Ecological effects of killing *Bacillus anthracis* on Gruinard Island with formaldehyde. Reclam. Reveg. Res. **6:** 271–283.
6. MANCHEE, R.J., M.G. BROSTER, A.J. STAGG & S.E. HIBBS. 1994. Formaldehyde solution effectively inactivates spores of *Bacillus anthracis* on the Scottish Island of Gruinard. Appl. Environ. Microbiol. **60:** 4167–4171.
7. DRAGON, D.C., R.P. RENNIE & B.T. ELKIN. 2001. Detection of anthrax spores in endemic regions of northern Canada. J. Appl. Microbiol. **91:** 435–441.

Implications of Tuberculosis in African Wildlife and Livestock

ANITA L. MICHEL

Tuberculosis Laboratory of the ARC-Onderstepoort Veterinary Institute, Onderstepoort 0110, South Africa

ABSTRACT: In most countries, tuberculosis caused by *Mycobacterium bovis* is mainly a disease of domestic cattle and can be controlled successfully by means of a test-and-slaughter program. Once the infection spills over into a wild animal species with maintenance host potential, conventional measures are no longer sufficient to provide effective control. In South Africa, African buffaloes (*Syncerus caffer*) represent the most important maintenance host for *M. bovis*. Apart from transmitting the disease to predators and scavengers that feed on them, buffalo also serve as a source of infection to other wildlife species through environmental contamination. In several countries, it was shown that an infected wildlife reservoir that interacts with livestock causes frequent herd breakdowns and substantial economic losses to the agricultural sector. The outbreak of tuberculosis in free-ranging wildlife populations thus poses a huge challenge on long-term management and control strategies to prevent spillover into other wildlife, especially endangered, wildlife species and domestic livestock.

KEYWORDS: *Mycobacterium bovis*; livestock; tuberculosis; wildlife; South Africa

INTRODUCTION

Tuberculosis in animals is a contagious disease caused by *Mycobacterium bovis*, a bacterium with a very wide host spectrum.[1] Infection with this pathogen is followed by a slow disease progression in which clinical signs are mostly limited to the advanced stages.[2] Excretion of infectious particles, which leads to transmission of the disease to other animals, appears to be dose-dependent and can commence relatively shortly after infection.[3]

Successful control leading to eradication of the disease has been accomplished in many countries applying test-and-slaughter schemes. In South Africa, bovine tuberculosis is thought to have been introduced by European settlers and their cattle towards the end of the eighteenth century.[4] Although complete eradication has not yet been achieved, the overall prevalence has remained relatively low.[5] Focal outbreaks with high herd prevalences occurred in various parts of the country and were most

Address for correspondence: Anita L. Michel, Tuberculosis Laboratory of the ARC-Onderstepoort Veterinary Institute, Private Bag x05, Onderstepoort 0110, South Africa. Voice: +27-12-5299384; fax: +27-12-5299127.

anita@moon.ovi.ac.za

Ann. N.Y. Acad. Sci. 969: 251–255 (2002). © 2002 New York Academy of Sciences.

probably the cause for the first outbreak of tuberculosis in wild animals, described in 1928.[6] In 1986 and 1990, *M. bovis* infection was diagnosed in the Hluhluwe-Um-folozi-Park[7] (HUP) and the Kruger National Park[8] (KNP), respectively. An epidemiological link between the infection in buffalo and cattle kept on a farm adjacent to the southern border of the KNP could be established by molecular typing of the *M. bovis* strains isolated from both species.[9,10]

HOST SPECTRUM AND TERMINOLOGY

Tuberculosis in cattle has been known even before classical times.[11] Owing to its close resemblance with the disease in humans and the close relationships between the causative agents, they were initially termed *M. tuberculosis typus bovinus* and *M. tuberculosis typus humanus*.[12] The disease was commonly known as bovine tuberculosis. During the twentieth century, the increasing number of reports published on this disease illustrated the extremely wide host spectrum of this organism. The most frequently affected species include cattle, goats, pigs, sheep, dogs, cats, farmed deer, and rarely horses, asses, and mules.[1,5,13,15] In domestic and wild species, both in zoological collections as well as under free-ranging conditions, tuberculosis caused by *M. bovis* has been diagnosed in a variety of species.[13–19]

In association with the more recent TB epidemic in the KNP and HUP, the following species were found to be infected: African buffalo (*Syncerus caffer*), lion (*Panthera leo*), cheetah (*Acinonyx jubatus*), chacma baboon (*Papio ursinus*),[20–22] greater kudu (*Tragelaphus strepsiceros*),[23] leopard (*Panthera pardus*), hyena (*Crocuta crocuta*) (Bengis, personal communication), large-spotted genet (*Genetta tigrina*), warthog (*Phacochoerus aethiopicus*) (Michel, unpublished data), bushpig (*Potamochoerus porcus*), and eland (*Taurotragus oryx*) (Cooper, personal communication).

It is suggested that these findings justify a revision of the terminology because the host spectrum does not only include end or spillover hosts of the infection, but also includes species with a proven potential to act as reservoirs of *M. bovis*.[9,24,25]

WILDLIFE-LIVESTOCK INTERFACE

Social herd structure, behavioral patterns, and a relatively high susceptibility to *M. bovis* make buffalo an optimum reservoir species that not only maintains the infection, but produces an increasing infection incidence.[9,26,27] Spillover of tuberculosis to other species is considered to have been triggered by the high prevalence levels observed in buffalo herds in the KNP. To date, the greater majority of these species can be contained within the infected ecosystem by adequate fences. Greater kudu, however, are known for their ability to cross fences of average height without difficulty, meaning that diseases such as tuberculosis can be spread across the border of the KNP. It might be argued, though, that the likelihood of such events is very limited. On the other hand, smaller mammals can extend their home ranges from a game sanctuary into agricultural land or vice versa since their movement is not, or not drastically, restricted by game fences. In the event of such an animal species becoming a wildlife reservoir, it can serve as a link in the transmission of *M. bovis* infection

TABLE 1. Implications of tuberculosis in domestic cattle versus African wildlife

Are the facts applicable?	Cattle	Wildlife
Socioeconomic impacts		
Zoonosis	Yes	Rarely
Loss in production (milk, fertility, condition, condemned carcasses)	Yes	N/A
Loss in market value and overseas trade	Yes	Yes
Transmission to other species	Yes	Yes
Maintenance potential	Yes	Yes
Spillover into healthy livestock populations	Yes	Yes
Impacts on control and conservation		
Exotic disease status	N/A	Yes
Effects on population dynamics	N/A	Yes
Diagnosis	Available	Very limited
Spillover into endangered species	N/A	Yes
Control	Achievable	Difficult to achieve
Eradication	Achievable	Unlikely

between wildlife and livestock. This wildlife-livestock interface is therefore of crucial importance in the management and control of tuberculosis in game reserves that are bordered by livestock farming communities. Similar scenarios have been reported from England and Ireland where a link was found between reinfection of cattle herds and the presence of infected colonies of badgers[24] (*Meles meles*), as well as from New Zealand where the role of the brushtail possums (*Trichosurus vulpecula*) in the epidemiology of tuberculosis in cattle has been well studied.[25]

A risk to human health posed by the zoonotic character of *M. bovis* is of additional concern in Africa as preference of unpasteurized milk or a lack of access to pasteurized milk is frequently observed in rural African communities.[28,29] Widespread immunosuppression caused by the soaring HIV/AIDS epidemic in Southern Africa[30] further increases the risk of developing clinical tuberculosis after exposure to *M. bovis*.

CONCLUSIONS

Governments and conservation bodies are challenged with the task to contain and control tuberculosis in affected and threatened free-ranging wildlife populations. The responsibility, however, is not limited to the conservation of a wide variety of wild animal species, but includes the prevention of spillover into domestic livestock. If tuberculosis can successfully establish itself in the wildlife-livestock interface, its spillover into livestock populations will unavoidably lead to high economic losses and public health hazard implications.

REFERENCES

1. O'REILLY, L.M. & C.J. DABORN. 1995. The epidemiology of *Mycobacterium bovis* infections in animals and man: a review. Tubercle Lung Dis. Suppl. **1:** 1–46.
2. FRANCIS, J. 1958. Pathogenesis and Pathology. *In* Tuberculosis in Animals and Man: A Study in Comparative Pathology, pp. 11–43. Cassell. London.
3. NEILL, S.D., S. HANNA, J.J. O'BRIEN & R.M. MCCRACKEN. 1988 (September). Excretion of *Mycobacterium bovis* by experimentally infected cattle. Vet. Rec. **24:** 340–343.
4. HENNING, M.W. 1956. Animal Diseases in South Africa. Third edition. Central News Agency. Pretoria.
5. HUCHZERMEYER, H.F.K.A., G.K. BRUECKNER, A. VAN HEERDEN *et al.* 1994. Tuberculosis. *In* Infectious Diseases of Livestock with Special Reference to Southern Africa, pp. 1425–1444. Oxford University Press. Cape Town/London/New York.
6. PAINE, R. & G. MARTINAGLIA. 1929. Tuberculosis in wild buck living under natural conditions. J. S. Afr. Vet. Med. Assoc. **1:** 87–91.
7. COOPER, D. 1998. Tuberculosis in wildlife in the Hluhluwe/Umfolozi complex. Presented at "The Challenges of Managing Tuberculosis in Wildlife in Southern Africa" Conference, Mpumalanga Parks Board Headquarters, Nelspruit (30–31 July 1998).
8. BENGIS, R.G., N.P.J. KRIEK, D.F. KEET *et al.* 1996. An outbreak of bovine tuberculosis in a free-living buffalo population in the Kruger National Park. Onderstepoort J. Vet. Res. **63**(1): 15–18.
9. DE VOS, V., J.P. RAATH, R.G. BENGIS *et al.* 2001. The epidemiology of tuberculosis in free ranging African buffalo (*Syncerus caffer*) in the Kruger National Park, South Africa. Onderstepoort J. Vet. Res. **68**(2): 119–130.
10. VOSLOO, W., A.D.S. BASTOS, A. MICHEL & G.R. THOMSON. 2001. Tracing of movement of African buffalo in Southern Africa through genetic characterisation of pathogens. OIE Sci. Tech. Rev. **20**(2): 630–639.
11. WEBB, G.B. 1939. Tuberculosis. Clio Medica. New York.
12. LEHMANN, K.B. & R. NEUMANN. 1907. Atlas und Grundriss der Bakteriologie und Lehrbuch der Speziellen Bakteriologischen Diagnostik. Fourth edition. Munich.
13. HUNTER, D.L. 1996. Tuberculosis in free-ranging, semi free-ranging, and captive cervids. Rev. Sci. Tech. Off. Int. Epizoot. **15:** 171–181.
14. THOREL, M.F., C. KAROUI, C.F. VARNEROT & V. VINCENT. 1998. Isolation of *Mycobacterium bovis* infection from baboons, leopards, and sea-lions. Vet. Res. **29:** 207–212.
15. THOEN, C.O. 1994. Tuberculosis in wild and domestic mammals. *In* Tuberculosis, Pathogenesis, Protection, and Control, pp. 157–162. Washington, District of Columbia.
16. BUSH, M., R.J. MONTALI, L.G. PHILIPS & P.A. HOLOBAUGH. 1990. Bovine tuberculosis in a Bactrian camel herd: clinical, therapeutic, and pathologic findings. J. Zoo Wildl. Med. **21:** 171–179.
17. MANN, P.C., M. BUSH, D.L. JANSSEN *et al.* 1981. Clinicopathologic correlations of tuberculosis in large zoo animals. J. Am. Vet. Med. Assoc. **179:** 1123–1129.
18. BRIONES, V., L. JUAN, C. SÁNCHEZ *et al.* 2000. Bovine tuberculosis and the endangered Iberian lynx. Emerg. Infect. Dis. **6**(2): 189–191.
19. SERRAINO, A., G. MARCHETTI, V. SANGUINETTI *et al.* 1999. Monitoring of transmission of tuberculosis between wild boars and cattle: genotypical analysis of strains by molecular epidemiology techniques. J. Clin. Microbiol. **37**(9): 2766–2771.
20. KEET, D.F., N.P.J. KRIEK, M-L. PENRITH *et al.* 1996. Tuberculosis in buffaloes (*Syncerus caffer*) in the Kruger National Park: spread of the disease to other species. Onderstepoort J. Vet. Res. **63**(3): 239–244.
21. KEET, D.F., N.P.J. KRIEK, M-L. PENRITH & A. MICHEL. 1998. Tuberculosis in free-ranging lions in the Kruger National Park. Proc. ARC-Onderstepoort OIE International Congress with WHO-Cosponsorship on Anthrax, Brucellosis, CBPP, Clostridial, and Mycobacterial Diseases, Berg-en-Dal, Kruger National Park.

22. KEET, D.F., N.P.J. KRIEK, R.G. BENGIS *et al.* 2000. The rise and fall of tuberculosis in a free-ranging chacma baboon troop in the Kruger National Park. Onderstepoort J. Vet. Res. **67**(2): 115–122.

23. BENGIS, R.G. & D.F. KEET. 1998. Bovine tuberculosis in free-ranging kudu (*Tragelaphus strepsiceros*) in the Greater Kruger National Park complex. *In* Proc. ARC-Onderstepoort OIE International Congress with WHO-Cosponsorship on Anthrax, Brucellosis, CBPP, Clostridial, and Mycobacterial Diseases, pp. 418–421. Sigma Press. Pretoria.

24. CHEESEMAN, C.L., J.W. WILESMITH & F.A. STUART. 1989. Tuberculosis: the disease and its epidemiology in the badger—a review. Epidemiol. Infect. **103**: 113–125.

25. MORRIS, R.S. & D.U. PFEIFFER. 1994. The epidemiology of *Mycobacterium bovis* infections. Vet. Microbiol. **40**: 153–177.

26. GRIMSDELL, J.J.R. 1969. Ecology of the buffalo, *Syncerus caffer*, in western Uganda. D.Ph. dissertation. Cambridge University.

27. RODWELL, T.C. 1999. The epidemiology of bovine tuberculosis in African buffalo. Ph.D. dissertation. University of California, Davis.

28. COSIVI, O., J.M. GRANGE, C.J. DABORN *et al.* 1998. Zoonotic tuberculosis due to *Mycobacterium bovis* in developing countries. Emerg. Infect. Dis. **4**: 59–70

29. DABORN, C.J. & J.M. GRANGE. 1993. HIV/AIDS and its implications for the control of animal tuberculosis. Br. Vet. J. **149**: 405–417.

30. DORRINGTON, R., D. BOURNE, D. BRADSHAW, *et al.* 2001. The Impact of HIV/AIDS on Adult Mortality in South Africa. Technical Report of the Burden of Disease Research Unit of the Medical Research Council, South Africa.

Mycobacterial Isolations in Captive Elephants in the United States

JANET B. PAYEUR,[a] J. L. JARNAGIN,[a] J. G. MARQUARDT,[a] AND D. L. WHIPPLE[b]

[a]National Veterinary Services Laboratories, United States Department of Agriculture, Ames, Iowa, USA

[b]National Animal Disease Center, United States Department of Agriculture, Ames, Iowa, USA

ABSTRACT: Interest in tuberculosis in elephants has been increasing over the past several years in the United States. Several techniques have been used to diagnose mammalian tuberculosis. Currently, the test considered most reliable for diagnosis of TB in elephants is based on the culture of respiratory secretions obtained by trunk washes.

KEYWORDS: tuberculosis; elephant(s); mycobacterial; guidelines

The interest in tuberculosis in elephants has been increasing over the past several years in the United States. Between 1994 and 2001, *Mycobacterium tuberculosis* (TB) was isolated from 24 captive elephants from 11 herds in California, Illinois, Arkansas, Missouri, Florida, and New Mexico. *Mycobacterium bovis* has been isolated from 1 captive elephant from the District of Columbia in 2000. At the time of diagnosis, 5 of these elephants resided in American Zoo and Aquarium Association–accredited zoos and 19 in private facilities. There had been known previous contact between 5 different herds of elephants. Five elephants demonstrated clinical signs that could be associated with TB. Clinical signs included chronic weight loss, anorexia, weakness, and (on occasion) dyspnea and coughing. *Mycobacterium tuberculosis* was isolated from 17 elephants premortem and 7 elephants postmortem, and *M. bovis* was isolated from 1 elephant postmortem.[1]

In 1997, a National Tuberculosis Working Group for Zoo and Wildlife Species in the United States formulated the Guidelines for the Control of Tuberculosis in Elephants. It specified criteria for the testing, surveillance, and treatment of elephants for tuberculosis.[2,3] In November 1997, these guidelines were implemented by the USDA Animal Care Staff in response to an outbreak of tuberculosis at an Illinois facility where 1 elephant died in 1994 and 2 elephants died in 1996. A fourth living elephant was culture-positive in October 1996. Twenty-two animal handlers were screened for tuberculosis and 11 had positive reactions to the intradermal injection

Address for correspondence: Dr. Janet B. Payeur, National Veterinary Services Laboratories, USDA, Ames, IA 50010.
janet.b.payeur@aphis.usda.gov

Ann. N.Y. Acad. Sci. 969: 256–258 (2002). © 2002 New York Academy of Sciences.

with *M. tuberculosis* purified protein derivative (PPD). One animal handler was smear-negative, culture-positive with active tuberculosis. DNA fingerprint comparison by IS*6110* and TBN12 typing showed that the isolates from the 4 elephants and the handler were the same strain of *M. tuberculosis*.[4] This event resulted in increased testing of all captive elephants owned by licensed exhibitors in the United States.[2]

Several techniques have been used to diagnose mammalian tuberculosis. Methods such as culture, acid fast smears, fluorescent smears, and nucleic acid amplification techniques (NAAT) directly detect the bacterial organism. Indirect methods such as serological assays, the gamma-interferon test, and the intradermal tuberculin test detect antigen-antibody or cellular reactivity to mycobacterial antigen. Intradermal tuberculin tests have correlated poorly with mycobacterial culture results, with high percentages of false-negatives in culture-positive animals. Currently, the test considered most reliable for diagnosis of TB in elephants is based on the culture of respiratory secretions obtained by trunk washes. Sterile saline is instilled into the trunk and then a sample for culture is recovered in a plastic bag or stainless-steel bucket. Three samples are collected on separate days. Elephant herds in the United States are tested by this method on an annual basis or more frequently if cases of TB have been detected or if the herd is known to have been previously exposed to TB.[1,3]

Over 5100 trunk washes or swabs from 539 elephants were submitted to the National Veterinary Services Laboratories (NVSL) in Ames, Iowa, from 1996 to the present. The most common mycobacterial species isolated were *M. avium* (129), *M. tuberculosis* (36), *M. tuberculosis* complex (4), *M. terrae* (9), *M. gordonae* (9), *M. scrofulaceum* (2), *M. ulcerans* (2), *M. fortuitum* (6), *M. gastri* (2), *M. chitae* (2), *M. phlei* (2), *M. xenopi* (1), *M. szulgai* (1), Runyon Group IV (14), *M. bovis* (2), and *Mycobacterium* species (76).

DNA fingerprinting has identified 5 different strains of *M. tuberculosis* from 11 elephants located in 6 different areas of the country. Test results indicated that the Illinois elephants were infected with a TB strain different from the one that infected the California, Florida, and Arkansas animals. The strains from the New Mexico and Missouri elephants have not been compared.[5]

Over 1100 NAAT [Gen Probe®–Amplified™ Mycobacterium Tuberculosis Direct Test (MTD)] have been performed. The MTD was positive on 13 elephants where *M. tuberculosis* was isolated, positive on 15 elephants where *M. tuberculosis* was not isolated, and positive on 1 elephant where *M. bovis* was isolated. *Mycobacterium tuberculosis* was isolated from 6 elephants that were negative on MTD. The advantages of NAAT include rapid turnaround time (3 h) and the capability of detecting low numbers of organisms. MTD is very specific for *M. tuberculosis* complex organisms, but mycobacterial species cannot be differentiated. Since both live and dead organisms are detected, MTD is of limited value in monitoring response to therapy.[1]

The current USDA Animal Care regulations (January 2000) require annual culture of all captive elephants held by licensed exhibitors in an effort to prevent future zoonotic outbreaks like the Illinois case. These guidelines can be found at http://www.aphis.usda.gov/ac/ElephTBGuidelines2000.html.[2]

Treatment and management procedures are listed in these guidelines. Current treatment protocols have been extrapolated from human treatment regimens and are still under investigation for efficacy in elephants. Anti-TB drugs recently used in elephants include isoniazid (INH), pyrazinamide (PZA), rifampin (RIF), and ethambutol (ETH). These drugs have been administered to elephants in food, by direct oral administration, and rectally. Oral delivery has been challenging as many elephants refuse oral medications. Anti-TB drug doses for individual elephants should be determined by measuring blood-level response.

The current recommended treatment for known infected elephants consists of INH and RIF daily for 2 months and then every other day for 10 months. A third drug, such as PZA, is given daily for the first 2 months of treatment. As a starting dose, INH can be given orally or rectally at a dose of 2.5–5.0 mg/kg. An INH blood level of 1–2 µg/mL is recommended for elephants. RIF can be initiated orally at a dose of 7.5–10.0 mg/kg orally. Human 2-h blood levels for this drug are 8–24 µg/mL. PZA can be initiated at a dose of 25–35 mg/kg orally or rectally. Human 2-h levels for PZA are 20–60 µg/mL. Supplementation with vitamin B_6 (pyridoxine) at a daily dose of 1 mg/kg is recommended to prevent possible peripheral neuropathy, a condition that has been associated with INH therapy in humans.[1,3] Elephants should be weighed before and throughout treatment. Side effects of treatment may include anorexia, lethargy, and colitis. Leukopenia has been observed in 1 elephant receiving INH and RIF. Currently, there are 3 elephants undergoing treatment for organisms that are resistant to INH (0.1 and 0.2 µg/mL). Each of the elephants had been on treatment previously. All culture-positive elephants ceased shedding organisms shortly after treatment was initiated and remained culture-negative during the treatment period.[1]

A complete postmortem examination should be performed on all elephants that die. A thorough search for TB lesions should be conducted even if TB is not suspected.[2] Seven elephants were found on necropsy to have TB lesions, while *M. tuberculosis* was cultured from the remaining 17 elephants from trunk washes.

Since elephants may be at risk of contracting TB from infected humans, handlers in close daily contact should undergo annual TB screening to minimize risks to the elephant's health. New employees should be tested prior to contact with elephants. Any facility with known TB culture-positive animals should develop an employee protection program. Zoos are encouraged to establish protocols for elephant-visitor interactions.[1,2,6]

REFERENCES

1. MIKOTA, S.K. *et al.* 2000. Tuberculosis in elephants in North America. Zoo Biol. **19:** 393–403.
2. MICHALAK, K. *et al.* 1998. *Mycobacterium tuberculosis* infection as a zoonotic disease: transmission between humans and elephants. Emerg. Infect. Dis. **4**(2): 283–287.
3. USDA. 2000. Guidelines for the Control of Tuberculosis in Elephants. APHIS, Animal Care, Washington, District of Columbia.
4. MONTALI, R.J. *et al.* 2001. *Mycobacterium tuberculosis* in zoo and wildlife species. Rev. Sci. Tech. Off. Int. Epizoot. **20**(1): 291–303.
5. WHIPPLE, D.L. *et al.* 2000. Reemergence of tuberculosis in animals in the United States. *In* Emerging Diseases of Animals, pp. 281–299. ASM Press. Washington, District of Columbia.
6. DAVIS, M. 2001. *Mycobacterium tuberculosis* risk for elephant handlers and veterinarians. Appl. Occup. Environ. Hyg. **16**(3): 350–353.

Bovine Tuberculosis in Michigan Wildlife

JANET B. PAYEUR,[a] S. CHURCH,[b] L. MOSHER,[b] B. ROBINSON-DUNN,[b]
S. SCHMITT,[c] AND D. WHIPPLE[d]

[a]National Veterinary Services Laboratories, United States Department of Agriculture,
Ames, Iowa, USA

[b]Michigan Department of Community Health, Lansing, Michigan, USA

[c]Michigan Department of Natural Resources, Lansing, Michigan, USA

[d]National Animal Disease Center, United States Department of Agriculture,
Ames, Iowa, USA

ABSTRACT: White-tailed deer in Michigan are now recognized as a reservoir
host of bovine tuberculosis (TB). It has been determined that the most likely
cause of bovine TB infection in the deer is from congregating in artificially high
numbers at feed sites. The presence of a wildlife reservoir of TB in Michigan
poses a serious threat to the control and eradication programs that are now in
their final stages in the United States.

KEYWORDS: tuberculosis (TB); bovine; deer; wildlife; Michigan

In 1975, a 9-year-old female white-tailed deer from Alcona County, Michigan, was
found to have lesions consistent with bovine tuberculosis (TB), and *Mycobacterium
bovis* was isolated. It was thought to be an isolated case and no further testing was
done on the surrounding livestock or deer.[1] Historically, bovine TB in wild deer has
been rare in the United States. Each of the 8 cases reported before 1995 was found
to be associated with exposure to infected cattle, bison, captive elk, or feral swine.[1,2]

In 1994, a hunter in southwestern Alpena County, Michigan, shot a 4-year-old
male whitetail deer, which had lesions consistent with TB, and *M. bovis* was isolated.
The deer was harvested approximately 10 miles from the site of the 1975 infected
deer. Michigan has been accredited as TB-free in cattle since 1979 and it was decided
to test the surrounding cattle and captive cervid herds. No evidence of bovine TB
was found. In the fall of 1995, surveillance of hunter-killed deer was initiated and
27/814 deer were found to be culture-positive for bovine TB. The wildlife surveys
have continued annually to monitor the prevalence of the disease.[1,3]

The Bovine TB Eradication Project was established as a multiagency partnership
to investigate the issues. The project consisted of personnel from the United States
Department of Agriculture (USDA); the Michigan Departments of Agriculture

Address for correspondence: Dr. Janet B. Payeur, National Veterinary Services Laboratories,
USDA, Ames, IA 50010.
janet.b.payeur@aphis.usda.gov

Ann. N.Y. Acad. Sci. 969: 259–261 (2002). © 2002 New York Academy of Sciences.

(MDA), Natural Resources (DNR), and Community Health (MDCH); and Michigan State University (MSU).[3]

Since 1995, wildlife surveys have been conducted by the DNR in the surrounding area. As of June 18, 2001, over 64,536 whitetail deer, 869 elk, and 1080 noncervids have been examined for bovine TB in project laboratories. The noncervid species have come primarily from the 5-county high-risk area (Alcona, Alpena, Montmorency, Oscoda, and Presque Isle). The species tested included badger (25), black bear (153), bobcat (53), coyote (290), feral cat (24), feral dog (1), gray fox (4), mink (3), opossum (260), otter (8), porcupine (1), raccoon (217), red fox (18), skunk (21), snowshoe hare (1), and weasel (1). From 1996 through 2000, a total of 71,262 deer carcasses and/or heads have been examined for TB lesions at deer check stations. Each of the cervid and noncervid carcasses and/or heads were examined grossly for lesions. Suspicious lymph nodes and tissues from cervids were submitted to the National Veterinary Services Laboratories (NVSL) or MDCH for culture and to MSU and NVSL for histopathology. A pool of tissues and lymph nodes from the head and thoracic regions of noncervid species were submitted to NVSL and MDCH for culture since many of these animals did not exhibit visible lesions.[3]

Michigan has approximately 1.3 million cattle on 17,000 farms and 200,000 goats, bison, and privately owned cervids. As of June 25, 2001, the USDA and MDA have skin-tested over 601,965 Michigan livestock and 11,400 privately owned cervid (deer and elk) for bovine TB. In the high-risk area, 41 TB-infected cows have been found in 14 beef herds and 2 dairy herds. Fourteen of these cattle herds have been depopulated or are in the process of being depopulated, and 2 are on the "test and remove" plan. Positive animals have been found in Alpena, Alcona, Presque Isle, and Montmorency Counties. These counties are considered the high-risk area.[3] No human cases of *M. bovis* have been traced to the TB-infected deer. As of May 23, 2001, 116 privately owned white-tailed deer have been tested and 14 were culture-positive for bovine TB from a herd of 325 deer.[3,4]

During these wildlife surveys, 340 white-tailed deer, 1 elk, 14 coyotes, 2 raccoons, 1 black bear, 2 red fox, 2 opossum, and 4 bobcats have been confirmed infected with *M. bovis* by the NVSL and/or MDCH. All of the infected wildlife have come from 12 northeastern Lower Peninsula counties in Michigan. The discovery of *M. bovis* in free-ranging carnivores is rare.[2] The last documented case was in a coyote in Montana, which was associated with an infected captive elk herd. There were no visible gross or microscopic lesions in this Montana coyote nor in several of the TB-positive Michigan coyotes, a raccoon, an opossum, the black bear, a bobcat, and the red fox. This is consistent with several reports of mycobacterial isolation in noncervid wildlife without visible lesions. It is thought that this might indicate a recent infection or be due to a resistance to tuberculosis.[2,5,6]

The MDCH and the USDA National Animal Disease Center (NADC) performed restriction fragment length polymorphism analysis. They have concluded that the index deer and subsequent deer, elk, carnivore, and bovine isolates have identical IS6110 and TBN12 patterns, indicating that the same strain of *M. bovis* is involved in the outbreak in cattle and wildlife. The most likely source of the infection in the carnivore and omnivore population was through the consumption of tuberculous white-tailed deer.[2,7]

White-tailed deer in Michigan are now recognized as a reservoir host of bovine TB. It has been determined that the most likely cause of bovine TB infection in the deer is from congregating in artificially high numbers at feed sites. Once the disease is eliminated from the deer, it is presumed that the disease should die out in the carnivorous and omnivorous species. As long as bovine TB exists in the free-ranging deer population, there will be some risk to local wildlife species that feed on bovine TB-infected deer carcasses or gut piles. Therefore, continued surveillance will be necessary.[1,2]

The goal of the TB eradication strategy is to eradicate the disease by decreasing the prevalence rate of bovine TB in white-tailed deer in the TB core area to less than 1% by the fall of 2003 and to have the disease eliminated in the wild deer herd by the fall of 2010. The prevalence rate for the hunter harvest in the TB core area was 2.3%, 4.4%, 2.5%, 2.2%, and 2.3% for the years 1996 to 2000, respectively. The wildlife strategy consists of deer management actions and wildlife disease surveys. Deer management actions such as a ban on feeding and increased deer harvest are used to eliminate bovine TB in wildlife, while wildlife disease surveys are used to monitor the prevalence of bovine TB and the geographical spread of the disease. Hunters are asked to examine deer from all areas of the state and to submit their deer heads for free TB testing from the 42-county intensive surveillance area.[1,3]

The presence of a wildlife reservoir of TB in Michigan poses a serious threat to the control and eradication programs that are now in their final stages in the United States. Recent risk assessments completed by the Centers for Epidemiology and Animal Health of the USDA have indicated that *M. bovis* will continue to exist in the free-ranging deer population of northern Michigan in 2010 even with aggressive efforts to eliminate the disease.[2,8]

REFERENCES

1. SCHMITT, S.M. *et al.* 1997. Bovine tuberculosis in free-ranging white-tailed deer from Michigan. J. Wildl. Dis. **33**(4): 749–758.
2. WHIPPLE, D.L. *et al.* 2000. Reemergence of tuberculosis in animals in the United States. *In* Emerging Diseases of Animals, pp. 281–299. ASM Press. Washington, District of Columbia.
3. ANONYMOUS. 2001 (March). Bovine tuberculosis in Michigan: activities report, Lansing, MI (http://www.bovinetb.com).
4. PALMER, M.V. *et al.* 2000. Naturally occurring tuberculosis in white-tailed deer. J. Am. Vet. Med. Assoc. **216**(12): 1921–1924.
5. BRUNING-FANN, C.S. *et al.* 2001. Bovine tuberculosis in free-ranging carnivores from Michigan. J. Wildl. Dis. **37**(1): 58–64.
6. BRUNING-FANN, C.S. *et al.* 1998. *Mycobacterium bovis* in coyotes from Michigan. J. Wildl. Dis. **34**(3): 632–636.
7. WHIPPLE, D.L. *et al.* 1997. Restriction fragment length polymorphism analysis of *Mycobacterium bovis* isolates from captive and free-ranging animals. J. Vet. Diagn. Invest. **9**: 381–386.
8. CORSO, B.A. 1999. Risks associated with *M. bovis* in Michigan free-ranging white-tailed deer: an update to the 1996 report. USDA, APHIS, VS, CEAH, Fort Collins, CO.

Bovine Tuberculosis in Michigan Wildlife and Livestock

STEPHEN M. SCHMITT,[a] DANIEL J. O'BRIEN, [a] COLLEEN S. BRUNING-FANN,[b] AND SCOTT D. FITZGERALD[c]

[a]Wildlife Disease Laboratory, Rose Lake Wildlife Research Station, Michigan Department of Natural Resources, East Lansing, Michigan 48823, USA

[b]Veterinary Services, Animal and Plant Health Inspection Service, United States Department of Agriculture, East Lansing, Michigan 48823, USA

[c]Animal Health Diagnostic Laboratory and Department of Pathology, College of Veterinary Medicine, Michigan State University, East Lansing, Michigan 48824, USA

ABSTRACT: Since 1994, the state of Michigan has recognized a problem with bovine tuberculosis (TB), caused by *Mycobacterium bovis*, in wild white-tailed deer from a 12-county area in northeastern Lower Michigan. A total of 65,000 free-ranging deer have been tested, and 340 have been found to be positive for *M. bovis*. The disease has been found in other wildlife species, and, in 1998, in domestic cattle, where to date 13 beef cattle and 2 dairy cattle herds have been diagnosed with bovine TB. Unfortunately, the situation is unique in that there have never been reports of self-sustaining bovine TB in a wild, free-ranging cervid population in North America. Scientists, biologists, epidemiologists, and veterinarians who have studied this situation have concluded that the most logical theory is that high deer densities and the focal concentration caused by baiting (the practice of hunting deer over feed) and feeding are the factors most likely responsible for the establishment of self-sustaining TB in free-ranging Michigan deer. Baiting and feeding have been banned since 1998 in counties where the disease has been found. In addition, the deer herd has been reduced by 50% in the endemic area with the use of unlimited antlerless permits. The measures of apparent TB prevalence have been decreased by half since 1997, providing hopeful preliminary evidence that eradication strategies are succeeding.

KEYWORDS: bovine tuberculosis; *Mycobacterium bovis*; white-tailed deer

Since 1994, the state of Michigan has recognized a problem with bovine tuberculosis, caused by *Mycobacterium bovis*, in wild white-tailed deer (*Odocoileus virginianus*) from a 12-county area in northeastern Lower Michigan (FIG. 1). A total of 64,423 free-ranging deer have been tested, and 340 have been found to be positive for *M. bovis* (TABLE 1). The disease has been found in other wildlife species, including 1 elk (*Cervus elaphus*), 13 coyotes (*Canus latrans*), 2 raccoons (*Procyon lotor*), 2 opossums (*Didelphis virginiana*), 2 bobcats (*Felis rufus*), 4 black bear (*Ursus americanus*), and 2 red fox (*Vulpes vulpes*) (TABLE 2), and, in 1998, in domestic cat-

Address for correspondence. Dr. Stephen M. Schmitt, Wildlife Disease Laboratory, Rose Lake Wildlife Research Station, Michigan Department of Natural Resources, East Lansing, MI 48823. Voice: 517-373-9358; fax: 517-641-6022.

schmitts@state.mi.us

Ann. N.Y. Acad. Sci. 969: 262–268 (2002). © 2002 New York Academy of Sciences.

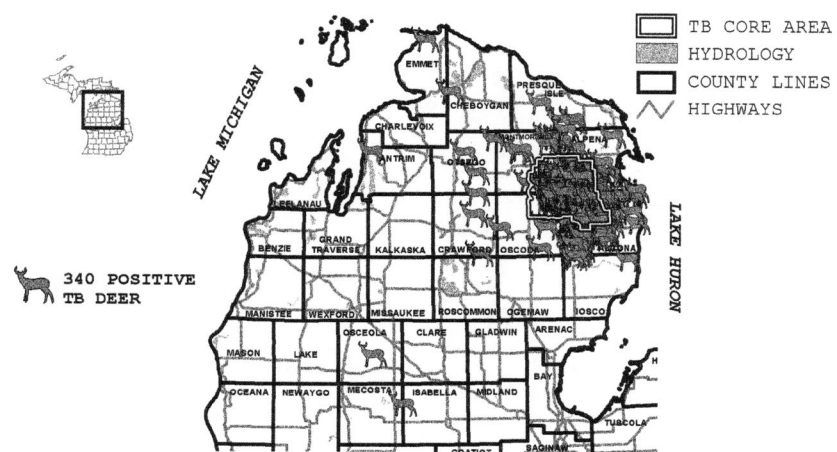

FIGURE 1. Location of *Mycobacterium bovis*–infected white-tailed deer in Michigan, 1975, 1994–2001.

tle, where to date 14 beef and 2 dairy cattle herds have been diagnosed with bovine tuberculosis.

Recognizing the potential economic and public health consequences of bovine tuberculosis to the state, the governor has issued orders to eradicate *M. bovis* from the state's deer population. Unfortunately, the situation is unique in that there have never been reports of self-sustaining bovine TB in a wild, free-ranging cervid population in North America. There are no existing control programs for bovine TB in wild deer, and there is much about bovine TB in deer that is currently unknown. Scientists, biologists, epidemiologists, and veterinarians who have studied this situation have concluded that the most logical theory is that high deer population densities and the focal concentration caused by baiting (the practice of hunting deer over feed) and feeding are the factors most likely responsible for the establishment of self-sustaining bovine TB in free-ranging Michigan deer.[1] By congregating deer into close contact with each other repeatedly, baiting and feeding provide ideal conditions for the transmission of bovine TB via both inhalation of infectious aerosols and ingestion of bovine TB–contaminated feed.[2]

The elimination of bovine TB from free-ranging deer is likely to be a difficult goal, but it is an extremely important one to accomplish. It will require the cooperation and collaboration of state and federal animal health and wildlife resource agencies. Animal health agencies do not have sufficient expertise in wildlife biology and management techniques to address the situation independently; the same can be said for wildlife resource agencies faced with diseases in domestic animal populations. Therefore, multiple agencies must rely on each other and work collaboratively to deal with the control of disease in wildlife; unilateral efforts cannot be expected to succeed. It should be understood that wildlife resource agencies want their free-ranging wildlife populations to be free of disease just as much as animal health agencies want domestic animals to be free of disease.[3]

TABLE 1. Summary of bovine tuberculosis testing of free-ranging white-tailed deer in Michigan by year

Year	Tested positive	Total tested
1975	1	1
1994	1	1
1995	27	814
1996	47	4471
1997	73	3705
1998	78	9067
1999	58	19,500
2000	53	25,857
2001 (ongoing)	2	1007
Total	370	64,423

TABLE 2. Summary of noncervid wildlife tuberculosis testing by species

Species	Tested	Positive
American badger (*Taxidea taxus*)	25	
Black bear (*Ursa americanus*)	153	4
Bobcat (*Felis rufus*)	53	4
Coyote (*Canus latrans*)	291	13
Feral cat (*Felis domesticus*)	25	
Feral dog (*Canis domesticus*)	1	
Gray fox (*Urocyon cinereoargenteus*)	4	
Mink (*Mustela vison*)	3	
Opossum (*Didelphis virginiana*)	261	2
Northern river otter (*Lutra canadensis*)	8	
Porcupine (*Erithizon dorsatum*)	1	
Raccoon (*Procyon lotor*)	220	2
Red fox (*Vulpes vulpes*)	18	2
Striped skunk (*Mephitis mephitis*)	21	
Snowshoe hare (*Lepis americanus*)	1	
Long-tailed weasel (*Mustela frenata*)	1	
Total	1086	27

A management strategy recommended by a multiagency committee composed of individuals with disease expertise and jurisdiction included surveying wildlife populations, testing livestock, educating the public about bovine TB, eliminating feeding and baiting of deer, reducing the deer density through legal hunting in areas of

Michigan where bovine TB has been found, and banning the transport of free-ranging deer from the infected area.

A comprehensive statewide program of surveillance of free-ranging deer populations is necessary to identify areas that will need intensified management practices, and to monitor the success of these practices. The continued evaluation of the prevalence of the disease allows the Michigan Department of Natural Resources to determine the reservoir of existing disease, define geographic areas of infection, and assess trends in disease occurrence. Such information will need to be collected for many years in order to interpret trends. The deer surveillance plan focuses on areas that are most likely to have bovine TB–positive free-ranging deer. The plan is science based, using past and present livestock infection rates, locations of livestock, areas of deer density, and appropriate sample sizes for statistical analysis. The plan is coordinated with surveillance of livestock conducted by the Michigan Department of Agriculture, and it is practical in terms of manpower, money, and laboratory capacities.

A strong education program is necessary to bring about public understanding of, develop support for, and encourage participation in the TB eradication project. Improved communication, both at the grassroots level and through statewide marketing, is vital to the success of the education program. Continued and enhanced contact with key audiences (i.e., livestock producers, industry representatives, the media, hunters, and recreational wildlife viewers) will lead to an understanding of the recommended strategies for *M. bovis* eradication in the white-tailed deer and livestock populations. Examples of ongoing education efforts include Michigan Department of Natural Resources/Michigan Department of Agriculture/Michigan State University extension training sessions, bovine TB brochures and newsletters, the annual Bovine TB in Michigan conference, a bovine TB web site, infomercials, satellite training sessions, and press packets.

Methods employed for eradicating bovine TB from free-ranging Michigan deer should decrease the transmission of bovine TB among deer. Reduction of transmission can be enhanced in two ways: reduction in the number of infected animals, and reduction in the amount of contact (direct or indirect) between infected and susceptible animals. Increasing the hunter harvest of deer will reduce the overall number of deer as well as reduce the average age of the deer population. Hunting regulations should be liberalized to remove greater numbers of antlerless deer to control deer populations and to remove greater numbers of adult males because a higher prevalence of bovine TB has been observed in adult male deer in Michigan (TABLE 3). The goal of liberalized hunting regulations should be a smaller deer herd with a younger age structure.

Elimination of baiting and supplemental feeding of deer will reduce the deer population as the herd density approaches the carrying capacity of the land, and will decrease contact among deer. Artificial feed supplies (baiting and supplemental feeding) increase the density of deer populations beyond the carrying capacity. Even if the deer herd density is not artificially inflated, the presence of feed and bait encourages unnatural congregation of the animals, thereby increasing contact among deer and enhancing the transmission of infectious agents. Large numbers of animals in close proximity for extended periods of time are more likely to inhale infected aerosolized droplets or to consume food contaminated by coughing and exhalation.[1]

TABLE 3. Bovine tuberculosis apparent prevalence for endemic area by year and various sex and age groupings

Year	Both sexes		Two years and older	
	All ages	Yearlings	Does	Bucks
1996	2.3%	1.3%	2.7%	4.0%
1997	4.4%	1.5%	4.7%	9.5%
1998[a]	2.4%	1.4%	1.9%	7.7%
1999[b]	2.2%	0.6%	2.8%	4.3%
2000[c]	2.3%	0.6%	2.1%	4.9%

[a]Feeding banned, baiting restricted, doe harvest increased.
[b]Continued feeding ban, baiting banned, doe harvest increased.
[c]Continued feeding ban, baiting banned.

The discovery of endemic tuberculosis in deer coupled with the wide host range of *Mycobacterium bovis*,[4] the causative agent of bovine TB, provided the impetus for a survey of other wild species present in the area.[5] Wildlife species selected for inclusion in the ongoing study are those noncervid mammalian species present in the area where deer have been found with bovine TB and whose population density was sufficient to allow collection. Species that have been tested in this survey are the badger (*Taxidea taxus*), black bear, bobcat, coyote, feral cat (*Felis domesticus*), feral dog (*Canis domesticus*), gray fox (*Urocyon cinereoargonteus*), mink (*Mustela vison*), opossum, otter (*Lutra canadensis*), porcupine (*Erithizon dorsatum*), raccoon, red fox, striped skunk (*Mephitis mephitis*), snowshoe hare (*Lepus americanus*), and long-tailed weasel (*Mustela frenata*). To date, 1080 noncervid animals have been tested, with 13 coyotes, 2 raccoons, 4 black bear, 4 bobcats, 2 red fox, and 2 opossums found or suspected to be infected with *Mycobacterium bovis* (FIG. 2). Since all six of these species are known to be opportunistic scavengers,[6] the most likely source of infection for these animals was through the consumption of tuberculous white-tailed deer.[7]

Cranial, thoracic, and abdominal lymph nodes, as well as any gross lesions, are collected routinely for histology and mycobacterial culture from all noncervid carcasses examined.[7] Designation as infected is based solely on positive culture results. The lack of any gross or microscopic lesions in the vast majority of Michigan noncervids tested thus far indicates that these animals were either infected recently (sufficient time had not elapsed to allow the development of lesions) or that the development of discernable lesions was impaired due to the relative resistance of these animals to tuberculosis.[4] Thus far, high numbers of bacteria have not been associated with lesions from the native Michigan noncervid wildlife. Without extensive lesion development containing enormous numbers of bacteria and an avenue of excretion of the bacteria from the body, successful disease transmission to other animals is doubtful.

The number of tuberculous noncervid wildlife, the variety of species involved, and the geographic spacing between the cases is more indicative of disease spillover from free-ranging deer, the primary reservoir to these noncervid wildlife species, rather than of endemic tuberculosis. Although it is currently thought that no wildlife

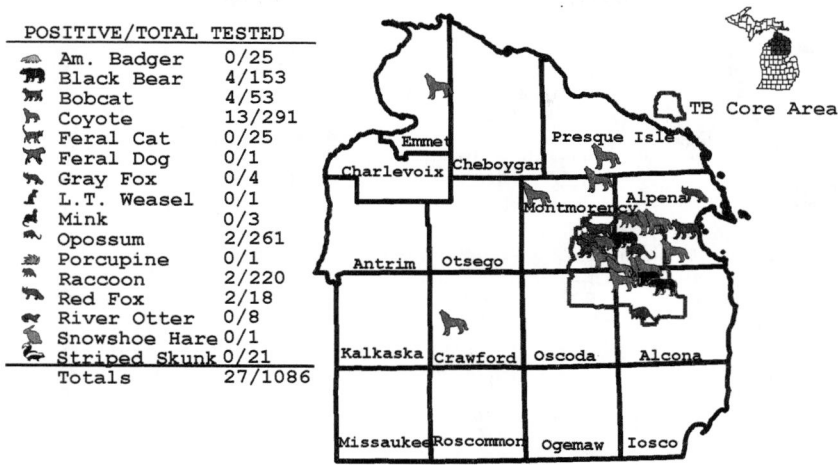

POSITIVE/TOTAL TESTED	
Am. Badger	0/25
Black Bear	4/153
Bobcat	4/53
Coyote	13/291
Feral Cat	0/25
Feral Dog	0/1
Gray Fox	0/4
L.T. Weasel	0/1
Mink	0/3
Opossum	2/261
Porcupine	0/1
Raccoon	2/220
Red Fox	2/18
River Otter	0/8
Snowshoe Hare	0/1
Striped Skunk	0/21
Totals	27/1086

FIGURE 2. Location of *Mycobacterium bovis*–infected noncervid wildlife in Michigan, 1996–2001.

other than white-tailed deer serve as a reservoir for tuberculosis in Michigan, continued and expanded wildlife surveys and experimental inoculation studies are in progress.

Michigan has a small elk population of approximately 1200 animals, whose range overlaps into the area of Michigan where TB-positive deer have been found. Since 1984, tightly controlled annual elk hunts have been held in Michigan, and almost 3500 elk have been harvested. All of the elk carcasses and gut piles were examined; no TB lesions were noted. With the discovery of bovine tuberculosis in the white-tailed deer population that shares much of the elk range, hunters were asked in 1996 to voluntarily turn in elk heads to be examined for bovine TB. Since 1998, hunter-harvested elk head submission has been mandatory. Along with road kills and other losses, a total of 848 elk have been tested for the disease from May 1996 to present. To date, 1 adult female elk has been confirmed positive for bovine TB, having exhibited a unilateral tonsil lesion. Analysis by restriction fragment length polymorphisms of DNA extracted from the TB isolate cultured from this elk indicates that it is the same strain found in infected cattle, deer, and other wildlife in the area. It is believed that the elk herd has recently, in the last several years, been infected with bovine TB.

In summary, the two main strategies for eradicating bovine TB from free-ranging Michigan deer are to minimize concentrations of deer by eliminating baiting and feeding and to reduce deer numbers through hunting to the biological carrying capacity. Baiting and feeding have been banned since 1998 in counties where the disease has been found. In addition, the deer herd has been reduced by 50% in the endemic area with the use of unlimited antlerless permits. The measures of apparent bovine TB prevalence have decreased by half since 1997, providing hopeful preliminary evidence that eradication strategies are succeeding.

REFERENCES

1. SCHMITT, S.M., S.D. FITZGERALD, T.M. COOLEY, et al. 1997. Bovine tuberculosis in free-ranging white-tailed deer from Michigan. J. Wildl. Dis. 33(4): 749–758.
2. WHIPPLE, D.L. & M.V. PALMER. 2000. Survival of Mycobacterium bovis on feeds used for baiting white-tailed deer (Odocoileus virginianus) in Michigan. In 49th Annual Wildlife Disease Association Conference Proceedings: 21. Wildlife Disease Association, Grand Teton National Park, Wyoming.
3. SALMAN, M.D., M. MILLER, J. CLIFFORD, et al. 2000. Report of the USAHA working group on tuberculosis: domestic animal/wildlife interface. In Proceedings: One Hundred and Fourth Annual Meeting of the United States Animal Health Association, Birmington, Alabama. Carter-Printing Company. Richmond, VA, pp. 659-660.
4. FRANCIS, J. 1958. Tuberculosis in Animals and Man. Cassell. London.
5. BRUNING-FANN, C.S., S.M. SCHMITT, S.D. FITZGERALD, et al. 1998. Mycobacterium bovis in coyotes in Michigan. J. Wildl. Dis. 34: 632–636.
6. BAKER, R.H. 1983. Michigan Mammals. Michigan State University Press. East Lansing, MI.
7. BRUNING-FANN, C.S., S.M. SCHMITT, S.D. FITZGERALD, et al. 2001. Bovine tuberculosis in free-ranging carnivores from Michigan. J. Wildl. Dis. 37: 58–64.

Increasing Risks of Introduction of Heartwater onto the American Mainland Associated with Animal Movements

MICHAEL J. BURRIDGE,[a] LEIGH-ANNE SIMMONS,[a] TREVOR F. PETER,[b] AND SUMAN M. MAHAN[b]

[a]Department of Pathobiology, University of Florida, P.O. Box 110880, Gainesville, Florida 32611-0880, USA

[b]University of Florida/USAID/SADC Heartwater Research Project, Central Veterinary Laboratory (Diagnostic and Research Branch), Box CY 551, Causeway, Harare, Zimbabwe

ABSTRACT: Opportunities to introduce heartwater onto the American mainland through animal movements include importation from Africa of tick-infested reptiles and of subclinically infected wild ungulates and importation of livestock from islands in the Caribbean infested with *Amblyomma variegatum* ticks. Measures to control importation of heartwater vectors on reptiles include importation bans of infested species, treatment of imported reptiles, and eradication of established infestations on the American mainland. Measures to control importation of infected wildlife must focus on improved methods, such as the PCR assay, of screening animals to prevent the entry of carriers of *Cowdria ruminantium*. Measures to control importation of infected animals from the Caribbean must be based on knowledge of the islands that are infected with *C. ruminantium* so that the risk of dissemination of heartwater can be established.

KEYWORDS: heartwater; *Cowdria ruminantium*; *Amblyomma* ticks; reptiles; Africa; Caribbean; America

INTRODUCTION

Heartwater is a disease that causes high mortality and heavy economic losses in domestic ruminants.[1] It is caused by infection with the rickettsia *Cowdria ruminantium*, which is transmitted by ticks of the genus *Amblyomma*.[2] The disease is widespread in sub-Saharan Africa and also occurs in the eastern Caribbean.[1] In 1997, Burridge[3] described the threat posed to the livestock and deer populations of the United States by heartwater. He listed four reasons why the threat should be considered seriously: (1) the risk of introduction of infected ticks from the Caribbean was ever present; (2) the risk of introduction of infected ticks on imported reptiles was becoming apparent; (3) the risk of introduction of infected wild game animals from

Address for correspondence: Dr. Michael J. Burridge, Department of Pathobiology, University of Florida, P.O. Box 110880, Gainesville, FL 32611-0880. Voice: 352-392-4700 ext. 3131; fax: 352-846-0246.
burridgem@mail.vetmed.ufl.edu

Ann. N.Y. Acad. Sci. 969: 269–274 (2002). © 2002 New York Academy of Sciences.

Africa was real; and (4) two tick species indigenous to the Americas had been shown to be experimental vectors of heartwater. In this article, information on the risks associated with animal movements is updated, and recommendations are made on measures to minimize these risks.

RISKS ASSOCIATED WITH INTERNATIONAL TRADE IN LIVE REPTILES

The risk of introduction of heartwater into the United States through the international trade in live reptiles was emphasized by the results of three of our recent studies. First, we found that two of the imported reptilian tick species that have been reported to be experimental vectors of heartwater, *A. marmoreum* and *A. sparsum*, have become established in Florida,[4,5] although subsequent actions have successfully eradicated the known established infestations.[5] Second, we demonstrated convincingly that *A. marmoreum* ticks that had originated from infested reptiles on premises in Florida are competent experimental vectors of *C. ruminantium*.[6] Finally, we showed that one shipment of ticks, imported from Zambia into Florida on leopard tortoises (*Geochelone pardalis*), was positive for *C. ruminantium* infection by PCR assay.[7] This finding was the first reported evidence of the introduction of *C. ruminantium*–infected ticks into the United States, and it demonstrated that the continued international dissemination of *A. sparsum* on tortoises exported from Africa posed a real risk for the spread of heartwater to the United States and elsewhere.

RISKS ASSOCIATED WITH INTERNATIONAL TRADE IN WILD GAME ANIMALS

Wild African ungulates have been imported into the United States for many years, and importations continue even though some are of species proven to be susceptible to heartwater. It has been known for some time that a wide range of wild ruminants are susceptible to *C. ruminantium* infection,[8] but only recently was it shown that many of the susceptible species can become subclinical carriers of *C. ruminantium*, capable of infecting ticks that later are able to transmit fatal infections to domestic livestock. Carrier species include the blesbok (*Damaliscus pygargus*), the black wildebeest (*Connochaetes gnou*),[9,10] the African buffalo (*Syncerus caffer*),[11] the eland (*Taurotragus oryx*), the giraffe (*Giraffa camelopardalis*), the greater kudu (*Tragelaphus strepsiceros*), the blue wildebeest (*Connochaetes taurinus*),[12] and the sable antelope (*Hippotragus niger*).[13] It is clear, therefore, that at least some species of wild ruminants from heartwater-endemic regions of Africa are capable, if imported, of introducing heartwater into the United States.

The United States Department of Agriculture (USDA) continues to utilize serological tests to screen animals, including wildlife species, for *C. ruminantium* infection using the indirect fluorescent antibody test and, more recently, also a competitive ELISA. However, it is well known that *Ehrlichia* spp. cross-react with *C. ruminantium* in the indirect fluorescent antibody test,[14-17] and concerns over use of this test for screening animals for importation into the United States have already been expressed.[14,18] The indirect fluorescent antibody test was compared with the competitive ELISA utilizing *C. ruminantium* antigens, and in both tests extensive cross-reactions were recorded with antibodies to ehrlichial infections.[17] It is evident, therefore, that positive serological responses are uninterpretable in current screening tests of individual animals for heartwater since it is impossible to determine whether they are due to exposure to *C. ruminantium* or exposure to some cross-reacting agent such as an *Ehrlichia* sp. Furthermore, recent studies in Zimbabwe have shown that some cattle known to be carriers of *C. ruminantium* infection can be seronegative,[19] demonstrating that even a negative serological response to current tests does not always indicate absence from *C. ruminantium* infection. Clearly current tests used by the USDA to screen wild ruminants for heartwater prior to importation from Africa are not adequate to prevent the introduction of subclinically infected animals.

RISKS ASSOCIATED WITH MOVEMENT OF ANIMALS FROM THE CARIBBEAN

Heartwater was confirmed in the Caribbean for the first time on the French island of Guadeloupe in 1980[20] and soon thereafter on the islands of Marie Galante[21] and Antigua.[22] However, the vector of heartwater in the Caribbean, *A. variegatum*, has spread as far north as Puerto Rico and as far south as Barbados and St. Vincent.[23] There is strong circumstantial evidence that much of the recent inter-island spread of *A. variegatum* has occurred through the movement of infested migratory birds, and in particular cattle egrets (*Bubulcus ibis*).[24] The potential for the cattle egret to introduce *A. variegatum* ticks, and thereby heartwater, into the United States was graphically demonstrated in 1992 when a cattle egret, banded on the heartwater-endemic island of Guadeloupe, was found on Long Key in Florida.[24]

By 1988, *A. variegatum* had spread to at least 18 islands in the eastern Caribbean.[23] There are no published reports of attempts to isolate *C. ruminantium* from *A. variegatum*-infested islands since heartwater was detected on Guadeloupe, Marie Galante and Antigua in the early 1980s. Consequently, it is not known definitively whether or not heartwater exists on 15 of the 18 *A. variegatum*-infested islands in the Caribbean, and yet cattle, for example, are still exported from at least one of the infested islands, St. Croix, to mainland America.

MEASURES TO MINIMIZE SPREAD OF HEARTWATER

Control of Importation of Ticks on Reptiles

In response to the findings that several exotic tick vectors of heartwater had been introduced into Florida on multiple occasions on imported reptiles,[25] the USDA requested and received in 1999 a crisis exemption from the Unites States Environmental Protection Agency to use certain permethrin and cyfluthrin products, registered for use on mammals, for tick control on reptiles and in reptile facilities. This crisis exemption provided state and federal authorities with acaricides to treat tick infestations on reptiles until such time as acaricides were registered for specific use on reptiles. Later, in response to the report providing evidence of *C. ruminantium* infection in ticks found on tortoises imported into Florida,[7] the USDA passed an interim rule in March 2000, prohibiting the importation into the United States of leopard tortoises, African spurred tortoises (*Geochelone sulcata*) and Bell's hinge-backed tortoises (*Kinixys belliana*).[26] This rule provided regulatory authority to prohibit the importation into the United States of three of the chelonian species most commonly found to be infested with tick vectors of heartwater.[27]

Treatment of imported tortoises, either at the port of entry or at the premises of the importer, is another measure that will assist the control of exotic ticks, including those that are potential vectors of heartwater. Recent studies have identified one permethrin product (Provent-a-Mite®, Pro Products, Mahopac, NY) as an acaricide formulation that is safe for reptiles, that can be administered easily either to reptiles or to their bedding and that will predictably kill reptilian ticks.[5]

The regulations and treatment measures mentioned above should greatly reduce the risk of introduction of tick vectors of heartwater into the United States. However, it is evident that numerous shipments of infested reptiles have already been imported, at least into Florida, and have become established on premises housing reptiles. There is a urgent need to eradicate these infestations in order to minimize the risk that exotic vectors of heartwater will spread to native fauna and become established as indigenous tick species. Protocols for exotic tick eradication have been developed in Florida, and trials, using a permethrin product (Provent-a-Mite®) for treatment of infested reptiles and a cyfluthrin product (Tempo®, Bayer Corp., Kansas City, MO) for treatment of the premises, have produced excellent results.[5]

Control of Importation of Infected Wildlife

Since at least some wild African ungulates can harbor subclinical *C. ruminantium* infections, it is imperative that any ungulates intended for importation into the United States be tested for heartwater before entry is permitted. Such testing must consider the *C. ruminantium* carrier status of any wild ungulates from heartwater-endemic regions of Africa. The only diagnostic test shown to be able to detect subclinical *C. ruminantium* infections is the PCR assay.[28] It is recommended that all wild ungulates being considered for importation from heartwater-endemic regions of Africa be tested for *C. ruminantium* infection by the PCR assay,[29] with those testing positive refused entry into the United States. A request was submitted to the USDA in December 1997 for validation of the PCR assay for diagnosis of *C. ruminantium* infection, but a decision is still pending. The more sensitive and specific PCR assay that detects *C. ruminantium* infection should be used to screen animals for heartwater prior to importation rather than the non-specific serological tests currently in use by the USDA that can detect only antibodies of uncertain origin. Such a change in the method of screening of animals for heartwater is necessary if subclinically infected wildlife are to be prevented from introducing heartwater into the United States. Furthermore, the Office International des Epizooties (OIE) in its Manual of Standards for Diagnostic Tests and Vaccines has stated that serological tests should not be used as a diagnostic method for heartwater at the individual animal level.[30]

Control of Importation of Animals from the Caribbean

A regional program to eradicate *A. variegatum* ticks, and thereby heartwater, from the Caribbean was developed in the early 1990s.[31] The eradication program was initiated in 1994 with the creation of the Caribbean Amblyomma Program, with eradication activities launched on anglophone islands in 1995. A separate eradication program was initiated by France on francophone islands. A recent report has indicated problems with progress of both eradication programs, with unexpected new foci of *A. variegatum* infestation appearing in the northern (St. Croix), central (Dominica) and southern (St. Vincent) regions of the Caribbean.[32] It is as important as ever, therefore, to determine which *A. variegatum*-infested islands are infected with heartwater to prevent the spread of the disease from the eastern Caribbean to the American mainland. It is recommended that *A. variegatum* populations be sampled on each infested Caribbean island to determine whether or not there is evidence of *C. ruminantium* infection on each island, using such techniques as the PCR assay, tick transmission trials and cell culture isolation. Ruminants should not be imported onto the American mainland from any island showing evidence of *C. ruminantium* infection, and tick eradication efforts should be intensified on all heartwater-infected islands to minimize the opportunities for dissemination of *C. ruminantium*-infected ticks.

REFERENCES

1. CAMUS, E., N. BARRÉ & G. UILENBERG. 1996. Heartwater (Cowdriosis). A Review (2nd edit.). Office International des Epizooties. Paris.
2. WALKER, J.B. & A. OLWAGE. 1987. The tick vectors of *Cowdria ruminantium* (Ixodoidea, Ixodidae, genus *Amblyomma*) and their distribution. Onderstepoort J. Vet. Res. **54:** 353–379.
3. BURRIDGE, M.J. 1997. Heartwater: an increasingly serious threat to the livestock and deer populations of the United States. *In* Proceedings of the 101st Annual Meeting of the United States Animal Health Association, pp. 582–597. Spectrum Press. Richmond, VA.
4. ALLAN, S.A., L.A. SIMMONS & M.J. BURRIDGE. 1998. Establishment of the tortoise tick *Amblyomma marmoreum* (Acari: Ixodidae) on a reptile-breeding facility in Florida. J. Med. Entomol. **35:** 621–624.
5. BURRIDGE, M.J., L.A. SIMMONS, T.F. PETER & S.M. MAHAN. 2002. Control and eradication of reptilian tick infestations, with particular reference to vectors of heartwater. Ann. New York Acad. Sci. **969:** in press.
6. PETER, T.F., M.J. BURRIDGE & S.M. MAHAN. 2000. Competence of the African tortoise tick, *Amblyomma marmoreum* (Acari: Ixodidae), as a vector of the agent of heartwater (*Cowdria ruminantium*). J. Parasitol. **86:** 438–441.
7. BURRIDGE, M.J., L.A. SIMMONS, B.H. SIMBI, *et al.* 2000. Evidence of *Cowdria ruminantium* infection (heartwater) in *Amblyomma sparsum* ticks found on tortoises imported into Florida. J. Parasitol. **86:** 1135–1136.
8. OBEREM, P.T. & J.D. BEZUIDENHOUT. 1987. Heartwater in hosts other than domestic ruminants. Onderstepoort J. Vet. Res. **54:** 271–275.
9. NEITZ, W.O. 1933. The blesbuck (*Damaliscus albifrons*) as a carrier of heartwater and blue tongue. J.S. Afr. Vet. Med. Assoc. **4:** 24-26.
10. NEITZ, W.O. 1935. The blesbuck (*Damaliscus albifrons*) and the black-wildebeest (*Connochaetes gnu*) as carriers of heartwater. Onderstepoort J. Vet. Sci. Anim. Ind. **5:** 35-40.
11. ANDREW, H.R. & R.A.I. NORVAL. 1989. The carrier status of sheep, cattle, and African buffalo recovered from heartwater. Vet. Parasitol. **34:** 261–266.
12. PETER, T.F., E.C. ANDERSON, M.J. BURRIDGE & S.M. MAHAN. 1998. Demonstration of a carrier state for *Cowdria ruminantium* in wild ruminants from Africa. J. Wildl. Dis. **34:** 567–575.
13. PETER, T.F., E.C. ANDERSON, M.J. BURRIDGE, *et al.* 1999. Susceptibility and carrier status of impala, sable and tsessebe for *Cowdria ruminantium* infection (heartwater). J. Parasitol. **85:** 468– 472.

14. LOGAN, L.L., C.J. HOLLAND, C.A. MEBUS & M. RISTIC. 1986. Serological relationship between *Cowdria ruminantium* and certain ehrlichia. Vet. Rec. **119:** 458–459.
15. DU PLESSIS, J.L., E. CAMUS, P.T. OBEREM & L. MALAN. 1987. Heartwater serology: some problems with the interpretation of results. Onderstepoort J. Vet. Res. **54:** 327–329.
16. JONGEJAN, F., L.A. WASSINK, M.J.C. THIELEMANS, *et al.* 1989. Serotypes in *Cowdria ruminantium* and their relationship with *Ehrlichia phagocytophila* determined by immunofluorescence. Vet. Microbiol. **21:** 31–40.
17. DU PLESSIS, J.L., J.D. BEZUIDENHOUT, M.S. BRETT, *et al.* 1993. The sero-diagnosis of heartwater: a comparison of five tests. Rev. Elev. Méd. Vét. Pays Trop. **46:** 123-129.
18. DILBECK, P.M., J.F. EVERMANN, T.B. CRAWFORD, *et al.* 1990. Isolation of a previously undescribed rickettsia from an aborted bovine fetus. J. Clin. Microbiol. **28:** 814-816.
19. SEMU, S.M., T.F. PETER, D. MUKWEDEYA, *et al.* 2001. Antibody responses to MAP 1B and other *Cowdria ruminantium* antigens are down regulated in cattle challenged with tick-transmitted heartwater. Clin. Diagn. Lab. Immunol. **8:** 388–396.
20. PERREAU, P., P.C. MOREL, N. BARRÉ & P. DURAND. 1980. Existence de la cowdriose (heartwater) à *Cowdria ruminantium* chez les ruminants des Antilles francaises (La Guadeloupe) et des Mascareignes (La Réunion et Ile Maurice). Rev. Elev. Méd. Vét. Pays Trop. **33:** 21–22.
21. UILENBERG, G., N. BARRÉ, E. CAMUS, *et al.* 1984. Heartwater in the Caribbean. Prev. Vet. Med. **2:** 255–267.
22. BIRNIE, E.F., M.J. BURRIDGE, E. CAMUS & N. BARRÉ. 1985. Heartwater in the Caribbean: isolation of *Cowdria ruminantium* from Antigua. Vet. Rec. **116:** 121–123.
23. BARRÉ, N., G. GARRIS & E. CAMUS. 1995. Propagation of the tick *Amblyomma variegatum* in the Caribbean. Rev. Sci. Tech. Off. Int. Epizoot. **14:** 841–855.
24. CORN, J.L., N. BARRÉ, B. THIEBOT, *et al.* 1993. Potential role of cattle egrets, *Bubulcus ibis* (Ciconiformes: Ardeidae), in the dissemination of *Amblyomma variegatum* (Acari: Ixodidae) in the eastern Caribbean. J. Med. Entomol. **30:** 1029–1037.
25. BURRIDGE, M.J., L.A. SIMMONS & S.A. ALLAN. 2000. Introduction of potential heartwater vectors and other exotic ticks into Florida on imported reptiles. J. Parasitol. **86:** 700–704.
26. ANONYMOUS. 2000. Importation and interstate movement of certain land tortoises. Fed. Register **65:** 15216–15218.
27. BURRIDGE, M.J. 2001. Ticks (Acari: Ixodidae) spread by the international trade in reptiles and their potential roles in dissemination of diseases. Bull. Entomol. Res. **91:** 3–23.
28. MAHAN, S.M., T.F. PETER, B.H. SIMBI & M.J. BURRIDGE. 1998. PCR detection of *Cowdria ruminantium* infection in ticks and animals from heartwater-endemic regions of Zimbabwe. Ann. N.Y. Acad. Sci. **849:** 85–87.
29. PETER, T.F., A.F. BARBET, A.R. ALLEMAN, *et al.* 2000. Detection of the agent of heartwater, *Cowdria ruminantium,* in *Amblyomma* ticks by PCR: validation and application to field ticks. J. Clin. Microbiol. **38:** 1539–1544.
30. ANONYMOUS. 2000. Manual of Standards for Diagnostic Tests and Vaccines. 4th edit. Office International des Epizooties. Paris.
31. GARRIS, G.I., N. BARRÉ, E. CAMUS & D.D. WILSON. 1993. Progress towards a program for the eradication of *Amblyomma variegatum* from the Caribbean. Rev. Elev. Méd. Vét. Pays Trop. **46:** 359–362.
32. PEGRAM, R. 2000. Eradication of the tropical bont tick from the Caribbean: the Caribbean *Amblyomma* Programme. *In* Proceedings of the 104th Annual Meeting of the United States Animal Health Association: 449–455. Carter Printing Company. Richmond, VA.

Buffalo-Associated *Theileria parva*: The Risk to Cattle of Buffalo Translocation into the Highveld of Zimbabwe

A.A. LATIF,[a] T. HOVE,[b] G.K. KANHAI,[c] AND S. MASAKA[c]

[a]*Faculty of Science, Midrand University, P.O. Box 2986, Halfway House 1685, South Africa*

[b]*University of Zimbabwe, P.O. Box 167 MP, Harare, Zimbabwe*

[c]*Veterinary Research Laboratory, P.O. Box 8108 Causeway, Harare, Zimbabwe*

ABSTRACT: There has been an increase in the introduction of game animals, including African buffaloes, into the Highveld of Zimbabwe to establish private game reserves on condition that they are confined in separate and secured paddocks. Owing to shortages of pastures cattle were grazed in buffalo-grazed paddocks resulting in outbreaks of buffalo-derived theileriosis. This paper reports the results of epidemiological observations carried out on two game reserves to assess the risk of buffalo translocation. The infection rate with *Theileria* parasites in ticks collected from buffalo-grazed pastures was high and produced fatal theileriosis in susceptible cattle. Similarly, adult *R. appendiculatus* ticks artificially fed as nymphs on the buffaloes produced fatal infections in susceptible cattle. *Theileria parva* (Boleni), the vaccine used to immunize cattle against theileriosis, and a buffalo-derived *T. parva* stabilate (BV-1) were inoculated in naïve buffaloes to study the *Theileria* carrier-state in these animals. The two buffaloes that had received the Boleni stabilate showed no clinical theileriosis reaction; however, the ticks derived from them produced a subclinical reaction in one susceptible calf. The buffalo which had received stabilate BV-1 developed fever, high schizont parasitosis for 10 days and 15% piroplasms parasitemia. *R. appendiculatus* ticks fed as nymphs on this buffalo produced fatal theileriosis reaction in a susceptible calf.

KEYWORDS: theileriosis; *Theileria parva*; corridor disease; African buffalo; Zimbabwe Highveld

INTRODUCTION

There has been a general belief that corridor disease (buffalo-derived *Theileria parva* infection in cattle) in Zimbabwe is confined to the African buffalo (*Syncerus caffer*) environments and that the present disease control measures limit possible cattle-buffalo contact. The number of corridor disease outbreaks reported in the early 1980s was about 10% of the total theileriosis outbreaks recorded.[1] Recently, there has been an increase in the introduction of game animals, including buffaloes, into

Address for correspondence: Dr. A.A. Latif, Faculty of Science, Midrand University, P.O. Box 2986, Halfway House 1685, South Africa. Voice: +2711 3152853; fax: +2711 3155977.
abdulal@ed.co.za

Ann. N.Y. Acad. Sci. 969: 275–279 (2002). © 2002 New York Academy of Sciences.

the Highveld to establish private game reserves. In 1992 10 farms have been autho-
rized to keep buffaloes on condition that they be confined in separate and secure paddocks (S.K. Hargreaves, personal communication, 1992). Owing to the drought
during 1990–1991 and consequent shortages of pasture, some farmers introduced
cattle into their buffalo-grazed paddocks. Three outbreaks of buffalo-derived theileriosis were reported,[2] which were considered to be the result of a breakdown in farm
management and not a national problem. Since corridor disease produces a carrier
state in buffalo and cattle,[3] the risk of transmission of pathogenic buffalo-derived
theileriosis through a breakdown in the present strict tick control or by cattle movement on the Highveld could disturb the present theileriosis control system. The
present paper shows the results of epidemiological observations carried out on two
game parks in the Highveld of Zimbabwe regarding the infectivity of ticks collected
from buffalo-grazed pastures to cattle and the carrier-state in buffaloes after infection with the *T. parva* Boleni stabilate. This stabilate was registered as a vaccine under the name Blovac for vaccination of cattle against theileriosis in Zimbabwe.[4]

MATERIALS AND METHODS

Infectivity of Cattle- or Buffalo-Derived T. parva Stabilates to Susceptible Buffaloes

Three buffaloes (aged 1–2 years) born and raised in captivity at the Mazowe Field
Station, Zimbabwe were used. They were serologically negative to *T. parva* schizont
antigen in the IFA test,[5] and no *Theileria* piroplasms were seen in their blood smears.
Their susceptibility was also confirmed by attempted *Theileria* tick pick-up using *R.
appendiculatus* nymphs and testing the infectivity of the adults from each buffalo in
one susceptible calf. The feeding of the adult ticks obtained from the three buffaloes
did not transmit *Theileria* infection in the susceptible calves as judged by parasitological and serological examination. Two of the buffaloes (nos. 24 and 25) were inoculated with 4.0 mL each (equivalent to 80 ticks) of the cattle-derived *T. parva*
Boleni stabilate.[2] The third buffalo (no. 29) was given 1.0 mL of the buffalo-derived
T. parva BV-1 stabilate.[2] The three buffaloes were monitored daily by taking rectal
temperatures, lymph node biopsy smears when these nodes became enlarged, and
thin blood smears. Tick pick-up *of Theileria* parasites using *R. appendiculatus*
nymphs was attempted when *Theileria* piroplasms were detected in blood smears of
the buffaloes. The infection rate in the adult ticks with *Theileria* parasites was
assessed,[6] and their infectivity was determined by feeding each of the three tick
batches on one susceptible calf.

Infection Rates in Ticks Collected from Game Parks

Four collections of unfed *R. appendiculatus* adults were made between January
and April,1991–1992 during the adult tick activity season[7] from two privately owned
game parks (Bally Vaughaun and Dombawera) in the Highveld. The game animals
in the parks included buffaloes, impalas (*Aepyceros melampus*), kudus (*Tragelaphus
strepiceros*), sable antelopes (*Hippotragus niger*), and others. Tick infection rate
with *Theileria* parasites was assessed and their infectivity in seven susceptible cattle

was determined. Four animals immunized using the cattle-derived *T. parva* Boleni stabilate together with two unimmunized controls were challenged with the ticks collected from the two game parks to assess their cross-immunity. The number of ticks applied was approximately 100. In addition, two Boleni-immunized cattle received a homologous stabilate challenge to ascertain their immunity. Clinical and parasitological monitoring of animals was carried out daily after tick application.

Attempted Parasite Pick-up and Transmission from Buffaloes

Tick pick-up using *R. appendiculatus* nymphs was carried out from four buffaloes kept in quarantine at Nyamandholwu, 50 km west of Bulawayo. Two of these animals (nos. 1 and 8) were found to harbor *Theileria* piroplasms; the other two buffaloes (nos. 5 and 10) did not show any piroplasms in their blood smears. The adult ticks obtained from each group of buffaloes were pooled and used to infect one susceptible calf.

RESULTS

There was no patent reaction in the two buffaloes that had received the cattle-derived *T. parva* Boleni stabilate. After a long search only one *Theileria* piroplasm parasite was seen in a blood smear from one of the two buffaloes (no. 25) on two different days. *Theileria* parasites were not detected in the salivary glands of *R. appendiculatus* adults that fed as nymphs on the ears of these two buffaloes. However, ticks derived from buffalo number 25 produced subclinical infection in a susceptible calf when they were fed in large numbers (600 engorged females were dropped from this animal). The tick batch obtained from the other buffalo (no. 24) did not transmit any infection to a susceptible calf. In contrast, buffalo number 29, which had received stabilate BV-1 developed a moderate theileriosis reaction. The schizont parasitosis persisted for 10 days, fever for 5 days; a piroplasm parasitemia of 15% was recorded. Adult ticks that had fed as nymphs on this buffalo showed a 40% infection rate, with eight infected acini per infected tick. The feeding of these ticks on a susceptible calf induced a fatal theileriosis reaction 19 days after infection.

Questing *R. appendiculatus* adults on grass tips were found in high numbers; up to 3000 ticks were easily picked by two collectors after a 2–3 hour sampling time from Bally Vaughaun Game Park. Ticks were regularly seen on animals and were also collected from grass on the game park during the months of January to the first week of June. The mean infection rate with *Theileria* in two out of the three tick batches was high, being 15% (11.6 infected acini per tick) and 34% (13.3 infected acini). These two tick batches, and the one that was not examined, were highly pathogenic, producing severe and fatal reactions in the six susceptible cattle. The only tick batch that was not infective to cattle had a low infection rate (1.8%).

All of the four Boleni-immunized cattle and the two unimmunized controls developed severe theileriosis infection following the challenge with tick batches collected from the two game parks. The Boleni-immunized cattle that were inoculated with a homologous challenge did not show any apparent reaction.

Buffaloes numbers 1 and 8, which had *Theileria* piroplasms in their blood smears, produced highly infected ticks, with a 24.7% infection rate and 54 infected acini per infected tick. The application of these ticks onto a susceptible calf produced fatal theileriosis infection. However, buffaloes number 5 and 10, which were free of piroplasm, produced uninfected ticks.

DISCUSSION

The present study showed that the cattle-derived *T. parva* Boleni, used to immunize cattle in Zimbabwe,[4] and a buffalo-derived stabilate could both produce a carrier state in buffaloes. The carrier parasites were transmissible to cattle, with the buffalo-derived stabilate producing fatal reactions. It would be interesting to study the serial passages of Boleni in buffalo/cattle to see whether the mild Boleni carrier parasites would revert to a pathogenic stock, most probably due to the very low infection rate in ticks. The carrier buffaloes are known to be more infective to ticks than carrier cattle.[8]

Previous experience had shown that cattle immunized using the cattle-derived *T. parva* Boleni stabilate resisted challenge with two buffalo-derived *T. parva* stabilates, Serengeti-transformed[9–12] and Ngong 1.[12] In contrast, the Boleni-immunized cattle in the present study were not protected against the challenge with infected ticks collected from buffalo-grazed pastures. However, Serengeti-transformed and Ngong 1 stabilates had been passaged through cattle for several years[13] and had probably lost some of the original parasite components.

Several epidemiological factors drawn from the present study could pose risks to the cattle industry through a breakdown in the present farm management, disruption in the strict tick control policy, and cattle movement. These factors include the unstable epidemiological state of *Theileria* in cattle in the Highveld. Ticks originating from buffaloes or buffalo-grazed pastures were highly pathogenic in cattle; the cattle-derived *T. parva* Boleni stabilate did not afford protection against buffalo-derived challenge; and infected buffaloes and cattle became *Theileria* carriers.

ACKNOWLEDGMENTS

This work was supported by the Food and Agriculture Organization FAO of the United Nations, funded by the Danish Government and Government of Zimbabwe.

REFERENCES

1. THOMSON, J.W. 1985. Theileriosis in Zimbabwe. *In* Immunization against Theileriosis in Africa. A.D. Irvin, Ed.: 48–57. The International Laboratory for Research on Animal Diseases (ILRAD). Nairobi.
2. ANON. 1993. Zimbabwe: studies on theileriosis and economics of tick control. 1. Epidemiology and immunization. Field Document No. 1 GCP/ZIM/013/DEN. Food and Agriculture Organization of the United Nations (FAO). Rome.
3. MARITIM, A.C., D.P., KARIUKI, *et al.* 1989. The importance of the carrier state of *Theileria parva* in the epidemiology of theileriosis and its control by immunization. *In* Theileriosis in Eastern, Central and Southern Africa. T.T. Dolan, Ed.: 121–128. The International Laboratory for Research on Animal Diseases (ILRAD). Nairobi.

4. KANHAI, G.K., R.G., PEGRAM, *et al.* 1997. Immunization of cattle in Zimbabwe using *Theileria parva* (Boleni) without concurrent tetracycline therapy. Trop. Anim. Health Prod. **29:** 92–98.

5. BURRIDGE, M.J. & C.D. KIMBER. 1972. The indirect fluorescent antibody test for experimental East Coast fever (*Theileria parva* infection of cattle): evaluation of a cell culture schizont antigen. Res. Vet. Sci. **13:** 451-455.

6. BLEWETT, D.A. & D. BRANAGAN. 1973. The demonstration of *Theileria parva* infection in infected *Rhipicephalus appendiculatus* salivary glands. Trop. Anim. Health. Prod. **5:** 27–34.

7. SHORT, N.J. & R.A.I. NORVAL. 1981. The seasonal activity of *Rhipicephalus appendiculatus* Newmann, 1901 (Acarina: Ixodidae) in the highveld of Zimbabwe Rhodesia. J. Parasitol. **67:** 77–84.

8. MARITIM, A.C., A.S. YOUNG, *et al.* 1989. *Theileria* parasites isolated from carrier cattle after immunization with *Theileria parva* by the infection and treatment method. Parasitology **99:** 139–147.

9. UILENBERG, G., N.M. PERIE, *et al.* 1982. Causal agents of bovine theileriosis in southern Africa. Trop. Anim. Health Prod. **14:** 127–140.

10. IRVIN, A.D., S.P. MORZARIA, *et al.* 1989. Immunization of cattle with a *Theileria parva* bovis stock from Zimbabwe protects against challenge with virulent *T. parva* and *T. p. lawrencei* stocks from Kenya. Vet. Parasitol. **32:** 271–278.

11. HOVE, T., F.L. MUSISI, *et al.* 1995. Challenge of *Theileria parva* (Boleni)-immunized cattle with selected East African *Theileria* stocks. Trop. Anim. Health Prod. **27:** 202–210.

12. CHUMO, R.S.C., E. TARACHA, *et al.* 1985. East coast fever field trial at Ngong, Kenya. *In* Immunization against Theileriosis in Africa. A.D. Irvin, Ed.: 79–81. The International Laboratory for Research on Animal Diseases (ILRAD). Nairobi.

13. PURNELL, R.E., A.S. YOUNG *et al.* 1974. Comparative infectivity for cattle of stabilates of *Theileria lawrencei* (Serengeti) derived from adult and nymphal ticks. J. Comp. Pathol. **84:** 523–537.

Effect of the Association of Cattle and Rusa Deer (*Cervus timorensis russa*) on Populations of Cattle Ticks (*Boophilus microplus*)

N. BARRÉ, M. BIANCHI, AND M. DE GARINE-WICHATITSKY

CIRAD-EMVT/IAC, Païta, New-Caledonia

ABSTRACT: The wild population of rusa deer (*Cervus timorensis russa*) in New Caledonia (South Pacific) is nearly as large as the cattle population. The cattle tick is widespread and occurs all year round. Opinions are divided on the role of deer in the biological cycle of the tick: i) Do they maintain a sustainable tick population that is secondarily available for cattle? ii) Do they decrease the infestation of the environment by collecting larvae on the pasture, but preventing their development to the engorged female stage? or iii) Do they contribute to both situations? An experiment was conducted in three groups of pastures, each seeded with 450 000 larvae/ha and allowed to be grazed only by cattle, only by deer, and by a mixed herd of deer and cattle (deer representing 30% of the biomass), at approximately the same stocking rate (470–510 kg/ha). After 15 months of exposure, the tick burden per weight unit of host was 42 ticks/kg for the steers-only herd and 0.01/kg for the deer-only herd. The steers in the "mixed group" harbored 7 times fewer ticks (6.2/kg) than the cattle-only group, and the deer in the "mixed group," 130 times more (1.3/kg) than the deer-only group. Five emergency acaricide treatments had to be applied in the cattle-only group, but none in the other groups. The long-term sustainability of a viable tick population on deer as well as the potential benefit resulting from the association of deer and susceptible cattle in the tick control of cattle are highlighted.

INTRODUCTION

The cattle tick is a major pest for livestock in most tropical countries. Control is usually based on a rational application of chemicals as one facet of an integrated control strategy. In areas that are small and isolated, an alternative option may be the eradication of ticks. However, in countries where cattle are in contact with wildlife —particularly wild ungulates—eradication may be difficult, with the presence of these secondary hosts complicating any eradication strategy.[1] In New Caledonia, where wild rusa deer are abundant (100–120 000 head,[2] nearly as many as cattle) and widespread (they have been recorded on 70% of the farms, Bianchi and Barré unpublished), the role of deer host in the maintenance of the tick cycle required further investigation. An initial series of experiments proved that rusa deer support female

Address for correspondence: N. Barré, CIRAD-EMVT/IAC, BP 25, Païta, New-Caledonia. Voice: 687437425; fax 687437426.

barre@iac.nc

Ann. N.Y. Acad. Sci. 969: 280–289 (2002). © 2002 New York Academy of Sciences.

ticks to the engorged stage, but they indicated that the success of engorgement was considerably lower on deer than on cattle.[3] Thus it seems that the majority of ticks attached on deer are "lost" for cattle and consequently eliminated from the epidemiological process. This may be highly beneficial for the primary susceptible host, i.e., cattle. In order to demonstrate such a mechanism, a long-term experiment was conducted in New Caledonia to evaluate the effect of the association of deer and cattle on the infestation of the latter host.

MATERIALS AND METHODS

Pastures and Herds

The experiment was conducted on a mixed cattle/deer farm, located at Port Laguerre in the municipality of Païta (22°1 south, 166°3 east) in the southern part of New Caledonia. Three groups of pastures were used for the three experimental herds, each represented by 4 paddocks through which the herds rotated. Two paddocks (A, B) contained forage grasses only (*Setaria sphacelata, Brachiaria decumbens, Chloris gayana, Panicum maximum*), the other 2 (C, D) contained the same grasses plus shrubs of legumes (*Leucaena, Calliandra*).

Three groups of animals, equivalent to the same stocking rate, were allowed to graze on the pastures in February 2000:

- Cattle-only group: 13 two-year old Charolais steers, for a total weight of 7110 kg placed on 14.4 ha (4 paddocks of 3.6 ha each); stocking rate at the beginning of the trial 494 kg/ha;

- Deer-only group: 38 adult and one-year old does, for a total weight of 1887 kg on 4 ha (4 paddocks of 1 ha each); stocking rate 472 kg/ha;

- Mixed deer/cattle group: 3 two-year old Charolais weighting 1580 kg and 11 one-year old stags weighting 447 kg placed on 4 ha (4 paddocks of 1 ha each); stocking rate 507 kg/ha.

Except for 2 of the paddocks (between the "deer-only" (paddock B) and the "mixed herd" (C)), paddocks were not adjacent. A large path separated the cattle-only group from the other groups. This path was used every 6 weeks to transfer steers and deer to the stock yard or to the deer yard.

The cattle and deer originated from the farm and had been subject to tick challenge (not checked, but considered medium-high for steers, nil-low for deer) before the start of the experiment.

Ticks Used for Infestation of Paddocks

In order to standardize the infestation of pastures they were artificially infested with larvae collected as engorged females in January 2000 from Charolais cattle on the Port Laguerre farm and kept in individual plastic tubes placed in an incubator (28°C, 87% RH) until use.

The layings of females were deposited regularly on the ground of paddocks C and A on 15 March and on 25 April 2000, respectively. A dose of 586 layings per ha was previously demontrated to generate a high infestation.[3] A lower dose (half the pad-

docks infested with 180 layings/ha, resulting in a density of 90 layings/ha, i.e
225 000 viable larvae/ha) was preferred in this current experiment in order to repro-
duce conditions of a more naturally induced infestation

Management of the Groups

After establishement of the three groups on their respective pastures in February
2000, rotations on paddocks were made simultaneously for the three groups every 3
weeks. At every other rotation (i.e., every 6 weeks), animals were driven to the stock
yard or deer yard for tick counts and weighing. Tick counts were always made on
both host species between 7:30 and 11:00 am. This procedure was followed routinely for 15 months until the end of the experiment in May 2001. In the deer-only group,
fawns were born in April–July (total of 9) and were weaned in October.

Tick Counts and Tick Burden Estimation

Cattle

The procedure was the same as described in Barré et al.[3] Ticks were classified
into three categories: small instars (immatures, non-engorged adults); "standard" females, 4–8 mm long and "engorged" females over 8 mm long, ready to drop off.
They were counted on 100 cm^2 on each of 27 anatomical sites and their numbers extrapolated to the surface of the whole body. At each sampling interval, ticks were
counted on the 3 cattle in the mixed group and on 5 of the 13 cattle in the cattle-only
group. These animals had been randomly chosen at the beginning of the trial. An acaricide treatment was applied if infestation was considered important and presumably fatal for animals.

Deer

Ticks were counted on every deer of the deer only and mixed group. Four sites
were investigated: ears, one side of the back line, tail, and perineum. The ticks were
collected and identified at the laboratory. From previous observations (Barré & Bianchi unpublished) where the sites of attachment of 21 800 Boophilus microplus on
17 deer were recorded, it was shown that these sample sites represented 8.91% of the
total ticks. This ratio was used to estimate the number of ticks per deer in the current
experiment: total ticks = 100 × number ticks on sampled sites/8.91.

Unit Used to Compare Infestation of Deer and Steers

Steers weighed 10 times more than deer, and their level of infestation was not directly comparable to that of deer. In order to facilitate comparisons between animals
of various size and weight, tick burdens were expressed per kg of host.

Checking Ticks on Pastures

In order to relate tick burdens on hosts to ticks present in the environment and to
check the presence of larvae on pastures, dragging with a flannelette cloth 1×1.2 m
was regularly performed on paddocks (on 3 lines of 100 m each, total of 512 lines

for the 15-month period), usually after the departure of animals in a paddock and before moving to the next one.

Statistical Analysis

Data were analyzed using SPSS software.[4] Only comparisons between groups (cattle-only vs. mixed), type of host (cattle vs. deer) or pasture infestation periods were made. Because tick burden variances between groups were frequently significantly different, we used a non-parametric method, the Mann-Whitney test. Weight gains were compared using a multivariate analysis (ANOVA).[4]

RESULTS

Density of Larvae on Pastures

There was large variation in the numbers of larvae collected by dragging between lines and between sampling intervals, probably resulting from a non-regular distribution of ticks on the ground and heterogeneity in grass height and species. Nevertheless, some rough information may be obtained from this technique. Residual infestation of the three pastures before a standardized artificial infestation was not different between the groups. Later on, larvae were collected throughout the year on pastures grazed by the cattle-only group (0.5–3.2 larvae/m^2) and the mixed group (0.25–0.8 larvae/m^2). Ticks were significantly more abundant on the former in May–June only. Larvae remained at a low density (0.2 larvae/m^2) on the deer-only pasture and disappeared after a few months. In the deer-only group, larvae were only collected on the 2 artificially infested paddocks, whereas the 4 paddocks (2 infested; 2 non-infested) used by the cattle-only herd and mixed herd remained infested throughout the experiment.

Tick Burden of Cattle and Deer (FIGURE 1)

Cattle-Only Group

Tick numbers increased regularly and dramatically after 6 months of exposure (43.5 ticks/kg of host in September). This peak corresponded to the second biological cycle after depositing the larvae in March/April, resulting in a significant production of engorged females (787 per steer; 1.6/kg) in June. Accordingly, the cattle were permanently and highly infested from September until the end of the experiment in May 2001, with lower infestations in February–March 2001, a period of high rainfall. The range of infestation was between 10 and 55 ticks per kg during most of the period of exposure. Production of engorged females was irregular, with most engorged (F8) females recorded in June (13.3% of the total ticks), September (4%), January (0.8 %) and May (4%), with very few to nil (February–March 2001) in the other months. The infestation was considered detrimental for the steers on five occasions and they were treated with an acaricide (Amitraz 12% EC) (arrows in FIGURE 2). One highly infested steer died in June. These treatments were obviously insufficient to control the infestation and to induce a decline in the epidemiological cycle. In May 2001, after more than one year of intense exposure to ticks, the tick burden was similar to that observed 8 months earlier.

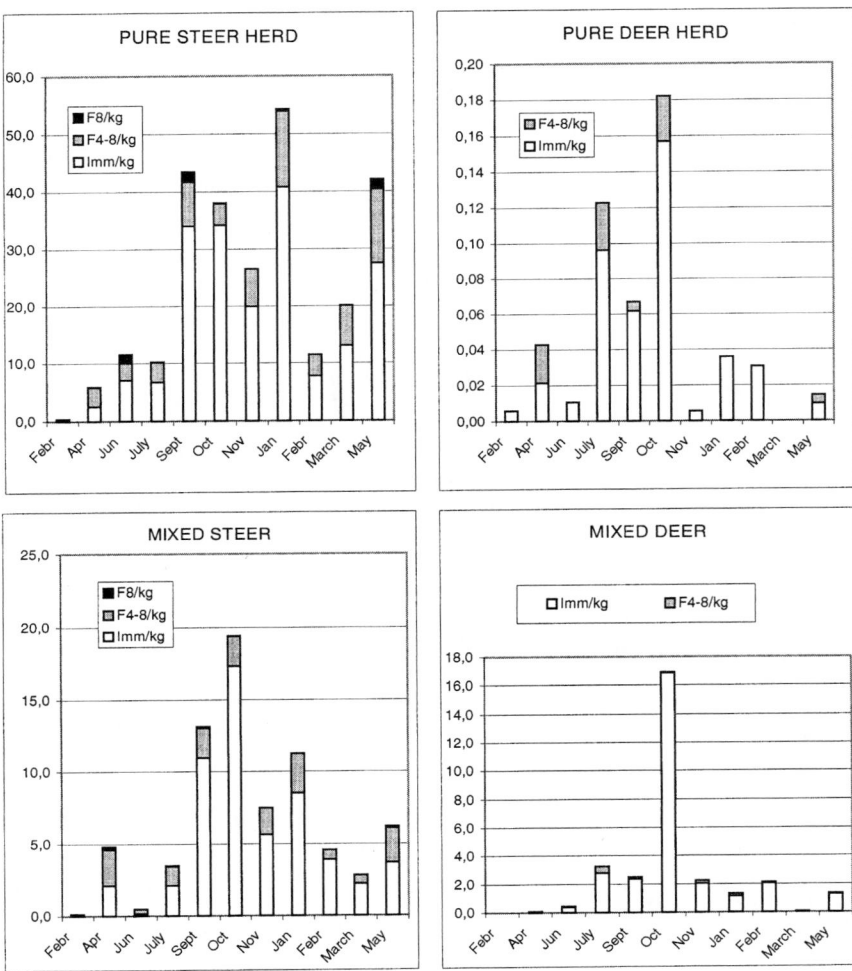

FIGURE 1. Mean number of ticks per kilogram of host on the 4 groups of hosts in the 3 experimental herds. Imm/kg: immatures and non-engorged adults/kg; F4–8: semi-engorged ("standard") females; F8: engorged females.

Deer-Only Group

Note that the scale for this group in FIGURE 1 is 300 time less than for the cattle only group. Only a few ticks, and always fewer than 0.2/kg, were collected, indicating a "low level" cycle. Ticks were observed on deer for the whole period, but were slightly more numerous in July–October. No engorged females were ever collected. Tick burdens between the deer-only and the cattle-only groups were highly significantly different (*P* always < 0.001, TABLE 1).

TABLE 1. Comparison of the mean infestation levels by the 3 categories of ticks recorded between the three groups of hosts

		April	June	July	September	October	November	January	February	March	May
Steers in cattle-only herd *vs.* steers in mixed herd	Imm	NS	<0.02	<0.03	<0.02	NS	NS	<0.02	NS	<0.02	<0.02
	F4–8	NS	<0.02	<0.03	NS	NS	NS	NS	<0.02	<0.02	<0.02
	F8	NS	NS	NS	NS	NS	NS	<0.02	NS	NS	<0.02
Deer in deer-only herd *vs.* deer in mixed herd	Imm	NS	<0.001	<0.001	<0.001	<0.001	<0.001	<0.001	<0.001	<0.001	<0.001
	F4–8	NS	<0.001	<0.001	<0.001	<0.001	<0.001	<0.001	<0.001	<0.001	<0.001
Deer in mixed herd *vs.* cattle in mixed herd	Imm	<0.001	NS	NS	<0.009	NS	<0.016	<0.01	<0.024	<0.006	<0.016
	F4–8	<0.004	NS	<0.009	<0.005	<0.003	<0.01	<0.004	<0.003	<0.000	<0.001
	F8	<0.000	NS	<0.003	<0.003	<0.003	NS	NS	NS	NS	<0.005

Mann-Whitney probability for differences; (no F8 in the deer groups).

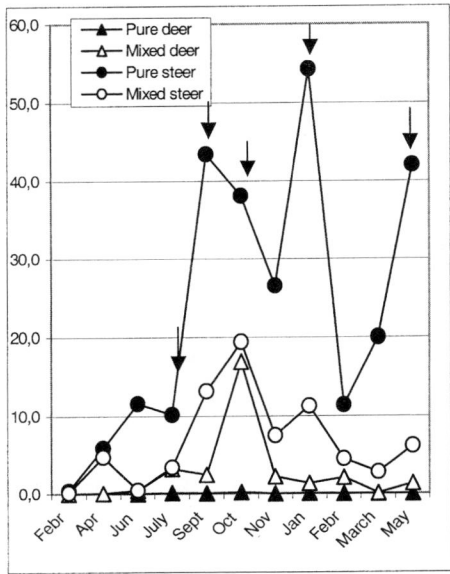

FIGURE 2. Mean number of ticks (all stages) per kg of host in the 3 herds (*arrow*: acaricide treatment in the pure steer herd).

Cattle in the Mixed Group

The infestation increased until a peak of 19.4/kg in October, the tick burden being generally between 3 and 13 ticks/kg. Few engorged F8 females were produced (0 to 0.2/kg) in April (4.1% of ticks), September (0.8%) and May (1.6%). Tick burdens on the cattle in the cattle-only and mixed group were generally different for at least one class of ticks (TABLE 1), except in October corresponding to the peak of infestation in the mixed group (FIG. 1). The health of the 3 steers of this group and their tick burden were never considered such as to justify acaricide treatment. Consequently, no treatment was applied on this group for the 15-month period of the experiment. After 15 months, the tick cycle was maintained, but the level of infestation remained moderate.

Deer in the Mixed Deer

The infestation was generally around 2–3 ticks/kg except in October, when it reached 16.9/kg. As for deer in the deer-only group, no engorged females were observed. The comparisons of tick burdens between these deer and the cattle are presented in TABLE 1.

Evolution of the Stocking Rate (FIGURE 3) and Weight Gain

Biomasses of cattle and deer in the 3 lots at the beginning of the experiment were quite close: 494 kg/ha for pure deer, 491kg/ha for pure steers, 507 kg/ha for the steer/

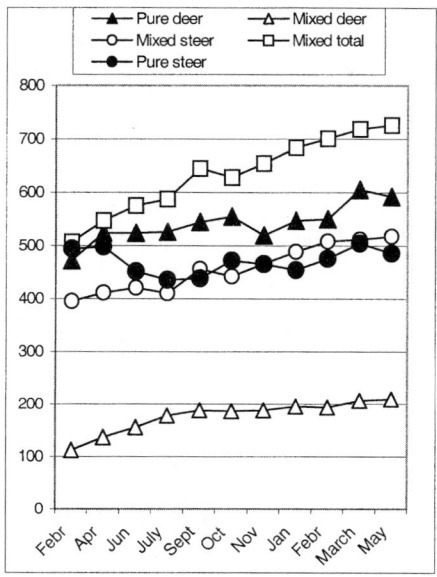

FIGURE 3. Evolution of the stocking rate (kg/ha) in the 3 herds.

deer group (112 kg/ha for stags, 395 kg/ha for steers). During the experiment, the stocking rate of deer decreased in November, when fawns were weaned and removed from the paddocks. In the cattle-only group, the death of a heavily infested steer explains the decline in June. However, the stocking rate in this group compared with the others never increased significantly. After 15 months, at the end of the trial, the weight gain per hectare was 120 kg in the deer group, 219 kg in the mixed group (97 kg for deer (stags), 122 kg for cattle) and −8 kg in the cattle-only group. The mean individual gain was 11.8 kg for does of the deer-only group (22.4 ± 4.9 kg for young does; 4.2 ± 5.7 kg for adults) and 35.7 ± 3.6 kg for stags in the mixed group. Growth of young does was not different (F = 0.82, P = 0.38) than for control does reared elsewhere on tick-free pastures, while growth of infested stags was reasonable but significantly lower than for control stags (F = 36.3, P < 0.001). Weight gain of cattle differed dramatically: 162.7 ± 34 kg for animals in the mixed group and only 42 ± 46.1 kg for animals in the cattle-only group of the same age (F = 17.6, P < 0.001 between both steer groups).

DISCUSSION

Despite similar pasture infestations by larvae and stocking rates, the establishment and development of the *Boophilus microplus* population in our three experimental herds were strikingly different.

In the cattle-only herd, the tick burden rapidly rose and remained at a high level for most of the experiment. At all but 2 of the 10 sampling intervals, a significant proportion of ticks (2.1%) were engorged females ready to drop off, giving evidence of a dynamic and sustainable parasitological cycle. Five acaricide treatments were considered necessary to prevent death in the cattle in this group. They were applied at intervals of 45–135 days, but were insufficient to depress the cycle and to prevent losses. After more than one year of exposure to ticks, a peak of infestation appeared, similar in intensity to those observed earlier, indicating that immunity was not yet established. The infestation of paddocks by larvae was found to be continuously high, and the spread of ticks from artificially infested paddocks to non-infested ones also indicated a well-established cycle. The productivity of steers in such a system was dramatically low: beginning at a standard stocking rate for New Caledonian agrosystems (about 1 head of cattle/ha), the weight gain obtained after 15 months was poor. This management system was not economically viable. It shows that the Charolais breed is particularly susceptible to the cattle tick and not well adapted to an environment characterized by a high parasitic pressure.

The situation in the deer-only group was completely different. During the whole experiment, the tick burden was low to nil, with no engorged female produced. It was apparent that this infestation was such that it had little, if any, detrimental effect on the growth of does. The density of larvae on pastures followed this general trend, with few larvae being collected. A long-term cycle in this host is probably not viable, the population declining naturally towards extinction.

The parasitic situation was intermediate in the mixed group. For cattle, the infestation was moderate and generated, albeit at a low rate, engorged females indicating a sustainable cycle. The continous presence of larvae on pastures, including the non-artificially infested paddocks, is in favor of such a cycle. However, and in comparison with the cattle-only group, the infestation level was much lower: for the whole period, each steer was infested with 3.5 fewer ticks of all stages (and 11.2 times fewer engorged females) than the steers in the cattle-only group. As a consequence, there was no reason to apply acaricides at any time during the 15-month period. In addition, the stocking rate increased regularly as well as individual body mass.

Deer in this group may be assumed to be responsible for the lowered infestation rate of the cattle in the mixed group. Deer were highly infested in this group, if we compare the data with the data recorded for the deer-only group. Similar to the deer-only group, no engorged females were observed on deer in the mixed group (amongst 1618 ticks collected over the duration of the experiment). This indicates that the larvae found on the deer originate from ticks that fed on steers. Further, ticks attached on deer are totally—or almost totally—unable to progress to the engorged stage and to continue the cycle. Thus the deer play the role of an epidemiological "cul de sac," able to trap ticks, but unsuitable as a host that supports ticks to the fully engorged stage. Deer would appear to deplete the source of contamination for coexisting susceptible steers. Despite significant infestations, deer weight gains remained high under mixed grazing.

These results are not conclusive on the role of deer in the maintenance—or not—of a wild *Boophilus* tick population. However, they open new prospects for the use of alternative hosts to control infestations in cattle. In New Caledonia, where deer are particularly abundant and often accused by farmers of competing with cattle for available grazing, their role in tick control may well require a reassessment. Their association with cattle and the sharing of food and parasites may possibly have globally beneficial consequences.

ACKNOWLEDGMENTS

The authors thank the staff of Port Laguerre station for their assistance and the New Caledonian Government for its support of this research work.

REFERENCES

1. GEORGE, J.E. 1990. Wildlife as a constraint to the eradication of *Boophilus* sp (Acari: Ixodidae). J. Agr. Entomol. **7**: 119–125.
2. CHARDONNET, P. 1988. Etude technique et économique de l'élevage de cerfs en Nouvelle-Calédonie. IEMVT-CIRAD, ADRAF, 278 pp.
3. BARRÉ, N., M. BIANCHI & L. CHARDONNET. 2001. Role of Rusa deer *Cervus timorensis russa* in the cycle of the cattle tick *Boophilus microplus* in New Caledonia. Exp. Appl. Acarol. **25**: 79–96.
4. SPSS, 1997. Base 8.0 for Windows. SPSS Inc. 444 N. Michigan Av. Chicago, IL 60611.

Ticks Associated with Armadillo (*Euphractus sexcinctus*) and Anteater (*Myrmecophaga tridactyla*) of Emas National Park, State of Goias, Brazil

GERVÁSIO H. BECHARA,[a] M.P.J. SZABÓ,[a] W.V. ALMEIDA FILHO,[a] J.N. BECHARA,[a] R.J.G. PEREIRA,[a] J.E. GARCIA,[a] AND MARCELO C. PEREIRA[b]

[a]*Faculdade de Ciências Agrárias e Veterinárias, Universidade Estadual Paulista, 14.884-900 Jaboticabal, SP, Brazil*

[b]*Instituto de Ciências Biomédicas, Depto. de Parasitologia, Universidade de São Paulo, 05.584-000 São Paulo, SP, Brazil*

ABSTRACT: This study was conducted in October 1998 and November 1999 in the Emas National Park (131,868 ha), a savanna-type cerrado region situated in the far south of Goias State, Brazil, near the geographic center of South America (15°–23° S; 45°–55° W). Animals were captured with the aid of nets and anesthetized (15 mg/kg ketamine + 1 mg/kg xylasine) in order to collect ticks for identification and to establish laboratory colonies. They included giant anteaters (*Myrmecophaga tridactyla*) (*n* = 4) and yellow armadillos (*Euphractus sexcinctus*) (*n* = 6). Free-living ticks (larvae, nymphs, and adults) were collected from the field by using a 1 × 2-m flannel cloth. Free-living ticks were identified as *Amblyomma* sp., *A. cajennense*, and *A. triste*. Adult ticks collected from anteaters were identified as *Amblyomma cajennense* and *A. nodosum* and from armadillos as *A. pseudoconcolor* and *A. nodosum*. The relevance of these host-tick relationships to possible mechanisms underlying emergence of tick-borne pathogens of importance to public health is discussed.

KEYWORDS: ticks; *Amblyomma* sp.; anteaters; *Myrmecophaga tridactyla*; yellow armadillos; *Euphractus sexcinctus*; Brazil

INTRODUCTION

Ticks have long been regarded as deleterious to the welfare of humans and domestic animals. Their harmful effects can take many different forms both because of the variety of the disease agents that ticks may transmit and because of their direct effects on host physiology.[1,2] The ever-growing cohabitation of wild and domestic animals as well as humans may lead to the emergence of new tick-host relationships and to the exchange of pathogens between hosts; it enhances the risk of unexpected

Address for correspondence: Dr. Gervásio H. Bechara, Faculdade de Ciências Agrárias e Veterinárias, Universidade Estadual Paulista, 14.884-900 Jaboticabal, SP, Brazil. Voice: 55-16-3209-2662; fax: 55-16-3202-4275.

bechara@fcav.unesp.br

Ann. N.Y. Acad. Sci. 969: 290–293 (2002). © 2002 New York Academy of Sciences.

infections.[3] Little information is available on ticks from wild animals in Brazil; a comprehensive survey of ticks collected from wild animals of the Pantanal region has been published.[4,5]

Emas National Park (131,868 ha) is a savanna-type cerrado region situated in the far south of Goias State, Brazil, near the geographic center of South America (15°–23° S; 45°–55° W). The climate is tropical; the highly seasonal rains give about 250 mm rainfall between October and March. The greater part of the park is covered by scattered bushland. The present work describes the identification of ticks from anteaters and armadillos of the Emas National Park region as a part of a more comprehensive study of established and emerging tick-host relationships and related disease processes.

MATERIALS AND METHODS

Location and period of collection. The study was conducted in October 1998 and November 1999 in Emas National Park.

Capture of wild animals. Giant anteaters (*Myrmecophaga tridactyla*) (*n* = 4) and yellow armadillos (*Euphractus sexcinctus*) (*n* = 6) were captured manually or with the aid of a net and anesthetized (15 mg/kg ketamine + 1 mg/kg xylasine, IM) for the collection of ticks.

Tick sample collection. Ticks from the anesthetized wild animals were collected with the aid of fine forceps or the tick remover Best Friend (Best Friend International, Nanterre) and stored in 70° alcohol until identification. Samples of off-host ticks in the field were obtained via the dragging technique by using a 1 × 2-m flannel cloth.

RESULTS

Free-living ticks were identified as *Amblyomma* sp., *A. cajennense*, and *A. triste*. Adult ticks collected from anteaters were identified as *Amblyomma cajennense* and *A. nodosum*; those collected from armadillos were identified as *A. pseudoconcolor* and *A. nodosum*. The individual results are presented in TABLE 1. Free-living ticks collected from the field by the dragging technique were identified as shown in TABLE 2.

DISCUSSION

Every animal captured in Emas National Park harbored ticks. In general, there was no predominance of the nymphal stage over the larval stage. Predominance of nymphs at the end of winter and spring has been described previously for *Amblyomma* sp. in South America,[6–8] but sampling should cover a whole year before useful conclusions can be reached.

All tick species belonged to the genus *Amblyomma*, which is not surprising inasmuch as this genus has 102 described species,[9] 33 of which are found in Brazil.[10] *A. cajennense* (Fabricius, 1787) was the tick species most frequently found by drag-

TABLE 1. Ticks collected from anteaters and armadillos in Emas National Park, State of Goias, Brazil in October 1998 and November 1999

Sample	Host	Tick identification
1	yellow armadillo	A (M,F) *A. pseudoconcolor* (++)
2	yellow armadillo	A (M,F) *A. pseudoconcolor* (+++)
3	yellow armadillo	4A (M,F) *A. nodosum*
4	yellow armadillo	A (M,F) *A. pseudoconcolor* (++)
5	yellow armadillo	A (M,F) *A. pseudoconcolor* (++)
6	yellow armadillo	A (M,F) *A. pseudoconcolor* (++)
7	giant anteater	A(M,F) *A. nodosum* (+)
8	giant anteater	1 (F) *Amblyomma* sp.
9	giant anteater	A (M,F) *A. cajennense* (+)
10	giant anteater	A (M,F) *A. nodosum* (+)

A = adults; M = male; F = female.

TABLE 2. Free-living ticks collected from Emas National Park

Sample	Place	Tick identification
1	Jacuba's bush	A (M,F) *A. cajennense* and *A. triste*
2	Jacuba's bush	nymphs of *Amblyomma* sp.
3	bush near the main house	nymphs of *Amblyomma* sp.
4	bush around Capybaras Lake	larvae of *Amblyomma* sp.
5	general bush	A (M,F) *A. cajennense*
6	general bush	A (M,F) *A. cajennense*

A = adults; M = male; F = female.

ging. Also, ticks of this species were recovered from a giant anteater, an observation similar to those made in wild animals captured in the Pantanal region.[4,5] This tick species is widely distributed in South America. In its immature stages it has low host specificity,[11] but adults are more common on equids and capybara.[12] *A. cajennense* is described as the main vector of the spotted fever agent *Rickettsia rickettsii* in Latin America.[13,14]

Amblyomma pseudoconcolor ticks were collected from yellow armadillos only, as observed in armadillos captured in the Pantanal region.[4,5] This tick species was originally described on armadillos (*Dasypus* sp.), which is considered the major host.[15] Ticks in immature stages can be found on wild birds.[16]

Although these observations of ticks from Emas National Park are interesting and valuable, it must be recognized that interpretation of results should take into account that sampling was restricted to the dry season, a relatively short tick collection time. Tick infestation should be evaluated in the wet season as well.

Host-tick relationships are important to public health, as they involve mechanisms underlying the emergence of tick-borne pathogens.

ACKNOWLEDGMENTS

The IBAMA kindly gave permission for the capture of animals. This research was supported by FAPESP, CNPq, and São Paulo State University.

REFERENCES

1. AESCHLIMANN, A. 1991. Ticks and disease: susceptible hosts, reservoir hosts and vectors. *In* Parasite-Host Associations: Coexistence or Conflict? C.A. Toft, A. Aeschlimann & L. Bolis, Eds.: 148–156. Oxford University Press. Oxford.
2. DE CASTRO, J.J. 1997. Sustainable tick and tickborne disease control in livestock improvement in developing countries. Vet. Parasitol. **71:** 77–97.
3. HOOGSTRAAL, H. 1981. Changing patterns of tickborne diseases in modern society. Ann. Rev. Entomol. **26:** 75–99.
4. BECHARA, G.H., M.P.J. SZABÓ, J.M.B. DUARTE, *et al.* 2000. Ticks associated with wild animals in the Nhecolandia Pantanal, Brazil. Ann. N.Y. Acad. Sci. **916:** 289–297.
5. CAMPOS PEREIRA, M., M.P.J. SZABÓ, G.H. BECHARA, *et al.* 2000. Ticks (Acari:Ixodidae) associated with wild animals in the Pantanal region of Brazil. J. Med. Entomol. **37:** 979–983.
6. GUGLIELMONE, A.A. *et al.* 1990. Ecological aspects of four species of ticks found on cattle in Salta, northwest Argentina. Vet. Parasitol. **35:** 93–101.
7. MANGOLD, A.J. *et al.* 1994. Seasonal variation of ticks (Ixodidae) in *Bos taurus* x *Bos indicus* cattle under rotational grazing in forested and deforested habitats in northwestern Argentina. Vet. Parasitol. **54:** 389–395.
8. OLIVEIRA, P.R. 1998. *Amblyomma cajennense* (Fabricius, 1787) (Acari: Ixodidae): avaliação de técnicas para estudo de dinâmica populacional e bioecologia em Pedro Leopoldo, Minas Gerais. PhD Thesis, Universidade Federal de Minas Gerais, Belo Horizonte, Brazil.
9. SONENSHINE, D.E. 1991. Biology of Ticks, Vol. 1: 25. Oxford University Press. New York.
10. ARAGÃO, H.B. & F. FONSECA. 1961. Notas de ixodologia. VIII. Lista e chave para os representantes da fauna ixodológica brasileira. Mem. Inst. Oswaldo Cruz **59:** 115–130.
11. LOPES, C.M.L. *et al.* 1998. Host specificity of *Amblyomma cajennense* (Fabricius, 1787) (Acari: Ixodidae) with comments on the drop-off rhythm. Mem. Inst. Oswaldo Cruz Rio **93:** 347–351.
12. CAMPOS PEREIRA, M. & M.B. LABRUNA. 1998. Febre maculosa: aspectos clínico-epidemiológicos. Clín. Vet. **12:** 19–23.
13. ACHA, P.N. & A. SZYFRES. 1986. Zoonosis y enfermedades transmisibles comunes al hombre y a los animales. Segunda edición. Org. Panamer. Salud **503:** 989.
14. DE LEMOS, E.R.S. *et al.* 1996. Primary isolation of spotted fever group Rickettsiae from *Amblyomma cooperi* collected from *Hydrochaeris hydrochaeris* in Brazil. Mem. Inst. Oswaldo Cruz Rio **91:** 273–275.
15. BOTELHO, J.R. *et al.* 1990. Interrelation of acari Ixodidae and hosts of Edentata of the Serra da Canastra, Minas Gerais, Brazil. Mem. Inst. Oswaldo Cruz Rio **84:** 61–64.
16. ARAGÃO, H.B. 1936. Ixodidas brasileiros e de alguns países limítrofes. Mem. Inst. Oswaldo Cruz Rio **31:** 759–844.

Control and Eradication of Chelonian Tick Infestations, with Particular Reference to Vectors of Heartwater

MICHAEL J. BURRIDGE,[a] LEIGH-ANNE SIMMONS,[a] TREVOR F. PETER,[b] AND SUMAN M. MAHAN[b]

[a]Department of Pathobiology, University of Florida, P.O. Box 110880, Gainesville, Florida 32611-0880, USA

[b]University of Florida/USAID/SADC Heartwater Research Project, Central Veterinary Laboratory (Diagnostic and Research Branch), Box CY 551, Causeway, Harare, Zimbabwe

ABSTRACT: Studies using the African tortoise tick (*Amblyomma marmoreum*) and leopard tortoises (*Geochelone pardalis*) demonstrated that cyfluthrin and permethrin were safe and efficacious acaricides for control of *Amblyomma* ticks on tortoises. A protocol was developed that successfully eradicated an *A. sparsum* infestation from a tortoise breeding facility in Florida. It involved treatment of all tortoises with a permethrin formulation, followed by treatment of the premises with a cyfluthrin formulation. Sentinel tortoises were later placed on the treated premises to establish successful tick eradication.

KEYWORDS: ticks; *Amblyomma marmoreum*; *Amblyomma sparsum*; tortoises; control; eradication; permethrin; cyfluthrin; heartwater

INTRODUCTION

In 1997, the exotic African tortoise tick *Amblyomma marmoreum* was identified in Florida outside importation facilities on a reptile breeding operation where it had become established.[1] Subsequent investigations found that at least 11 exotic tick species had been imported into Florida on reptiles, with at least seven species disseminated to reptile breeding facilities, zoos, wildlife theme parks, pet stores, wildlife care centers, and collections of private hobbyists.[2,3] These findings demonstrated an unregulated flow of exotic ticks into the United States through Florida. This was cause for concern given that the international trade in live reptiles was increasing and that two of the imported ticks (the large reptile tick *A. sparsum* and the tropical bont tick *A. variegatum*) were known vectors of heartwater,[4] a fatal disease of domestic and wild ruminants in sub-Saharan Africa and the eastern Caribbean.[5] This concern was heightened when *A. marmoreum* was confirmed as a capable vector of heartwater[6] and when *A. sparsum,* infesting a shipment of leopard

---

Address for correspondence: Dr. Michael J. Burridge, Department of Pathobiology, University of Florida, P.O. Box 110880, Gainesville, FL 32611-0880. Voice: 352-392-4700, ext. 3131; fax: 352-846-0246

burridgem@mail.vetmed.ufl.edu

Ann. N.Y. Acad. Sci. 1: 294–296 (2002). © 2002 New York Academy of Sciences.

tortoises (*Geochelone pardalis*) imported into Florida from Africa, were found to be infected with *Cowdria ruminantium*,[7] the causative agent of heartwater.

Since no acaricide was registered in the United States for use on reptiles, these findings prompted immediate studies to identify an acaricide that would kill tick infestations on reptiles, and especially tortoises, in a safe and efficacious manner. Also, since it was clear that numerous shipments of infested reptiles had been imported into Florida and that some had become established on premises housing tortoises, there was an urgent need to develop methods for eradication of these exotic tick infestations. This article summarizes the results of studies conducted to define methods for control and eradication of the exotic tick vectors of heartwater that had been introduced to Florida.

CONTROL OF CHELONIAN TICK INFESTATIONS

When it became evident that exotic reptilian ticks, and especially *A. marmoreum*, were being introduced repeatedly into Florida on imported reptiles,[2] a search was conducted for information on acaricides to control these tick species. Two research notes from South Africa gave short reports on the use of carbaryl and amitraz to treat *A. marmoreum*–infested tortoises.[8,9] The first note[8] gave a retrospective report of an owner's treatment of a pet tortoise with carbaryl solution, and the second note[9] summarized an experiment using amitraz to induce detachment of *A. marmoreum* to facilitate a tick survey. Neither report evaluated scientifically either the efficacy or the safety of the use of acaricides to treat tick-infested tortoises.

With so little previous data available, the acaricides chosen for investigation were those registered for use on other domestic animal species in the United States. They were amitraz, carbaryl, chlorpyrifos, cyfluthrin, fipronil, lindane, permethrin, and pyrethrins, with five (amitraz, carbaryl, chlorpyrifos, cyfluthrin, and permethrin) also tested for toxicity on leopard tortoises. The tick species chosen for the study was *A. marmoreum*; a tick colony established in Zimbabwe from adults and nymphs collected in Florida was used. The results of the study showed that only cyfluthrin and permethrin produced 100% tick mortality at a dilution of 0.01% in acetone, with both producing high mortality (80%) when used in dilutions up to 0.0001%. The only side effect of any duration was eye irritation, which was seen only with carbaryl and chlorpyrifos.

ERADICATION OF CHELONIAN TICK INFESTATIONS

During investigations of exotic tick infestations in Florida, it became evident that numerous shipments of infested reptiles had been imported and that at least two exotic tick species, *A. marmoreum* and *A. sparsum*, both known vectors of heartwater, had already become established as breeding populations. *A. marmoreum* had become established on three premises containing exotic tortoise species. On one premises, African spurred tortoises (*Geochelone sulcata*) had introduced *Amblyomma marmoreum*; on another, leopard tortoises were the initial host, from which the ticks spread to Aldabra giant tortoises (*Geochelone gigantea*), yellow-footed tortoises (*Geochelone denticulata*), a Galapagos giant tortoise (*Geochelone elephantopus*), and domestic dogs. *Amblyomma sparsum* had become established on one tortoise-breeding premises where the hosts were leopard tortoises. Consequently, protocols were developed and tested for eradication of these tick infestations in order to minimize the risk that such exotic vectors of heartwater would spread to native fauna and thus become established as indigenous tick species, as had happened in past years in Florida with the iguana tick *Amblyomma dissimile*[10] and the rotund toad tick *A. rotundatum*.[11]

The protocol finally adopted required all tortoises on the infested premises to be treated by spraying with a permethrin product (Provent-a-Mite™, Pro Products, Mahopac, NY) specifically formulated for use on reptiles[12] and then removed to a tick-free area. Next, the premises was sprayed on two occasions two weeks apart by a licensed pest control company with a cyfluthrin product (Tempo®, Bayer Corporation, Kansas City, MO) specifically formulated for premises treatment, ensuring that all surface areas, including housing and burrows, were treated. Finally, one week after the second premises treatment, sentinel tortoises, such as Hermann's tortoises (*Testudo hermanni*), which roam freely and whose skin area is easy to inspect, were placed on the treated premises for 10 days. If the sentinel tortoises remained free of ticks, the infestation was considered to have been eradicated from the premises. Using this protocol, the *A. sparsum* infestation was eradicated successfully from a reptile facility in Florida, with sentinel tortoises remaining tick-free when introduced again four months after premises treatment.

REFERENCES

1. ALLAN, S.A., L.A. SIMMONS & M.J. BURRIDGE. 1998. Establishment of the tortoise tick *Amblyomma marmoreum* (Acari: Ixodidae) on a reptile-breeding facility in Florida. J. Med. Entomol. **35:** 621–624.
2. BURRIDGE, M.J., L.A. SIMMONS & S.A. ALLAN. 2000. Introduction of potential heartwater vectors and other exotic ticks into Florida on imported reptiles. J. Parasitol. **86:** 700–704.
3. SIMMONS, L.A. & M.J. BURRIDGE. 2000. Introduction of the exotic ticks *Amblyomma humerale* Koch and *Amblyomma geoemydae* (Cantor) (Acari: Ixodidae) into the United States on imported reptiles. Int. J. Acarol. **26:** 239–242.
4. BURRIDGE, M.J. 2001. Ticks (Acari: Ixodidae) spread by the international trade in reptiles and their potential roles in dissemination of diseases. Bull. Entomol. Res. **91:** 3–23.
5. CAMUS, E., N. BARRÉ & G. UILENBERG. 1996. Heartwater (Cowdriosis). A Review. 2nd edit. Office International des Epizooties. Paris.
6. PETER, T.F., M.J. BURRIDGE & S.M. MAHAN. 2000. Competence of the African tortoise tick, *Amblyomma marmoreum* (Acari: Ixodidae), as a vector of the agent of heartwater (*Cowdria ruminantium*). J. Parasitol. **86:** 438–441.
7. BURRIDGE, M.J., L.A. SIMMONS, B.H. SIMBI, *et al.* 2000. Evidence of *Cowdria ruminantium* infection (heartwater) in *Amblyomma sparsum* ticks found on tortoises imported into Florida. J. Parasitol. **86:** 1135–1136.
8. WALKER, J.B. & J.D. BEZUIDENHOUT. 1973. Treatment of tick-infested tortoises. J. S. Afr. Vet. Assoc. **44:** 381.
9. PETNEY, T.N. & M.M. KNIGHT. 1988. The treatment of ticks on tortoises using amitraz. J. S. Afr. Vet. Assoc. **59:** 206.
10. BEQUAERT, J. 1932. *Amblyomma dissimile* Koch, a tick indigenous to the United States (Acarina: Ixodidae). Psyche **32:** 45–47.
11. OLIVER, J.H., M.P. HAYES, J.E. KEIRANS & D.R. LAVENDER. 1993. Establishment of the foreign parthenogenetic tick *Amblyomma rotundatum* (Acari: Ixodidae) in Florida. J. Parasitol. **79:** 786–790.
12. POUND, R. 2000. Mite and tick control for reptiles. United States Patent No. 6,121,318.

Eradication of the Tropical Bont Tick in the Caribbean

Is the Caribbean *Amblyomma* Program in a Crisis?

RUPERT G. PEGRAM,[a] EDWARD F. GERSABECK,[b] DAVID WILSON,[c] AND JORGEN W. HANSEN[d]

[a]*Caribbean Amblyomma Program, Bridgetown, Barbados*

[b]*International Services, USDA/APHIS, Riverdale, Maryland 20737, USA*

[c]*Veterinary Services, USDA/APHIS, Riverdale, Maryland 20737, USA*

[d]*Parasitic Diseases Group, FAO/AGAH, Rome, Italy*

ABSTRACT: The progress and problems in the Caribbean *Amblyomma* Program (CAP) are reviewed since its inception in 1995. During 1998, there were funding and administrative management problems. USDA resolved the acute funding crisis, and after three years of negotiation, the CAP has now secured an additional euro 1.5 million from the European Community. Changes in administration in 1998 included the withdrawal of IICA from the program, and the transition during the decentralization of administrative and financial management from FAO headquarters to the Regional Office for Latin America and the Caribbean, based in Chile. A general overview of technical progress and one case study, St. Kitts, is presented. One major concern that emerged during 2000 is that the elimination of the small remaining tropical bont tick (TBT) "hot spots" in both St. Kitts and St. Lucia remained elusive. Why is this so? Egrets? Alternative residual hosts? Or is it fatigue in both technical and administrative management functions? Of even greater concern is the finding of two, apparently new, foci in St. Croix (USVI) in the north and St. Vincent in the south. A critical overview of the program has identified one major remaining constraint—an appropriate management support function at both regional and, in some countries, at the national level. A proposal for a revised management strategy, coupled with the identification of a future strategy to succeed the CAP, namely a Caribbean Animal Resources Management (CARM) Program.

KEYWORDS: tropical bont ticks; Caribbean islands; *Amblyomma*; Caribbean *Amblyomma* Program

Address for correspondence: Dr. Rupert G. Pegram, FAO, Caribbean *Amblyomma* Program, Bridgetown, Barbados.
rupertgp@caribsurf.com

Ann. N.Y. Acad. Sci. 969: 297–305 (2002). © 2002 New York Academy of Sciences.

INTRODUCTION

Sources of Current Information

A general introduction to the Caribbean *Amblyomma* Program (CAP), including a comprehensive "Country Profiles" document,[1] can be found at the project Web site (www.capweb.org). Recent updates on the status of CAP are available at the Food and Agriculture Organization (FAO) Web site in the Recent FAO News & Highlights items[2] (www.fao.org/news/1999/99tick-e.htm and www.fao.org/news/1999/991001-e.htm); "Where CAP is working" and "Putting a CAP on the tropical Bont tick," and in New Agriculturist "Focus on Livestock Health—Eradicating a Tick in Time" (www.new-agri.co.uk/00-06/focuson.html).[3] For those without internet access, over-view articles are available in the *FAO World Animal Review*,[4] *Bayer Public Health*,[5] and previous STVM proceedings.[6-8]

The Caribbean countries involved include Anguilla, Antigua and Barbuda, Barbados, Dominica, Montserrat, St. Kitts and Nevis, St. Lucia, and St. Maarten for eradication activities, and Haiti, Dominican Republic, British Virgin Islands, Netherlands Antilles, St. Vincent, Grenada, and Trinidad and Tobago for surveillance. Representatives from each country, and each agency or organization, are all members of the *Amblyomma* Program Council, the overall governing body. The USDA, the EU–CAFP (Caribbean Agriculture and Fisheries Program), and the International Fund for Agriculture Development (IFAD), as well as being the primary donors to CAP, all provide technical support to FAO's role as the lead technical implementing agency. A Regional Coordination Unit (RCU) manages day-to-day operations at the field level.

TECHNICAL PROGRESS AND CONSTRAINTS

General Situation

Field operations started in late 1995 on the northern islands. In 1998–1999, tropical bont tick (TBT) eradication was almost completed on four islands—Dominica, Montserrat, St. Kitts, and St. Lucia—but the elimination of remaining "hot spots," although few in number, is remaining elusive. Why is this so?

- Egrets? This seems unlikely epidemiologically as a primary cause, but we are also now faced with unexpected new foci in St. Croix (north), Dominica (central), and St. Vincent (south). Where are these ticks coming from?

- Alternative residual hosts? Dogs, donkeys, and so on, or small populations of untreated feral ruminants?

- Program management (technical and administrative) and "fatigue?"

It may well be a combination of factors, but the last one is of major concern, particularly in the eradication countries. Since the midterm review in September 1997, some of the management constraints that were identified have continued during the past three years. At the RCU level, the most important constraint is related to a lack of an internal, independent, but unified management support structure. At the national level, a parallel observation can be made: the two countries that performed most consistently and effectively are St. Lucia and St. Kitts. They were managed by animal health officers who were committed to their respective national units with no other official major public or private activities.

In late 1999, the project refocused technical activities on the seven main TBT-eradication islands (Anguilla, Antigua, Barbados, St. Kitts and Nevis, St. Lucia, and St. Maarten). It deferred the important surveillance activities in adjacent islands (BVI, Dominican Republic, Haiti, Netherlands Antilles in the north, and Grenada, St. Vincent and Trinidad and Tobago in the south) for a further year, pending EU inputs and additional staff. Even under the restricted field program, the RCU staff spends over 75% of their time on administrative and financial management [budget issues, contracts, purchase and control, and donor (EU) negotiations]. Technical support to the national programs therefore has been inadequate, but at the last APC, the USDA agreed in principle that the RCU required at least one additional senior staff member.

Summary of the Status of National Programs

Anguilla: One major hot-spot area remains. It is under intensive treatment. However, the program is short of staff and there are concerns regarding uncontrolled movement of livestock in and out of the infested hot-spot area.

Antigua: After almost two years of management problems, and lack of focus and commitment, the Antigua national program was suspended in December 2001, pending the availability of additional funding and a formal demonstration of commitment. Overall compliance figures for treatment over the three-year period rarely exceeded 50%.

Barbados: There was a marked decrease in surveillance activities during the second half of 2000. Only 111 animals were examined during the main TBT season (July–September) compared to 4728 animals examined during the same period in 1999. There were seven positive cases from the 111, indicating an infestation level of 6%, compared to 0.1% over the same period in 1999.

Dominica: A new outbreak was reported in the north of the island in July/August 2000.

Montserrat: During 2000, one positive case involving one male tick was reported.

Nevis: Nevis suffered severe setbacks in 1998–1999, partly due to hurricanes. However, they have now recovered, and new staff and a pound for stray livestock were made available in the second half of 2000. At that time they resumed collection of quantitative surveillance data.

St. Kitts: St. Kitts stopped blanket treatment in July 1998 and should have been declared provisionally TBT-free by mid-1999. The difficulty in elimination of the hot spots is difficult to understand, but management changes occurred at a critical time, and moreover, it seemed that no one was prepared to take action against two blatantly uncooperative livestock owners. The past two rounds of surveillance (October 2000–March 2001) have indicated that the country may now be considered TBT-free.

St. Lucia: Overall St. Lucia continued on track, but they found a new focus in the southern peninsula when they had been so near to being declared provisionally TBT free. An emergency reaction plan to resolve the problem was put in place, and the area is being destocked through a slaughter and partial compensation policy.

St. Maarten: There is an urgent need to review the program in light of the continued level of TBT findings associated with TBT infestations in St. Maarten. Acaricide supplies on the French side of the island have been erratic and treatment very inconsistent.

St. Vincent: A completely new focus has been reported from St. Vincent. While this report increases the confidence of the national surveillance and awareness program, it is of concern that after 10 years, new islands can be found infested with the TBT. The source of entry of the ticks cannot be identified.

St. Croix (USVI): Although not part of the CAP *per se*, the outbreak was reported to RCU. Again, it is of concern to find a new outbreak, and it also raises the question: Can a focus remain undetected for several years? If it is a new introduction, like St. Vincent, where did it come from?

The St. Kitts Case: The Current Situation

Mandatory treatment of all livestock ended in July 1998. In 1999–2000, eradication activities continued in TBT foci (hot spots). The four (4) locations were in areas of the interface between St. Peter/St. George's and St. Mary's districts, Trinity District, and St. John's district. Surveillance continued throughout the island. A summary of surveillance data is shown in TABLES 1 and 2. On advice from the USDA chief biometrician, the protocol was modified in the second half of 1999 to increase the number of properties inspected. This was deemed necessary in view of the very heterogeneous nature of the environment and of the animal husbandry systems prevalent in the islands. Consequently, the number of properties inspected in later survey rounds increased three- to fourfold, although the actual number of animals inspected decreased slightly. The efficacy of this revised strategy is clearly demonstrated in that the number of infested properties/animals detected increased in the second half of 1999. While this may have shown increased confidence in the data, it demonstrated that the hot-spot areas remained infested.

In total, some 799 properties were surveyed during the period 1998 to 1999. In the last six months of 1999, 447 (over 50%) properties were surveyed. The number of contacts (properties) at its highest point was 887. Overall, almost 40% (5587) of the estimated livestock population (14,753) was examined. However, it must be noted that because properties and animals were selected at random from the database for each survey cycle, some properties and animals may have been selected more than once. In fact, this was done purposely in instances where *A. variegatum* were found on a property in one cycle. Thereafter, they were intentionally included in the next cycle.

Very low numbers of ticks were reported during the first half of 2000, indicating that the hot spots remained. Some 40 egrets were also examined from near two hot-spot sites, but no immature tick stages were found. We believe that the most important factor is staff fatigue, and loss of motivation. At the end of 1999, significant staff changes occurred in St. Kitts. Furthermore, during 2000, intervention at two farms where owners were very uncooperative and treatment was not carried out at regular prescribed intervals was deferred for almost 12 months.

TABLE 1. St. Kitts Tropical Bont Tick Eradication Program: chronological analysis (1998–2001)

Period 1998–1999	Cycle number	Number[a] of contacts	Animals examined	TBT[a] positive	Number males	Number females
Apr.–June '98	2	82	969	3	5	3
July–Sep. '98	3	77	855	1	2	0
Oct.–Dec. '98	4	47	558	1	4	0
Jan.–Mar. '99	5	77	915	2	1	1
Apr.–June '99	6	69	949	1	1	0
July–Sep. '99	7	182	749	5	11	11
Oct.–Dec. '99	8	265	592	2	3	7
Subtotals		**799**	**5,587**	**15**	**27**	**22**
2000–2001						
Jan.–Mar. '00	9	164	488	3	3	2
Apr.–June '00	10	140	350	3	3	0
July–Sep. '00	11	197	607	1	1	0
Oct.–Dec. '00	12	195	899	0	0	0
Jan.–Mar. '01	13	151	394	0	0	0
Apr.–June '01	14	109	294	0	0	0
Subtotals		**956**	**3,032**	**7**	**7**	**2**
Totals		**1,755**	**8,619**	**22**	**34**	**24**

NOTE: From mid-2000, increased attention was paid to surveillance in the hot-spot areas.
[a]Tropical bont tick.

TABLE 2. St. Kitts Tropical Bont Tick Eradication Program: host analysis (1998–1999)

Host	Estimated population	Number examined	%	TBT positive	%	Number males	Number females
Cattle	3,384	1,311	39	10	0.007	21	14
Sheep	6,331	2,156	34	1	<0.001	1	0
Goats	5,038	2,120	42	4	0.002	5	8
Totals	14,753	5,587	38	15	0.003	27	22

CAP MANAGEMENT ISSUES

Funding

FAO/trust funds (TF) originating from the SECNA Program (ODA, GTZ, and USA) were available during 1994–1998. FAO/IFAD funds became available in 1997. The FAO accounts were managed by the FAO-R office in Barbados, and later, the FAO-SRO. The CAP-RCU and USDA were concerned over the difficulties associat-

TABLE 3. St. Kitts Tropical Bont Tick Eradication Program: Geographical analysis (1998–1999)[a]

Parish	Host	No. of contacts	Estimated population	Animals examined	TBT positive	No. male	No. female	Survey no.
Christ Church	Cattle		262	187	0	0	0	
	Sheep		802	334	0	0	0	
	Goats		257	174	0	0	0	
	Subtotal	**93**	**1,321**	**695**	**0**	**0**	**0**	
Trinity	Cattle		404	162	3	5	3	2,7
	Sheep		680	186	0	0	0	
	Goats		1,230	369	2	3	7	8
	Subtotal	**123**	**2,314**	**717**	**5**	**8**	**10**	**2,7,8**
St. Anne	Cattle		74	63	0	0	0	
	Sheep		1,127	275	0	0	0	
	Goats		374	170	0	0	0	
	Subtotal	**82**	**1,575**	**508**	**0**	**0**	**0**	
St. John	Cattle		744	341	3	7	0	2,5
	Sheep		1,426	410	0	0	0	
	Goats		643	241	0	0	0	
	Subtotal	**157**	**2,813**	**992**	**3**	**7**	**0**	**2,5**
St. Mary	Cattle		278	74	3	8	10	6,7
	Sheep		611	333	0	0	0	
	Goats		447	297	0	0	0	
	Subtotal	**152**	**1,336**	**704**	**3**	**8**	**10**	**6,7**
St. Paul	Cattle		180	107	0	0	0	
	Sheep		249	156	0	0	0	
	Goats		433	80	0	0	0	
	Subtotal	**43**	**862**	**343**	**0**	**0**	**0**	
St. Peter & St. George	Cattle		1,442	377	1	2	1	7
	Sheep		1,436	462	1	1	0	7
	Goats		1,654	789	2	2	2	3,5
	Subtotal	**237**	**4,532**	**1,628**	**4**	**4**	**2**	**3,5,7**
	Grand Totals	**887**	**14,753**	**5,587**	**15**	**27**	**22**	

[a]Since the protocol was modified in the second half of 1999, the number of properties inspected in SIDs 7 and 8 increased three- to fourfold. In total some 799 properties were surveyed during the period under review. The number of contacts (properties) at its highest point was 887.

ed with IICA management of project funds, especially post-1996. During the same period, USDA funds were managed via IICA. In 1998, however, USDA identified an additional $1.94 million for the CAP via a USA/FAO TF, and it was then decided to route their annual contribution also via FAO. At this time, their previous, existing, and pledged commitments total about US$ 5.0 million.

In 1996–1997, the EU provided approximately euro 0.75 million, mainly for purchase of insecticide and two vehicles. A request was then made for an additional euro 1.5–2.0 millon. This was approved in 1999, but thereafter, prolonged negotiations took place regarding contractual and disbursement procedures. Eventually, an agreement was reached under a Memorandum of Understanding between FAO and the EU-CARIFORUM signed in May 2000, and funds became available in March 2001.

Additional funds are also available under the current EU-CARIFORUM Caribbean Agriculture and Fisheries Program (CAFP) for livestock health and quarantine activities and for CSF control. Collectively the various components could be packaged more economically and effectively, with particular attention to TBT, CSF, screw-worm, and the interrelated quarantine project, and marketed as a "Caribbean Animal Resources Management program."

Major benefits and technical justification include the following:

- Cost-effectiveness, especially of field operations in the Dominican Republic and Haiti.
- Increased sustainability.
- Establishing a regional core database on livestock statistics and health.
- Strengthening veterinary quarantine and emergency preparedness.
- Marketing of a more favorable package to farmers.

Earlier, the USDA proposed that future projects in the Caribbean use the CAP model, as it currently functions very cost-effectively. The fact that it already exists and operates in 18 islands/countries could be presented as strong justification to implement a regional Caribbean Animal Resources Management (CARM) program (disease and pest eradication, emergency preparedness, and quarantine) under a unified management coordination unit. Moreover, the USDA is cofunding complementary programs for CSF in the Dominican Republic and NWS in Jamaica. Moreover, the wider program would fit conceptually into the joint FAO/USDA draft proposal for post-CAP activities. Implementation commonalties include:

- Same major donors (USDA and EU).
- Same 16 CARIFORUM countries, plus British and Dutch dependencies.
- Same national agriculture ministries and livestock departments.

Coordination and Overall Management

The organization chart (FIG. 1) shows the complexity of the current CAP management structure and of trying to synthesize it into a unified approach.

One issue addressed at the 2000 meeting of the APC is further clarification of the respective roles of the APC, the EU, the FAO, the USDA, and the RCU. There is a

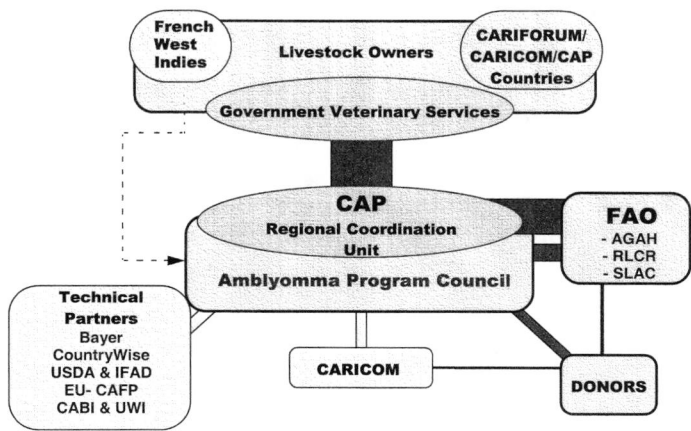

FIGURE 1. Caribbean *Amblyomma* Program (CAP) organizational chart.

need to reemphasize the conclusions of earlier meetings and agreements that stated that the RCU is the focal point for all activities, correspondence, and discussions pertaining to the CAP, and the APC is the focal point for all decisions. Most importantly in this respect are the requirements, as stated by Lindquist,[9] for successful area-wide eradication control programs:

- Prevent political control of the program.
- Establish an independent organization to operate the program.

It was also noted during that conference that some programs have failed, not because of inappropriate technologies, but because of conflicting political and institutional agendas.

Thus, the main agencies should be requested to accept their respective roles of equal, strategic partners. No single agency or organization, or an individual representing them, should claim "seniority" status on administrative, financial, political, or technical grounds.

REFERENCES

1. CAP. 2000. Country Profiles, document. (www.capweb.org)
2. FAO-CAP. 1999. Where CAP is working and Putting a CAP on the tropical Bont tick. (www.fao.org/news/1999/99tick-e.htm and www.fao.org/news/1999/991001-e.htm)
3. New Agriculturist. 2000. Focus on Livestock Health—Eradicating a Tick in Time. (www.new-agri.co.uk/00-06/focuson.html)
4. PEGRAM, R.G. *et al.* 1996. Eradicating the tropical bont tick from the Caribbean. FAO World Anim. Rev. **87:** 56–65
5. PEGRAM, R.G., J.J. DE CASTRO & D.D. WILSON. 1998. The Caribbean *Amblyomma* Programme. Public Health (Bayer) **14:** 60–67.

6. PEGRAM, R.G., J.J. DE CASTRO & D.D. WILSON. 1997. The CARICOM/FAO/IICA Caribbean Amblyomma Programme. Ann. N.Y. Acad. Sci. **849:** 343–348.
7. PEGRAM, R.G., J.W. HANSEN & D.D. WILSON. 2000. Eradication and surveillance of the tropical bont tick in the Caribbean: an international approach. Ann. N.Y. Acad. Sci. **916:** 179–185.
8. PHILLIP, K. ST.C. 2000. Tropical bont tick (*Amblyomma variegatum*) eradication in the Caribbean. Ann. N.Y. Acad. Sci. **916:** 320–325.
9. LINDQUIST, D.A. 2000. Pest management strategies: area-wide and conventional. *In* International Conference on Area-wide Control of Insect Pests, K.-H. Tan, Ed.: 13–19. International Atomic Energy Agency.

Adult Tick Burdens and Habitat Use of Sympatric Wild and Domestic Ungulates in a Mixed Ranch in Zimbabwe

No Evidence of a Direct Relationship

M. DE GARINE-WICHATITSKY

CIRAD-EMVT, Programme ECONAP, Projet "Santé et Environnement" TA30/F, 34398 Montpellier Cedex 5, France, and

IAC, Programme Elevage et Faune Sauvage, Station de Port Laguerre, BP 25, 98890 Païta, New Caledonia

ABSTRACT: Ticks do not usually infest sympatric hosts species according to their availability in a given environment, and it has been suggested that habitat use by hosts is a major determinant of tick burdens. The knowledge of such infestation patterns and their relationship with host habitat use is important for the control of the vectors of some major stock diseases in Africa, particularly in the context of mixed game/cattle ranching. In a ranch of Zimbabwe, we monitored the number of adult ticks found on cattle and wild ungulates. Tick burdens were measured weekly during one year on 12 heifers of an experimental herd (no acaricide used), and on wild ungulates occasionally shot for meat. Adult ticks were not evenly distributed among wild hosts, and infestation patterns corresponded to observations made by several authors in similar conditions. However, these infestation patterns could not be related to habitat use by ungulates, which had been previously monitored by road transect at the scale of the ranch, as these authors found a high niche overlap and no habitat segregation between ungulate species. In an attempt to relate habitat use by Brahman and Simmental heifers with the number of adult ticks collected during one day of grazing, we followed the heifers and recorded their position and activity (one or two days per week; each recording session was 7 h 30 min on average, for a total of 940 hours of survey). No correlation was found between the number of ticks collected and the distance (or time spent) traveled in each vegetation type or the number of grooming episodes. The possible role of other behavioral and physiological parameters is discussed, and the results are compared with those found for other tick–host associations.

KEYWORDS: tick burdens; wild ungulates; domestic cattle; Zimbabwe

Address for correspondence: Dr. M. De Garine-Wichatitsky, IAC, Programme Elevage et Faune Sauvage, Station de Port Laguerre, BP 25, 98890 Païta, New Caledonia. Voice: 687-43-74-25; fax: 687-43-74-26.

m.degarine@iac.nc

Ann. N.Y. Acad. Sci. 969: 306–313 (2002). © 2002 New York Academy of Sciences.

INTRODUCTION

Compared to standard extensive livestock production systems, the association of livestock and wildlife on the same pastures in Africa bears both benefits and costs, the latter being mainly the consequences of health problems.[10] Among these, ticks and tick-borne diseases are a major constraint to improved livestock production in Africa and to the coexistence of wildlife and livestock.[11–14]

Although host preference of ticks is variable according to the tick species considered,[15–17] ticks of large ungulates do not usually infest sympatric hosts species according to their availability in a given environment. It has been suggested that habitat use by hosts is a major determinant of ungulate tick burdens,[1,2] including different cattle breeds grazing on the same pastures,[18] and under certain circumstances, this could have important consequences for the management of livestock regarding the control of ticks and tick-borne diseases.[19,20] However, the mechanisms of host–tick contact have seldom been described. This paper presents the result of a study on habitat use and tick burden of wild and domestic ungulates in a mixed ranch in Zimbabwe.

MATERIALS AND METHODS

Study Site

This work was conducted on an extensive ranch (Kelvin Grove Ranch, Agricultural and Rural Development Authority) located in the highveld of Zimbabwe (Mashonaland west province; 18°36′08″–18°43′24″ south latitude and 30°00′16″–30°05′57″ east longitude). The ranch is situated between 1100 and 1180 m in altitude, and the average annual rainfall is around 750 mm. Three major seasons prevail: [9,21] wet season (November to April); cool-dry season (May to July); and hot-dry season (August to October). The total surface of the ranch is 9400 ha, divided into 30 paddocks of approximately equivalent size.

The vegetation of the ranch is a wooded savanna to woodland, with four major communities: Miombo woodland (*Brachystegia* spp. and *Julbernardia globiflora*), Mopane woodland (*Colophospermum mopane*), Terminalia bush savanna, (*Terminalia sericea*), and some patches of Acacia bush savanna on richer soils (*Acacia nilotica* and *Dichrostachys cinerea*).[9] A vegetation map was established using aerial photograph and ground truthing. All our records were incorporated into a geographical information system (GIS, Mapinfo Software).

Wild Ungulates

Wild ungulates (including impala, *Aepyceros melampus*; wildebeest, *Connochaetes taurinus*; greater kudu, *Tragelaphus strepsiceros*; eland, *Taurotragus oryx*; and zebra, *Equus burchellii*) range freely over the whole area of the ranch. They represent approximately 50% of the biomass of large ungulates of the ranch[22] and are occasionally shot for meat and trophy hunting. Whenever possible, adults ticks were counted from the whole body surface of the animals shot during three hunting seasons from May to October, 1996 to 1998). Previous studies have investigated habitat use and feeding behavior of both wild and domestic herbivores in the Kelvin Grove Ranch.[9,23]

Livestock and Experimental Herd of Heifers

Cattle (*Bos taurus, Bos indicus,* and cross-bred) are raised extensively for the purpose of meat production. They are dipped with acaricides (Amitraz, Taktik N.D) on a weekly basis during the rainy season and every fortnight during the dry season.

An experimental herd of 12 heifers (6 Brahman and 6 Simmental), which was not treated with acaricides during the course of the study (February 1997 to February 1998), was established. Once a week, these animals were immobilized, and all the adult ticks were counted, removed, and preserved for further identification at the laboratory (Tick Research Unit, Veterinary Research Laboratory, Harare). Two heifers (1 Brahman and 1 Simmental) were randomly chosen and checked for ticks again in the morning before their release in a paddock. They grazed freely for 7h30 on average, and their position (GPS and map) and activity (including the number of grooming episodes) were recorded at regular intervals (every 10 to 20 minutes). In the evening, the heifers were driven back to the stock yard where they were immobilized, and the number of ticks collected during the day was measured. Between February 1997 and 1998, we carried out 65 recording sessions, for a total of 940 hours of surveys.

Ticks

Tick species encountered are those commonly found on large ungulates in the region and included mainly *Rhipicephalus appendiculatus, R. zambeziensis, R. evertsi evertsi, Hyalomma marginatum rufipes, H. truncatum,* and *Boophilus decoloratus.* Adult ticks were removed and preserved for further identification at the laboratory. The distribution of tick larvae in the vegetation of the ranch has also been described during another study.[11,24]

Statistical Methods

Details of the procedures are presented in De Garine-Wichatitsky[11] and follow the recommendations of Sokal and Rolf.[25] Whenever possible, we used parametric tests (ANOVA, Scheffé paired comparisons) but often had to use nonparametric tests (Kruskall-Wallis, Mann-Whitney, or Wilcoxon) because tick infestation levels were usually not normally distributed, even after log transformation.

RESULTS

Tick Burdens of Wild Ungulates

FIGURE 1 presents the results of the tick counts carried out on the wild ungulates shot during the dry season (May to October). Infestations were significantly different between ungulate species for *H. m. rufipes* and *H. truncatum* (Kruskal-Wallis; $P = 0.003$ and $P = 0.024$ respectively), and for *R. e. evertsi* and the total number of adult ticks collected (ANOVA, $P < 0.001$), eland and zebra being significantly more infested than kudu and impala. The number of *B. decoloratus* was not significantly different between ungulate species (ANOVA, $P > 0.05$), and very few *R. appendiculatus* were collected during this period.

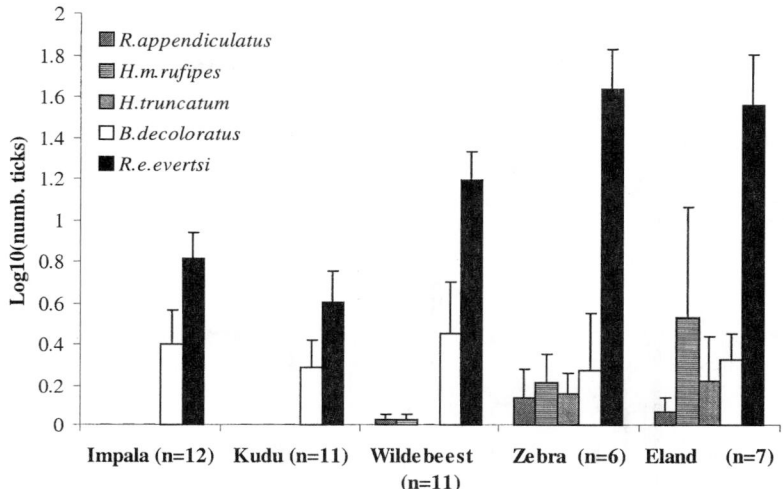

FIGURE 1. Infestation of wild ungulates by adult ticks during the dry season (May to October) of three consecutive years (1996 to 1998). Mean number of ticks per animal (Log_{10} $(X + 1)$). Error bars indicate the standard error of the mean. See text for significant differences.

Previous studies on habitat use of wild and domestic ungulates of the Kelvin Grove Ranch[9,22] revealed selective use of the available habitats. Habitat preferences were similar between species, and there was an important niche overlap, although it was variable according to season and the species of ungulates considered. Another study carried out in the area during which recent tracks and dungs were recorded on 255 different sites revealed that more than 60% of the sites checked had recently been visited by two or more species of ungulates.[11,24]

Tick Burdens of Heifers of the Experimental Herd

Weekly counts (52 counts between February 1997 and February 1998) of the number of adult ticks collected from the heifers in this study showed important seasonal variations for *R. appendiculatus, R. zambeziensis, H. m. rufipes*, and *H. truncatum*, which were more abundant during the rainy season, and *B. decoloratus* and *R. e. evertsi,* which were found throughout the year. Simmental heifers always carried significantly more ticks than Brahman heifers, and this was true for all species of ticks (Wilcoxon, 52 pairs, $P < 0.01$).

FIGURE 2 presents the number of adult ticks collected by the heifers during one day of grazing. Although few ticks were collected overall, the seasonal variations were similar to those found for the weekly counts. Of significance is that the number of ticks collected from Brahman heifers was not significantly smaller than for Simmental, except for the number of adult *R. appendiculatus,* which showed a marginal significance (Wilcoxon, 65 pairs, $P < 0.05$).

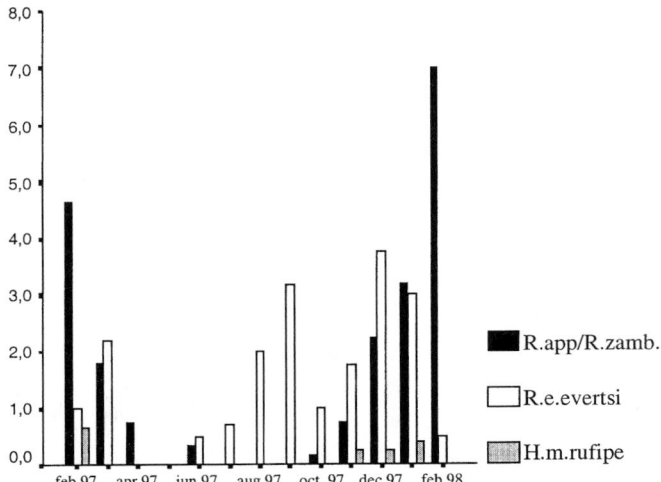

FIGURE 2. Seasonal variations of the number of ticks collected by heifers during one day grazing. Data for Brahman and Simmental heifers pooled together. Mean number of adult ticks (*R. app/R. zamb.* = *R. appendiculatus/R. zambeziensis)* collected every month (total of 130 counts) between February 1997 and February 1998.

Habitat Use and Activity of Heifers

The distance traveled by the heifers during one day of grazing was not significantly different according to season (ANOVA, $P < 0.05$), and all vegetation types were used. During the dry season, there was a preference for Acacia bush savanna, but no difference was found between habitat use by Brahman and Simmental heifers. We found no significant correlation between the number of adult ticks collected and the total distance traveled during the survey or the distance traveled within each vegetation community (*R. appendiculatus/R. zambeziensis, n* = 43; *R. e. evertsi, n* = 61; *H. m. rufipes, n* = 19; and total number of ticks, *n* = 61; Spearman correlation, $P < 0.05$).

The frequency of grooming episodes (oral grooming, scratching) was not correlated with the number of adult ticks collected from heifers during one day of grazing (Spearman correlation, $P < 0.05$). The number of episodes of oral grooming or scratching during the surveys was not significantly different between the two breeds (Mann-Whitney, $P < 0.05$).

DISCUSSION

Ticks, like most parasites, do not infest the host according to their availability in a given environment. For wild African ungulates, some species accumulate more tick species and are more heavily infested than others.[2] Although our sample size

TABLE 1. Infestation by adult ticks of Brahman and Simmental heifers of the experimental herd

	R. eve		H. m. ruf		H. tru		R. ap/R. za		B. dec	
	Mean	S.E.	Mean	S.E.	Mean	S.E.	Mean	S.E.	Mean	S.E.
Brahman (n = 284	26.39	1.17	3.03	0.33	0.14	0.04	5.14	0.61	1.04	0.04
Simmental (n = 289)	35.06	1.43	6.07	0.59	0.35	0.06	9.82	1.11	9.15	1.10
Wilcoxon Z	5.564		5.247		3.227		2.615		5.638	
P	0.0001**		0.0001**		0.001*		0.009*		0.0001**	

Mean number of ticks (S.E.) measured weekly between February 1997 and February 1998. Paired comparisons (Wilcoxon, 52 pairs); probability corrected for multiple tests

ABBREVIATIONS: *R. eve* = *Rhipicephalus e. evertsi*; *H. m. ruf* = *Hyalomma marginatum rufipes*; *H. tru* = *H. truncatum*; *R. ap/R. za* = *R. appendiculatus/R. zambeziensis*; *B. dec* = *Boophilus decoloratus*; S.E. = standard error; *P* = probability; corrected significance level: * = *P* < 0.05; ** = *P* < 0.001.

was limited and restricted to the dry season, our conclusions are similar to those obtained by other authors in the region.[4–7] As for cattle, it is well known that imported *Bos taurus* breeds are more heavily infested by African ticks than *Bos indicus* breeds.[26–29] Indeed, this is what we found for Brahman (*Bos indicus*) and Simmental (*Bos taurus*) heifers during our study.

The hypothesis that differences in tick burdens, both within and between species, could be related to differences in habitat use[1,2,19,30,31] or to differences in grooming rate,[32–34] is not confirmed by our study. Habitat use by wild and domestic ungulates in Kelvin Grove[9] did not show a segregation between ungulate species (or between cattle breeds), which could explain the observed differences in tick burdens. We were unable to establish a direct relationship between the use of a given vegetation and the number of ticks collected by heifers during one day of grazing. Grooming rates were not measured for wild ungulates. There was no significant correlation for heifers between the number of tick collected and the number of grooming episodes, and the frequency of grooming episodes was not significantly different between Brahman and Simmental heifers.

Under particular circumstances where domestic hosts have contrasting habitat preferences and infesting ticks are restricted to particular habitats,[19,30] it might be possible to manage herds in order to minimize host–tick contact or to optimize the use of acaricides to destroy ticks collected during the periods at risk.[35] Our results show that habitat use might be of secondary importance for tick burdens of sympatric wild and domestic ungulates at the scale of the ranch where the study took place, and we were not able to draw similar conclusions.

ACKNOWLEDGMENTS

I would like to thank G. Uilenberg, F. Monicat, F. Renaud, and D. Cuisance for their help at various stages during the course of this study. I also thank S. Ducornez,

N. Vittrant, and B. Butete for their valuable help in data collection. W. Mazhowu and M. Chiswa (Veterinary Research Laboratory Tick Unit, Harare), and I. G. Horak (University of Pretoria) kindly contributed to tick identification. I am grateful to L. Mhlanga, N. Kombani, and the staff of ARDA Battlefield complex for their collaboration, and to the CIRAD-EMVT team in Zimbabwe for their support. This study was funded by CIRAD and the French Ministry for Education and Research (Fellowship MESR No. 96091).

REFERENCES

1. DE GARINE-WICHATITSKY, M., H. FRITZ & S. DUCORNEZ. 1995. Habitat use as a factor influencing cattle tick burdens. Proceedings of the 2nd International Conference on Tick-borne Pathogens at the Host-Vector Interface. Kruger National Park, South Africa. Vol. 2: 429–437.
2. GALLIVAN, G.J. & I.G. HORAK. 1997. Body size and habitat as determinants of tick infestations of wild ungulates in South Africa. S. Afr. J. Wildl. Res. 27: 63–70.
3. COLBORNE, J.R.A. 1988. The role of wild hosts in maintaining tick populations on cattle in the southeastern lowveld of Zimbabwe. M.Sc. Thesis. University of Zimbabwe, 200 pp.
4. HORAK, I.G., F.T. POTGIETER, J.B. WALKER, et al. 1983. The ixodid tick burdens of various large ruminant species in South African nature reserves. Onderstepoort J. Vet. Res. 50: 221–228.
5. HORAK, I.G., V. DE VOS & M.R. BROWN. 1983. Parasites of domestic and wild animals in South Africa. XVI. Helminth and arthropod parasites of blue and black wildebeest (*Connochaetes taurinus* and *Connochaetes gnou*). Onderstepoort J. Vet. Res. 50: 243–255.
6. HORAK, I.G., L.J. FOURIE, J.M. V. ZYL & Z.-J.M. VAN. 1995. Arthropod parasites of impalas in the Kruger National Park with particular reference to ticks. Onderstepoort J. Vet. Res. 25: 123–126.
7. HORAK, I.G., J. BOOMKER, A.M. SPICKETT & V. DE VOS. 1992. Parasites of domestic and wild animals in South Africa. XXX. Ectoparasites of kudus in the eastern Transvaal Lowveld and the eastern Cape Province. Onderstepoort J. Vet. Res. 59: 259–273.
8. MINSHULL, J.I. 1981. Seasonal occurrence, habitat distribution and host range of four ixodid ticks species at Kyle recreational park in south eastern Zimbabwe. Zimbabwe Veterinary J. 12: 58–63.
9. FRITZ, H., M. DE GARINE-WICHATITSKY & G. LETESSIER. 1996. Habitat use by sympatric wild and domestic herbivores in an African savanna woodland: the influence of cattle spatial behaviour. J. Appl. Ecol. 33: 589–598.
10. BOURN, D. & R. BLENCH. 1999. Can livestock and wildlife co-exist? An interdisciplinary approach. ODI. London. 261 pp.
11. DE GARINE-WICHATITSKY, M. 1999. Écologie des interactions hôtes-vecteurs: analyse du système tiques-ongulés sauvages et domestiques en zone tropicale. Ph.D. Thesis. Université de Montpellier II. Montpellier, 302 pp.
12. PEGRAM, R.G., R.J. TATCHELL, J.J. DE CASTRO, et al. 1993. Tick control: new concepts. World Animal Rev. 74–75: 2–11.
13. UILENBERG, G. 1995. International collaborative research: significance of tick-borne hemoparasitic diseases to world animal health. Vet. Parasitol. 57: 19–41.
14. UILENBERG, G. 1992. Veterinary significance of ticks and tick-borne diseases. *In* Tick Vector Biology. B. Fivaz, T. Petney, et al., Eds.: 24–33. Springer-Verlag. Berlin.
15. HOOGSTRAAL, H. 1956. African Ixodoidea. I. Ticks of the Sudan. Cairo, Egypt, 1101 pp.
16. MOREL, P.C. 1969. Contribution à la connaissance de la distribution des tiques (Acariens, Ixodidae et Amblyommidae) en Afrique éthiopienne continentale. Thèse de Doctorat. Faculté des Sciences d'Orsay, Paris, 388 pp.
17. OLIVER, J.H. 1989. Biology and systematics of ticks (Acari: Ixodida). Annu. Rev. Ecol. Syst. 20: 397–430.

18. BARNARD, D.R. 1989. Daily pickup rates of the lone star tick (Acari: Ixodidae) by pastured beef cattle. Ann. Entomol. Soc. Am. **82**: 446–449.
19. FOURIE, L.J. & O.B. KOK. 1992. The role of host behaviour in tick-host interactions: a domestic host-paralysis tick model. Exp. Appl. Acarol. **13**: 213–225.
20. BARNARD, D.R. 1991. Mechanisms of host-tick contact with special reference to *Amblyomma americanum* (Acari: Ixodidae) in beef cattle forage areas. J. Med. Entomol. **28**: 557–564.
21. NORVAL, R.A.I., J.B. WALKER & J. COLBORNE. 1982. The ecology of *Rhipicephalus zambeziensis* and *Rhipicephalus appendiculatus* (Acarina, Ixodidae) with particular reference to Zimbabwe. Onderstepoort J. Vet. Res. **49**: 181–190.
22. FRITZ, H. 1995. Etude des systèmes mixtes d'herbivores sauvages et domestiques en savane africaine: structure des peuplements et partage de la ressource. Ph.D. Thesis. Université Paris 6, Paris, Vol. 1, 86 pp.
23. FRITZ, H. & M. DE GARINE-WICHATITSKY. 1996. Foraging in a social antelope: effects of group size on foraging choices and resource perception in impala. J. Anim. Ecol. **65**: 736–742.
24. DE GARINE-WICHATITSKY, M., T. DE MEEÛS, J.-F. GUÉGAN & F. RENAUD. 1999. Spatial and temporal distributions of parasites: can wild and domestic ungulates avoid African tick larvae? Parasitology **119**: 455–466.
25. SOKAL, R.R. & F.J. ROHLF. 1981. Biometry. The Principles and Practices of Statistics in Biological Research. W.H. Freeman and Company. New York, 859 pp.
26. NORVAL, R.A.I., R.W. SUTHERST & J.D. KERR. 1996. Infestations of the bont tick *Amblyomma hebraeum* (Acari: Ixodidae) on different breeds of cattle in Zimbabwe. Exp. Appl. Acarol. **20**: 599–605.
27. RECHAV, Y., J. DAUTH & D.A. ELS. 1990. Resistance of Brahman and Simmentaler cattle to southern African ticks. Onderstepoort J. Vet. Res. **57**: 7–12.
28. RECHAV, Y. & M. KOSTRZEWSKI. 1991. Relative resistance of six cattle breeds to the tick *Boophilus decoloratus* in South Africa. Onderstepoort J. Vet. Res. **58**: 181–186.
29. SPICKETT, A.M., D. DE KLERK, C.B. ENSLIN & M.M. SCHOLTZ. 1989. Resistance of Nguni, Bonsmara and Hereford cattle to ticks in a bushveld region of South Africa. Onderstepoort J. Vet. Res. **56**: 245–250.
30. BARNARD, D.R. 1989. Habitat use by cattle affects host contact with the lone star ticks (Acari: Ixodidae), J. Econ. Entomol. **82**: 854–859.
31. HART, B.L. 1990. Behavioral adaptations to pathogens and parasites: five strategies. Neurosci. Biobehav. Rev. **14**: 273–294.
32. MOORING, M.S., J.E. BENJAMIN, C.R. HARTE & N.B. HERZOG. 2000. Testing the interspecific body size principle in ungulates: the smaller they come the harder they groom. Anim. Behav. **60**: 35–45.
33. OLUBAYO, R.O., J. JONO, G. ORINDA, *et al.* 1993. Comparative differences in densities of adult ticks as a function of body size on some East African antelopes. Afr. J. Ecol. **31**: 26–34.
34. NORVAL, R.A.I. 1992. Host susceptibility to infestation with *Amblyomma hebraeum*. Insect Sci. Appl. **13**: 498–494.
35. BARNARD, D.R. 1986. Aspects of the bovines host-lone star tick interaction process in forage areas. *In* Morphology, Physiology and Behavioural Biology of Ticks. J.R. Sauer & J.A. Hair, Eds.: 187–199. Ellis Horwood. Chichester.
36. RICE, W. 1989. Analyzing tables of statistical tests. Evolution **43**: 223–225.
37. HOLM, S. 1979. A simple sequentially rejective multiple test procedure. Scand. J. Stat. **6**: 65–70.

Tick-Borne Diseases (TBDs) of Dairy Cows in a Mediterranean Environment

A Clinical, Serological, and Hematological Study

P. TASSI, G. CARELLI, AND L. CECI

Department of Animal Health and Welfare, Faculty of Veterinary Medicine, University of Bari, Valenzano, Italy

ABSTRACT: A longitudinal study of tick-borne diseases (TBDs) in Southern Italy was carried out by monitoring two dairy farms (A and B) located in the Apulia Region. On each farm ten calves and ten heifers were observed monthly from May 1999 to February 2001 for clinical signs and blood parameters; antibodies against *Babesia bigemina* and *Anaplasma marginale* using an ELISA test were also monitored for the first eight months of the study. Totals of 28 and 14 cases of TBDs were observed in the complete herds of Farms A and B, respectively. Timing of disease appearance, categories of animals affected and changes in blood parameters are discussed.

Keywords: tick-borne diseases; cattle diseases; babesiosis

INTRODUCTION

Although *Babesia* spp. have been recognized since the end of 19th century,[1] and TBDs were well described at the beginning of the 20th century in Italy,[2] there is still scanty information about these parasite species, their vectors, distribution, incidence and impact on livestock production. More recently, several reports indicate that *Babesia* spp. (mainly *B. bigemina*) are widespread on dairy farms in the central and southern parts of the country,[3,4] and acute or subclinical cases due to *B. bigemina*, *A. marginale* and/or *Theileria buffeli*, alone or together, have been described.[3,5–8] Lack of knowledge, however, exists concerning the clinical manifestation and epidemiology of the diseases in these environments; arthropod vectors that may be involved in their transmission are also not known. This paper describes the results of one 22-month longitudinal study carried out with the purpose of gathering information on the clinical aspects and epidemiology of the diseases under field conditions.

Address for correspondence: (Temporary address) Dr. P. Tassi, Onderstepoort Veterinary Institute, Private Bag X05, 0110 Onderstepoort, RSA.
paolo@moon.ovi.ac.za

Ann. N.Y. Acad. Sci. 969: 314–317 (2002). © 2002 New York Academy of Sciences.

METHODS

Two dairy farms (designated A and B) with about 140 Friesian and/or Brown Swiss animals each, located in the Apulia Region and in which clinical cases due to *A. marginale*, *B. bigemina* and *T. buffeli* had previously been recognized, were chosen for the study. On each farm, ten calves, three months old or younger, kept in fenced areas, and ten heifers, 12 to 18 months old, with permanent access to pasture, were chosen at random, observed monthly for clinical signs, sampled for complete blood count (from May 1999 to February 2001) and monitored serologically (from May 1999 to December 1999) for antibodies against *B. bigemina* and *A. marginale* using an ELISA test (ILRI, Nairobi) based on recombinant antigens p200 and MSP5 of the two organisms, respectively. At the onset of the study and again about 12 months later all milking animals in the two herds were sampled for complete blood counts and for serological tests. Ticks were also collected monthly from animals.

RESULTS

Farm A

The screening for TBDs on the whole herd at the beginning of the study revealed seroprevalences of 82% (64/78) and 86% (67/78) for *B. bigemina* and *A. marginale,* respectively. After 12 months, seroprevalences were 60.5% (46/76) and 69.7% (53/76) for the two organisms, respectively. The ten calves remained healthy, and all but one were negative on ELISA until October 1999, although nine of them showed a low and erratic *A. marginale* parasitemia; all remained negative for *B. bigemina* on blood smears examination, but four were inconsistently positive on the ELISA, and one permanently. From June 2000, when they were already heifers, seven of them showed signs of babesiosis with packed cell volumes (PCVs) between 24 and 14%, and parasites were seen on blood-smear examination. In two of the heifers *A. marginale* was also present and all were treated with diminazene and tetracyclines. From June to July 1999 all the heifers became positive for *A. marginale* on the ELISA and seven of them showed subclinical anaplasmosis during June–August 1999 with PCVs ranging between 20.9 and 16.7%; all of them recovered slowly without treatment. Between May 1999 and February 2001, 28 cases of TBDs were observed in the complete herd of Farm A, 18 of which were caused by *A. marginale*, 8 by *B. bigemina* and 2 by a mixed infection. Tick collections revealed that *Rhipicephalus bursa* was the most abundant species, followed by *Hyalomma marginatum* and *Haemaphysalis parva*.

Farm B

At the start of the study the seroprevalences for *B. bigemina* and A. *marginale* were 69.9% (51/73) and 87.7% (64/73), respectively; 80% of the blood smears were also positive for *Theileria* sp. After 12 months, the seroprevalences were 53.3% (48/90) and 81.1% (73/90) for the two organisms, respectively. On Farm B, as on Farm A, the ten calves remained healthy during the study and only one of them was shown to be positive on the ELISA for *A. marginale*, although this organism was present in blood smears of four of the calves on a few occasions. In three calves *Th. buffeli* was also recognized. All the heifers remained consistently negative on the ELISA for *A. marginale* and *B. bigemina* throughout 1999. Six of them developed acute clinical anaplasmosis following parturition, which occurred between August 2000 and February 2001. They required treatment with tetracyclines. Between May 1999 and February 2001, a total of 14 cases of TBDs were observed in the complete herd of Farm B, ten of which were caused by *A. marginale*, three by *A. marginale* and *Th. buffeli*, and one by *A. marginale, B. bigemina,* and *Th. buffeli. R. bursa, H. marginatum* and *Ixodes ricinus* were found in low numbers on this farm.

DISCUSSION

The survey showed a high prevalence and a high incidence of TBDs in the two farms monitored. During a period of almost two years a total of 42 clinical cases was recorded. Some differences were observed in the behavior of the diseases between the two farms. Although *A. marginale* seems to play a major role on both farms, *B. bigemina* appears to pose a serious risk mainly on Farm A, while *Th. buffeli*, which was not found on Farm A, was found to have a high prevalence on Farm B.[9] In accordance with the common observation that young animals rarely show clinical symptoms of TBDs, on both farms calves less than 1 year old remained healthy and they were also negative on the ELISA test. However, clinical cases of babesiosis and/ or anaplasmosis appeared in most of the same animals of the Farm A during June–August of the following year, when they had become heifers. Differences between the two farms were observed for the heifers; in Farm A the heifers seroconverted both for *Anaplasma* and *Babesia* during May–June, increasing their titers in July–August; seven out of 10 developed clinical symptoms of TBDs. It must be underlined that the summer months coincide with the maximum abundance of *R. bursa* adults. Heifers on Farm B remained substantially negative on the ELISA tests conducted during the first 8 months of the trial, but they did develop clinical symptoms during the summer and winter of the following year. In Farm A infection occurred during the first year while ticks were present on the animals, while on Farm B signs of disease were also recognized in winter when no vectors were present. Although the role of vectors cannot be underestimated in the transmission of TBDs, other stress factors may account for the appearance of clinical disease. These may include parturition, high production levels, climatic influences[10] and farm management,[5] which may be associated with outbreaks of TBDs when ticks are not present. This was also the case in the present study on Farm B where six animals showed clinical anaplasmosis following parturition and the misuse of oxytocin as a stimulant for milk production.[11]

REFERENCES

1. GUGLIELMI, G. 1899. Un caso di malaria nel cavallo. La Clinica Veterinaria 220–223; 229–233.
2. CARPANO, M. 1927. Le infezioni da emoprotozoi endoglobulari dei bovini in Italia. La Clinica Veterinaria **50:** 389–400.

3. SAVINI, G., A. CONTE, G. SEMPRONI, *et al.* 1999. Tick-borne diseases (TBD) in ruminants of central and southern Italy. Parassitologia **41** (Suppl. 1): 95–100.
4. PROSPERI, S., R. BALDELLI, R. FIORAVANTI RODAR, *et al.* 1990. Pascoli a rischi sanitari per il bovino. Nota II: Indagine sierologica per Brucellosi, Febbre Q, Clamidiosi a Babesiosi. Obiettivi a Documenti veterinari **11**: 59–61.
5. CECI, L., G. CARELLI, M. SASANELLI, *et al.* 1994. Theileriosi a anaplasmosi bovina in Puglia da probabile trasmissione iatrogena. Proc. Congr. Soc. Italiana delle Scienze veterinarie **48**: 1353–1355.
6. CECI, L., G. CARELLI & M. SASANELLI. 1995. Su di un focolaio di babesiosi bovina da *Babesia bigemina* osservato in Puglia. Proc. Congr. Soc. Italiana delle Scienze veterinarie **49**: 729–730.
7. CARACAPPA, S., F. PRATO, V. DI MARCO, *et al.* 1997. Malattie da zecche in bovini siciliani. Proc. Congr. Soc. italiana di Buiatria **39**: 371.
8. CECI, L., G. CARELLI & P. TASSI 2000. Theileriosi in Puglia da *Theileria buffeli:* caso clinico, indagine clinico-epidemiologica d'allevamento a tipizzazione biomolecolare. Proc. Soc. italiana di Buiatria **32**: 311–320.
9. STOCKHMAN, S.L., A.M. KJEMTRUP, P.A. CONRAD, *et al.* 2000. Theileriosis in a Missouri beef herd caused by *Theileria buffeli:* case report, herd investigation, ultrastructure, phylogenetic analysis, and experimental transmission. Vet. Pathol. **37**: 11–21.
10. CECI, L., G. CARELLI, P. TASSI, *et al.* 1999. Aspetti epidemiologici a clinici di un focolaio di babesiosi bovina da *Babesia bigemina* verificatosi in inverno. Proc. Congr. Soc. italiana di Buiatria **31**: 311–318.
11. NOSTRAND, S.D., D.M. GALTON, H.N. ERB, *et al.* 1991. Effects of daily exogenous oxytocin on lactation milk yield and composition. J. Dairy Sci. **74**: 2119–2127.

Tick Reference Collection of the Late Dr. P.C. Morel

A Tool for Tick Taxonomists and Veterinarians

S. DUCORNEZ,[a] M. DE GARINE-WICHATITSKY,[b,c] N. BARRÉ,[b,c]
G. UILENBERG,[b] AND J.L. CAMICAS[d]

[a]32, rue Bataille, Vallée des Colons, 98800 Nouméa, Nouvelle-Calédonie

[b]CIRAD-EMVT, Programme ECONAP, Projet "Santé et Environnement", TA30/F, 34398
Montpellier Cedex 1, France

[c]IAC, Programme Elevage et Faune Sauvage, B.P. 25, 98890 Païta, Nouvelle-Calédonie

[d]IRD Centre de Montpellier, B.P. 5045, 34032 Montpellier Cedex, France

ABSTRACT: Host preference of ticks is an important, but still controversial,
subject. Recent developments in molecular biology provide new opportunities
to test some hypotheses about host preference in a given environment if appropriate specimens are available. Since the unique collection gathered by Dr. P.C.
Morel could help achieve this goal, we present an overview of the samples available in his collection.

KEYWORDS: P.C. Morel; tick collection; Africa

Although major works and excellent reviews have been published on the subject
(e.g., refs. 1 and 2), host preference of ticks is still a controversial issue, and the conclusions drawn for the lesser known species in tropical regions are likely to evolve
as more records of tick collections are published.[3] The knowledge of these patterns
of infestation is an important parameter to consider for the control of major vectors
of stock diseases, particularly in the context of mixed game/cattle ranching taking
place in several regions of the world.[4] The recent developments of molecular biology
offer new opportunities to test some hypotheses about host preference of ticks within
a given environment, provided that appropriate specimens are available. In addition
to making a major contribution to tick taxonomy, the unique collection gathered by
Dr. P.C. Morel could contribute to this goal. We present hereafter an overview of the
samples available in his collection.

Address for correspondence: Dr. M. De Garine-Wichatitsky and Dr. S. Ducornez, IAC, Programme Elevage et Faune Sauvage, Station de Port Laguerre, BP 25, 98890 Païta, Nouvelle-
Calédonie. Voice: 687-43-74-25; fax: 687-43-74-26.
  m.degarine@iac.nc

Ann. N.Y. Acad. Sci. 969: 318–322 (2002). © 2002 New York Academy of Sciences.

TABLE 1. List of genera, number of species per genus, and total number of samples for each genus represented in the tick collection of P.C. Morel

	Number of species per genus represented in the collection	Total number of existing species per genus[5]	Number of samples in the collection
ARGASINA			
Argasidae			
Argasinae			
Argas	10	44	109
Carios	3	12	34
Ogadenus	4	7	18
Ornithodorinae			
Alectorobius	21	78	95
Alveonasus	4	7	12
Antricola	1	13	1
Microargas	0	1	0
Nothoaspis	0	1	0
Ornithodoros	7	13	63
Otobius	1	2	14
Parantricola	1	1	1
NUTTALLIELLINA			
Nuttalliellidae			
Nuttalliella	0	1	0
IXODINA			
Ixodidae			
Eschatocephalinae			
Ceratixodes	1	2	3
Eschatocephalus	2	2	22
Lepidixodes	1	1	3
Pholeoixodes	8	32	73
Scaphixodes	6	31	26
Ixodinae			
Ixodes	44	168	526
Amblyommidae			
Amblyomma	75	113	1628
Anocentor	1	2	16
Anomalohimalaya	0	3	0
Aponomma	9	23	155
Boophilus	4	5	599
Cosmiomma	1	1	1
Dermacentor	21	33	144
Haemaphysalis	39	163	466
Hyalomma	22	30	1221
Margaropus	1	3	4
Nosomma	0	1	0
Rhipicentor	2	2	6
Rhipicephalus	59	74	1906
Total	**348**	**869**	**7146**

Number of species listed by Camicas *et al.*[5] are taken as a reference. Each sample may comprise one to several dozen individual ticks.

TABLE 2. Overview of the diversity of hosts on which the samples of the collection have been collected: number of host species and samples for humans, domestic and wild animals, and laboratory reared and free-living specimens

	Number of samples	Number of host species
Humans	64	—
Domestic animals		—
Camel	55	—
Cat	53	—
Cattle	1914	—
Dog	390	—
Donkey	12	—
Dromedary	152	—
Goat	67	—
Horse	113	—
Pig	20	—
Poultry	14	—
Rabbit	35	—
Wild animals		
Mammalia		
Artiodactyla	626	49
Carnivora	280	42
Chiroptera	11	3
Edentata	109	5
Hydracoidea	7	3
Insectivora	70	9
Macroscelidea	10	1
Marsupiala	87	6
Monotrema	2	1
Perissodactyla	112	3
Pholidota	45	3
Primates	19	10
Proboscidea	25	1
Rodentia and Lagomorpha	549	37
Scandentia	18	0
Tubulidentata	3	1
Batrachia	18	1
Aves	190	57
Reptilia	303	23
Laboratory-reared	48	—
Free-living specimens		
Soil	30	—
Vegetation	54	—
Burrow	33	—
Nest	6	—
Cave	16	—
Human habitation	19	—
Henhouse	22	—
Others	76	—
Host unknown	1469	—
Total	**7146**	**255**

DESCRIPTION OF THE COLLECTION

General Information

For more than 40 years, the late Dr. P.C. Morel devoted his life to the study of tick biology and taxonomy, mainly in tropical regions of the world. During his career, he collected or received from renowned tick systematicians, veterinarians, or biologists (e.g., A. Aeschlimann, H. Hoogstraal, and J.B. Walker) a unique collection of tick samples. A total of 7634 samples have been recorded, each sample consisting of one tick to several dozen. P.C. Morel identified or confirmed 7146 samples, and the following information is available for most of them: tick species; stage, date, and location of collection; host species; and name and function of collector. This collection is kept in Montpellier at the CIRAD-EMVT laboratories where P.C. Morel spent most of his professional life.

Genus and Species of Ticks Represented

Following the list established by Camicas *et al.* 1998,[5] a total of 348 species or subspecies are represented in the collection (TABLE 1). This total represents 40% of the species or subspecies described by 12/31/95.[5] Eleven paratypes of species described by P.C. Morel or P.C. Morel *et al.*, and ten species described by other authors are also included in the collection. In addition, specimens of two new species[6] that were about to be described by P.C. Morel when he died, and five additional putative species of *Amblyomma* spp. are preserved in the collection.

Host Information

Host species consist mainly of domestic animals (cattle, horse, dromedary, goat, sheep, donkey, cat, and dog), but humans and numerous species of wild mammals, birds, and reptiles are also well represented, along with some samples of free-living stages. TABLE 2 presents an overview of the diversity of hosts on which the ticks have been collected.

Geographical Distribution

Most of the specimens have been collected in Africa (mainly Western, Central, and Northern Africa) and South America, but some come from other parts of the world, including Europe, the Middle East, and Asia. The details concerning the location of samples collected are currently being analyzed.

DISCUSSION

The unique collection of specimens gathered by the late P.C. Morel has been restored by CIRAD-EMVT in Montpellier. When the collection has been fully inventoried and the information entered in a database, it will be made accessible to the scientific community. For instance, the data could be included in the tick museum database established by ICTTD-2,[7] and some samples could be used for genetic analysis of ticks from various locations and various hosts, and for diachronic analysis of ticks at the same location after several decades.

ACKNOWLEDGMENTS

We would like to thank J. Domenech, F. Monicat, and D. Cuisance (CIRAD-EMVT) for their help in the preparation of the draft of this paper.

REFERENCES

1. MOREL, P.C. 1969. Contribution à la connaissance de la distribution des tiques (Acariens, Ixodidae et Amblyommidae) en Afrique éthiopienne continentale. Thèse de Doctorat. Faculté des Sciences d'Orsay. Université de Paris, Orsay, 388 pp.
2. HOOGSTRAAL, H. & A. AESCHLIMANN. 1982. Tick-host specificity. Bull. Société Entomologique Suisse **55:** 5–32.
3. OLIVER, J.H. 1989. Biology and systematics of ticks (Acari: Ixodida). Annu. Rev. Ecol. Systematics **20:** 397–430.
4. BOURN, D. & R. BLENCH. 1999. Can livestock and wildlife co-exist? An interdisciplinary approach. ODI. London, 251 pp.
5. CAMICAS, J.-L., J.-P. HERVY, F. ADAM & P.C. MOREL. 1998. Les tiques du monde. ORSTOM éditions. Paris, 233 pp.
6. PAPADOPOULOS, B., W. BÜTTIKER, P.C. MOREL & A. AESCHLIMANN. 1991. Ticks (Acarina, Fam. Argasidae & Ixodidae) of Oman. Fauna of Saudi Arabia **12:** 200–208.
7. JONGEJAN, F. 2000. ICTTD-2 Newsletter on ticks and tick-borne diseases of livestock in the tropics n°1.

Epizootiology of Sixty-Four Amphibian Morbidity and Mortality Events in the USA, 1996–2001

D. EARL GREEN, KATHRYN A. CONVERSE, AND AUDRA K. SCHRADER

United States Geological Survey, National Wildlife Health Center, Madison, Wisconsin 53711 USA

ABSTRACT: A total of 44 amphibian mortality events and 20 morbidity events were reviewed retrospectively. The most common cause of amphibian mortality events was infection by ranaviruses (Family: Iridoviridae). Ranavirus epizootics have abrupt onset and affect late-stage larvae and recent metamorphs. Mortality events due to ranavirus infections affected only widespread and abundant amphibian species, and there was a clear association with high population densities. Chytrid fungal infections accounted for seven mortality events in postmetamorphic anurans only. Chytrid epizootics are insidious and easily overlooked in the field. While both ranavirus and chytrid fungal epizootics were associated with >90% mortality rates at affected sites, only the chytrid fungal infections were linked to multiple amphibian population declines. Three primitive fungal organisms in the newly erected clade, Mesomycetozoa, caused morbidities and mortalities in anurans and salamanders.

KEYWORDS: amphibians; ranavirus; "red leg" disease; iridovirus infections; frogs; toads

INTRODUCTION

Amphibian population declines, extirpations of populations, and species extinctions have increased in the last 25 years.[1–5] While some declines, extirpations, and extinctions are easily attributed to loss of habitat, many have occurred in relatively protected, remote, or pristine locations. Some population declines, extirpations, and extinctions have been preceded by documented mortality events,[6–8] but the cause of most mortality events was not confirmed by appropriate diagnostic tests. Other amphibian species have declined and disappeared insidiously; it is unclear in these cases whether field casualties were missed because of insufficient monitoring, because of efficient removal of carcasses by scavengers, because sick amphibians died in cryptic refugia, or whether there were no morbidities or mortalities preceding the declines.

Address for correspondence: Dr. D. Earl Green, DVM, National Wildlife Health Center, 6006 Schroeder Road, Madison, WI 53711.
david_green@usgs.gov

Ann. N.Y. Acad. Sci. 969: 323–339 (2002). © 2002 New York Academy of Sciences.

Spontaneous morbidity and mortality events (MME) in free-living amphibians are infrequently and poorly documented. The majority of published mortality events in amphibians have been attributed to "red leg" disease associated with *Aeromonas hydrophila*, but nearly all reports prior to 1990 have no supporting histological findings, and virus cultures consistently were not attempted. In the United States, Wolf *et al.*[9] documented an iridovirus mortality event in bullfrogs (*Rana catesbeiana*) and demonstrated the susceptibility of numerous other amphibian species to the virus, which was named tadpole edema virus. Iridovirus epizootics were not reported in the United States for another 28 years until mortality events in Sonora tiger salamanders (*Ambystoma stebbinsi*) were documented in Arizona.[10] The seminal work of Cunningham *et al.*[11] correlated bacterial and virus cultures with histology and emphasized the importance and morphological variations of iridovirus infections in numerous mortality events in Great Britain.

Throughout the 1990s, amphibian mortality events in numerous countries were associated with worrisome and persistent population declines. Berger *et al.*[12] correlated mortality events in Panama and Australia with a newly recognized chytrid fungal infection of the amphibian epidermis. The fungus was identified and named *Batrachochytrium dendrobatidis*.[13] Epizootic chytridiomycosis has been detected in recent years throughout the United States and in some cases involved multiple declining and threatened species.[14–17]

In 1996, in response to public concerns about high malformation rates in young postmetamorphic amphibians in Minnesota, USA,[18] the National Wildlife Health Center, U.S. Geological Survey, expanded its diagnostic capability to include amphibians. With each succeeding year, increasing numbers of amphibian MME have been reported and investigated. Sixty-four amphibian MME investigated between 1996 and early 2001 are included in this retrospective epizootiological investigation. The causes of these MME are presented as well as epizootiological features of the major amphibian diseases.

MATERIALS AND METHODS

Pathology reports and associated epizootiological files on 64 amphibian MME were reviewed (TABLES 1 and 2). Only cases in which amphibians were submitted for diagnostic examination were selected. Each event or case consisted of one to 84 amphibians; some cases included a few sympatric fish, reptiles, and invertebrates. Cases that consisted of only one or two submitted amphibians were included in this study only if the species was in decline or if population survey data were available to indicate either prevalence of the disease or magnitude of population decline. Casualties involving amphibian eggs and embryos are excluded.

Routine diagnostic examinations of each amphibian casualty event included necropsy under a dissecting microscope, virus cultures on fathead minnow cell line at 25°C, aerobic bacterial cultures, parasite identification, and histological examinations. Submitters were interviewed (telephone or e-mail) by a wildlife disease specialist to determine onset of casualties, casualty numbers, population size, duration of event, sympatric species, and effect on population size.

TABLE 1. Amphibian morbidity events in the United States, 1996–2001, investigated by the U.S. Geological Survey, National Wildlife Health Center

Number	Affected spp.	Life Stage	Location	Onset Date	Estimated Sick	Disease or Diagnoses
1	Tiger salamander	Larva	North Dakota	August 1996	>95%	Dermal metacercariae[b]
2	Green frog	RM	Wisconsin	June 1997	2%	Malformations
3	Mink frog	RM	Minnesota	July 1997	Unk	Malformations
4	Northern leopard frog	Larva	Maine	July 1998	>75%	Intestinal coccidiosis
5	Northern leopard frog	RM	Minnesota	July 1998	Unk	Malformations
6	Grotto salamander	Larva	Missouri	August 1999	100%	Dermal metacercariae
7	Western toad, Pacific treefrog	Larva	Oregon	Est. July 1999	5%	Hypopigmentation, Giantism
8	Barton Spring salamander[a]	Larva	Texas	April 2000	10%	Malformations (scoliosis)
9	Spring salamander	Larva	Tennessee	March 2000	<5%	Dermosporidiosis
10	Santa Cruz long-toed salamander, California red-legged frog	Larva	California	May 2000	Unk	Trauma, Chytrid fungus

TABLE 1. Amphibian morbidity events in the United States, 1996–2001, investigated by the U.S. Geological Survey, National Wildlife Health Center —(Continued)

Number	Affected spp.	Life Stage	Location	Onset Date	Estimated Sick	Disease or Diagnoses
11	Western toad, Bullfrog, Pacific tree-frog, Foothills yellow-legged frog	Larva	California	June 2000	Unk	Dermal metacercariae, malformations & Chytrid fungus
12	Pacific giant salamander, Rough-skin newt	Larva & Adult	California	July 2000	<10%	Dermal metacercariae
13	Bullfrog	Larva	New Hampshire	July 2000	50%	Malformations, Iridovirus
14	Blue-spotted salamander	RM	Indiana	Nov. 2000	5%	Dermal metacercariae
15	American toad	Adult	Virginia	Nov. 2000	Unk	Suspect Dermosporidiosis
16	Pacific treefrog	RM	California	Dec. 2000	Unk	Malformations
17	Barton Spring salamander[a]	Larva	Texas	March 2001	10%	Dermal metacercariae
18	Red-spotted newt, Four-toed salamander	Adult	Tennessee	April 2001	<5%	Dermal filariasis
19	American toad	Adult	Virginia	May 2001	<5%	Dermosporidiosis
20	Green frog	RM	Vermont	August 2000	Unk	Ichthyophonus

ABBREVIATIONS: RM, recent metamorph; Unk, unknown (unreported).
[a]Barton Spring salamander, Eurycea sosorum n. sp.
[b]Dermal metacercaris were ususally identified as Clinostomum sp.

TABLE 2. Amphibian mortality events in United States, 1996–2001, investigated by the U.S. Geological Survey, National Wildlife Health Center

Number	Affected spp.	Life Stage	Location	Onset Date	Estimated Dead	Etiology
1	Tiger salamander	Larva	Colorado	Aug. 1996	>200	Iridovirus
2	Tiger salamander	Larva	North Dakota	May 1998	>200	Iridovirus
3	Mink frog, Northern leopard frog	RM	Minnesota	June 1998	>200	Iridovirus
4	Spotted salamander	Larva	Maine	July 1998	100	Iridovirus
5	Tiger salamander	Larva	Utah	Sept. 1998	>200	Iridovirus
6	Bullfrog	RM	Indiana	June 1998	100	ND
7	Wood frog	Larva	North Dakota	July 1998	>200	Iridovirus
8	Bullfrog	Larva	Ohio	April 1999	50	Anchorworm
9	Bullfrog	Adult	Illinois	May 1999	20	Ichthyophonus
10	Wood frog	Larva	Maine	July 1999	50	Iridovirus
11	Northern leopard frog	Adult	Colorado	May 1999	20	ND
12	Tiger salamander	Larva	Idaho	June 1999	150	Iridovirus & selenosis
13	Wood frog	Larva	Maine	July 1991	>200	Iridovirus
14	Spotted salamander, Pickerel frog	Larva	Tennessee	June 1999	100	Iridovirus
15	Pickerel frog	RM	New Hampshire	July 1999	25	Iridovirus
16	Boreal toad	Adult	Colorado	Aug. 1999	20	Chytrid fungus

TABLE 2. Amphibian mortality events in United States, 1996–2001, investigated by the U.S. Geological Survey, National Wildlife Health Center —(*Continued*)

Number	Affected spp.	Life Stage	Location	OnsetDate	Estimated Dead	Etiology
17	Boreal toad	Adult	Colorado	May 1999	32	Chytrid fungus
18	Bullfrog	RM	Massachusetts	Aug. 1999	>200	Iridovirus
19	Bullfrog	Larva	New Hampshire	Sept. 1999	>200	Dermocystidium-like fungus
20	Tiger salamander	Larva	Wyoming	July 1999	>200	Iridovirus
21	Northern leopard frog	Adult	North Dakota	Nov. 1999	150	Chytrid fungus
22	Wood frog, Bullfrog, Spotted salamander	Larva	North Carolina	April 2000	>200	Iridovirus & Dermocystidium-like fungus
23	Southern leopard frog	Adult	North Carolina	Jan. 2000	Unk	Chytrid fungus
24	Tiger salamander	Larva	North Dakota	June 2000	>200	Iridovirus
25	Mink frog, Green frog, Northern leopard frog	Larva	Minnesota	June 2000	>200	Iridovirus & Dermocystidium-like fungus
26	Wood frog, Spotted salamander	Larva	Massachusetts	June 2000	>200	Iridovirus
27	Pickerel frog	RM	Maine	July 2000	100	Iridovirus
28	Mink frog	Larva	Minnesota	June 2000	>200	Iridovirus
29	Bullfrog	Larva	California	June 2000	>200	ND
30	Spring peeper	Larva	Maine	June 2000	>200	Iridovirus
31	Boreal toad	Adult	Wyoming	July 2000	Unk	Chytrid fungus
32	Green frog	Larva	Maine	Aug. 2000	>200	Iridovirus

TABLE 2. Amphibian mortality events in United States, 1996–2001, investigated by the U.S. Geological Survey, National Wildlife Health Center —*(Continued)*

Number	Affected spp.	Life Stage	Location	OnsetDate	Estimated Dead	Etiology
33	Mudpuppy	Adult	New York	July 2000	>200	ND
34	Bullfrog	Larva	Maine (Smith Pond)	Aug. 2000	>200	Iridovirus
35	Bullfrog	Larva	Maine (Cedar Lake)	Aug. 2000	>200	Iridovirus
36	Bullfrog	Larva	Maine (Peasant Lake)	Aug. 2000	>200	Iridovirus
37	Tiger salamander	Larva	Idaho	Aug. 2000	100	Iridovirus & selenosis
38	Mountain yellow-legged frog	RM	California	Aug. 2000	>200	Chytrid fungus
39	American toad, Bullfrog	Adult & larva	Maine	July 2000	100	ND
40	Wyoming toad	Adult	Wyoming	Sept. 2000	25	Chytrid fungus
41	California red-legged frog	Adult	California	Oct. 2000	Unk	ND, suspect chytrid
42	Wood frog, Red-spotted newt	Adult	Tennessee	Feb. 2001	100	ND, suspect weather
43	Southern leopard frog	Larva	Mississippi	March 2001	>200	Dermocystidium-like fungus
44	Wood frog	Adult	Maryland	May 2001	Unk	Ichthyophonus

ABBREVIATIONS: RM, recent metamorph; Unk, unknown (unreported); ND, not determined.

RESULTS

There were 20 morbidity events (disease outbreaks) involving 8 species of frogs, 2 species of toads, and 10 species of salamanders in 13 states (TABLE 1). In 15 cases (75%), only one species was involved, and in all cases, multiple species of amphibians were present at the site. The larval stage was the affected life stage in 55% of cases; postmetamorphs constituted the other half of cases. Recent metamorphs (those amphibians that completed metamorphosis within 30 days of capture) constituted 30% of morbidity events and were about twice as likely as adults to be involved in disease outbreaks.

Onset of nonlethal disease outbreaks in amphibians occurred from March to December; 55% of all cases were detected and submitted in a three-month time frame: June, July, and August; 30% of cases were detected and submitted in July. No disease outbreaks were recorded in January, February, September, and October, but three events occurred in November and December.

Fourteen amphibian morbidity events were attributed to only one etiology or disease process; multiple etiological agents were detected in six cases. The most common reason for submission of live amphibians was musculoskeletal deformities (malformations); it was the only cause for submission of six cases and was a factor in a mixture of etiologies in four other cases. The cause of musculoskeletal defects in most cases was not determined.

The second most common disease associated with morbidity events was infection by dermal metacercaria. The contributing biologist's principal concern or complaint in free-living amphibians was the presence of multiple distinct nodules and lumps in the skin. Dermal metacercaria, most often identified as *Clinostomum* sp., occurred in salamanders in five of six cases, and one case consisting of multiple species of tadpoles.

Small skin nodules, crusty ulcers, or skin pustules due to infection by *Dermosporidium* spp. were the main complaint in three cases, each consisting of only one affected amphibian from extensively surveyed populations. Hence, in each case, prevalence of infection was <5%. Two of three cases were first detected and submitted in the spring (March to May). Dermosporidiosis was not detected as an incidental, clinically silent, or lethal infection in the other amphibians (61 cases) in this study. Many amphibians with dermal metacercarial infections were submitted because dermosporidial infection was suspected.

Other diseases associated with amphibian morbidity events included runting in tadpoles due to intestinal coccidiosis, tail and limb trauma associated with invasive species of crayfish, swellings of the body wall associated with filarial nematodes, and swollen dorsal pelvic musculature due to infection by *Ichthyophonus fungus* (TABLE 1).

Mortality Events

The 44 mortality events are shown in TABLE 2. The number of recovered or dead amphibians counted in each case varied from 20 to several thousand. Seventeen species of amphibians were involved in these mortality events: 4 species of salamanders, 10 species of frogs, and 3 toad species. These mortality events occurred in 18 states. Seven die-offs involved two or more amphibian species, and multiple casualties in multiple species were suspected in another four die-offs (data not shown). Three distinct life stages of amphibians were involved in these die-offs: 25 (57%) events occurred principally in larvae; 6 (14%) involved mostly recent metamorphs (<30 days from completion of metamorphosis), and 12 (27%) events occurred mostly in adults. One mortality event involved a mix of larvae and adults. Most mortality events in larvae involved tadpoles and larval salamanders in late stages of development, such as Gosner stages 40 to 45,[19] which is a period of metamorphic climax. No mortality events involved recently hatched larvae (i.e., larvae <2 weeks posthatching).

The etiologies for these 44 amphibian mortality events were determined by virus, bacterial, and fungal cultures; toxicological analyses; and histological examinations. The main etiologies of these amphibian die-offs were (1) iridovirus infections (family, Iridoviridae; genus, *Ranavirus*), (2) combined iridovirus infection and selenium intoxication, (3) infection by the pathogenic amphibian chytrid fungus (*Batrachochytrium dendrobatidis*), (4) systemic infection by an unreported and previously unrecognized yeast-like fungal infection consistent with the mesomycetozoan organism, Dermocystidium, (5) fungal infections by a second mesomycetozoan, Ichthyophonus, (6) infection by the copepod, *Lernea* (anchorworms), and (7) not determined.

Iridovirus infections were the sole cause of 21 (48%) mortality events and were a factor in 4 (9%) additional die-offs with multiple etiologies. Recent metamorphs and larvae were the life stages involved in 24 of 25 mortality events in which iridoviruses were isolated or identified histologically. Iridovirus die-offs affected nine species of frogs and salamanders; only two amphibian species suffered iridoviral die-offs in the western half of the United States (west of 97th meridian), while eight species were affected in eastern states. In the western United States, each iridovirus mortality event involved only one amphibian species; seven western die-offs affected only larval tiger salamanders (*Ambystoma tigrinum*), and one case involved only wood frog tadpoles (*Rana sylvatica*). Multiple sympatric species of frogs and toads were present at western casualty sites involving tiger salamanders, but concurrent morbidities and mortalities in anurans were not observed. In 15 iridovirus-associated die-offs in Minnesota and four other eastern states, all events involved late stage tadpoles and recent metamorphs; three die-offs involved concurrent mortalities in frogs (tadpoles) and salamanders. Postmetamorphs of two months of age or greater were not affected in any iridoviral mortality events except one case in which multiple infectious agents were found.

Onset of each iridoviral die-off is shown in TABLE 2 and FIGURE 1. Twenty-two of 25 die-offs (88%) associated with iridovirus infections began in the months of June, July, and August. No iridoviral mortality events began in the months of October through March, and only one mortality event each occurred in April, May, and September. Daily casualty numbers in iridovirus die-offs are seldom available; however, casualty counts at each survey (data not shown) indicate the number of sick and dead amphibians ranged from as low as three to several hundred daily. Onset was often sudden; several biologists reported apparently normal populations on one day, and two or three days later, casualties consisted of hundreds or thousands of larvae. Duration of mortality events (data not shown) ranged from 5 to about 50 days; longer die-offs consistently involved multiple species of frogs, or frogs and salamanders. Total casualties at a site consistently exceeded 90%; recruitment was consistently zero or negligible.

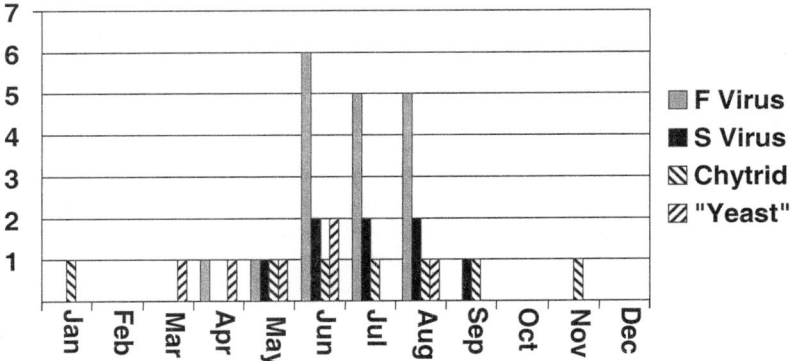

FIGURE 1. Date of onset of mortality events in amphibians due to four infectious diseases. F virus, ranavirus mortality events in frogs; S virus, ranavirus mortality events in salamanders; "Yeast," dermocystidium-like fungal mortality events. Y axis is the number of mortality events.

Iridovirus mortality events in multiple amphibian species have recurred for five consecutive years at one site in Minnesota, and massive die-offs of larvae for three consecutive years at sites in Tennessee and North Carolina are associated with iridovirus epizootics (not all years shown in TABLE 2, because submissions were solicited). There are insufficient annual field data on other mortality sites to estimate the probability of recurring annual die-offs at iridovirus casualty sites.

Chytrid fungus infections were considered the cause of seven mortality events in five states. Mortality events occurred only in frogs and toads; affected species included northern leopard frogs (*Rana pipiens*), southern leopard frogs (*R. sphenocephala*), mountain yellow-legged frogs (*R. muscosa*), boreal toads (*Bufo boreas*), and Wyoming toads (*B. baxteri*); the latter three species are considered in serious decline. Chytrid fungus-associated mortality events occurred only in postmetamorphic frogs and toads (recent metamorphs to breeding age adults); no mortality events involving larvae and salamanders were detected, although larval morbidity occurred.[17]

A temporal pattern of onset of chytrid fungal epizootics was not evident: the seven die-offs began on six different months. Daily casualty numbers were very low, often reported as one sick or dead amphibian per two or three visits (or surveys) of a site. The maximum casualty number in one season of surveys and collections at a site in Colorado was 32, but the population suffered a severe decline in 12–18 months. Population declines were >95% at three additional sites in Colorado and California with chytrid fungus infections in boreal toads and mountain yellow-legged frogs, respectively. Duration of chytrid fungus-associated mortality events could not be determined because date of onset often was undetected and daily casualty numbers usually were less than one. However, casualties due to chytrid fungal infection were usually detected in the second year, except where populations were extirpated. Numbers of breeding age adults in the first year after a chytrid epizootic usually were reduced by >90%. Recurrence of chytrid epizootics at a site probably is an inaccurate concept; chytrid epizootics probably persist or continue steadily from year to year.

A previously unreported severe systemic fungal infection was considered the sole cause of two mortality events and contributed to tadpole mortalities in two other die-offs in which multiple factors were present. The infection is identified by lethargic tadpoles with abdominal distension, and prominently enlarged and pale liver, spleen, pronephroi, and mesonephroi. Massive numbers of spherical, 6–9 micron diameter nonbudding yeast-like organisms are present in blood vessels, sinuses, sinusoids, and lymphatics. The organisms resemble the mesomycetozoan fungus, Dermocystidium. The infection occurred only in ranid tadpoles in Minnesota, Mississippi, North Carolina, and New Hampshire.

Onset of mortality events associated with dermocystidium-like mesomycetozoan fungi had no pattern; the four mortality events occurred in four different months. Mortalities in recently metamorphosed frogs and adult frogs were not observed at the two casualty sites in which the fungus was the only detected etiology, but at one site, no recent metamorphs were found following the die-off, and at the other site, numbers of recent metamorphs were severely reduced. These observations suggest that this fungal infection causes a >95% mortality rate in this population of tadpoles, and greatly impairs recruitment that year. Recurrences have not been investigated.

Ichthyophonus fungal infections, also a mesomycetozoan fungus, were the cause of two amphibian mortality events. In both cases, adult bullfrogs and wood frogs were found lethargic, unresponsive to prodding, and thin. Massive numbers of ovoid to elongate fungal organisms were present within myocytes throughout the body. Both mortality events occurred in May, but actual numbers of casualties were not reported. Other recent metamorphs and adult amphibians at the sites with much milder infections were considered normal appearing. Hence, Ichthyophonus fungal infection may occur more often as a endemic disease in a population, with morbidity exceeding mortalities. An insufficient numbers of die-offs attributed to Ichthyophonus have been investigated to determine its affects on populations and the likelihood of annual recurrence.

The cause of seven mortality events was not determined. In four cases, failure to determine the cause was attributed to the decomposed condition of the carcasses. Although intoxications were suspected in these events, toxicological analyses were consistently unrewarding. An additional two mortality events in tiger salamanders in Idaho were attributed to combined iridovirus infection and toxic levels of selenium in the tissues (selenosis). Only two mortality events of undetermined cause involved two or more species of amphibians and other vertebrates and invertebrates; all other die-offs involved one amphibian species. Distribution of mortalities by life stage showed four die-offs in adult amphibians only, one in adult and larval anurans, and one in recent metamorphs; hence, 71% of mortality events of undetermined cause affected postmetamorphic amphibians. Onset of mortality events of unknown cause ranged from February to October; four die-offs (57%) began in the months of June and July. Seven species were involved, with bullfrogs being involved solely or partially in three die-offs. Impact on the amphibian populations and recurrences have not been determined due to sufficient data and insufficient elapsed time since the die-offs.

Declining, threatened, or endangered (DTE) amphibians of six species, Santa Cruz long-toed salamanders (*Ambystoma macrodactylum croceum*), Wyoming toad

(*Bufo baxteri*), boreal toad (*B. boreas*), California red-legged frog (*Rana aurora draytoni*), foothills yellow-legged frog (*R. boylii*), and mountain yellow-legged frogs (*R. muscosa*) were involved in eight morbidity or mortality events (TABLES 1 and 2). Detected diseases in DTE amphibians in these events were chytrid fungus infection (five events), parasitism by dermal metacercaria (one case), and suspected trauma by introduced species of crayfish (one case); in one case involving *Rana aurora draytoni*, the cause was not determined because of advanced decomposition of the carcasses. Iridoviruses and mesomycetozoan fungi were not detected in any DTE amphibians involved in MME.

DTE species endemic to the eastern United States have not been submitted for diagnostic examinations or health screening. However, sympatric amphibians from three historic breeding sites of four eastern DTE amphibians, Blanchard's cricket frog (*Acris crepitans blanchardi*), flatwoods salamander (*Ambystoma cingulatum*), and gopher frogs (*Rana c. capito* and *R. c. sevosa*) have had infections by chytrid fungi, anchorworms, and mesomycetozoan fungi, but iridoviruses were not detected.

DISCUSSION

Five infectious diseases, consisting of one virus, three fungi, and a copepod parasite, were the sole cause or concurrent factor in 37 of 44 mortality events. Iridoviral and chytrid fungal etiologies were the cause of 32 (73%) of amphibian mortality events, and our findings are consistent with recent published literature.[10,12,20,21] However, literature prior to 1995 suggests that red leg disease due to *Aeromonas hydrophila* or other gram-negative bacilli has been the cause of most amphibian die-offs in the United States. Red leg disease was not the cause of any of 64 amphibian MME in this study, nor was it considered a contributing factor in any die-offs. This suggests that most published amphibian die-offs attributed to red leg disease, in which virus cultures and histological examinations were not reported, are suspect. Diagnoses in these 64 cases indicate red leg disease and other forms of bacterial septicemia are an infrequent cause of amphibian MME and, furthermore, suggest red leg disease may be a frequently misused and overused diagnosis in amphibian medicine and herpetological epizootiology.

Viruses in the family, Iridoviridae, genus, *Ranavirus*, were the most frequent cause of amphibian mortality events, accounting wholly or partially for 25 of 44 (57%) die-offs. Unlike reports from Europe[11,22] in which casualties involved adult ranids, all iridoviral mortality events in the United States involved late stage anuran and caudate larvae, and recent metamorphs. Die-offs of tiger salamanders and bullfrogs due to iridovirus epizootics have been reported previously;[9,10,20] this report documents iridoviral casualties in eight additional species, including spotted salamanders (*Ambystoma maculatum*), eastern red-spotted newt (*Notophthalmus viridescens*), northern leopard frogs, green frogs (*Rana clamitans*), mink frogs (*R. septentrionalis*), pickerel frogs (*R. palustris*), wood frogs, and spring peepers (*Pseudacris crucifer*).

Our data show that iridovirus mortality events occurred only in widespread and abundant amphibian species. To date, iridoviruses have not been isolated from species in decline, but many DTE species have not been examined in sufficient numbers to make firm conclusions. While iridoviral casualty rates at a site are usually >90%, recruitment is negligible, and annual recurrences are known, none of the affected amphibian species are considered in decline, nor have they achieved threatened or endangered status. Because all iridoviral die-offs of American amphibians to date have involved fairly widespread and abundant species, iridoviral epizootics may be a disease of dense populations and a hazard of crowding. Iridoviral die-offs in western states (west of the 97th meridian) consistently involved only one species, while die-offs in eastern states involved numerous species of anurans and caudates at the same site. This distinct pattern suggests that at least two species or strains of *Ranavirus* are involved in amphibian iridoviral mortality events.

In most regions of the United States, amphibians migrate and congregate at breeding ponds in the months of February through May. Only three iridovirus mortality events began in the months of April and May, and no iridoviral die-offs involved adult amphibians in breeding condition. These observations indicate that many adult amphibians may be resistant to, or have acquired immunity to, iridoviruses. However, the source of virus in massive mortality events involving thousands of larvae remains unknown. Recurrence of iridoviral die-offs at multiple sites for two to five consecutive years suggests there are carrier animals, or the virus persists in water, soil, or sediment. Because some amphibians, such as bullfrogs and green frogs are summer breeders and deposit eggs at a time when the larvae of spring-breeding amphibians are in metamorphic climax, and because it is known that the Lucke tumor herpesvirus of northern leopard frogs is shed in massive quantities only during spawning,[23] iridovirus carrier animals or persistently infected amphibians need to be investigated. Wolf *et al.*[9] observed an inverse relationship between age of tadpoles and mortality rates due to tadpole edema virus, and concluded that some individuals survive infections and develop immunity.

Key epizootiological features of iridoviral die-offs are the following: onset of die-offs usually is in the months of June, July, and August when many larvae are metamorphosing; the number of casualties per survey of a site varies greatly from less than 10 to several thousand; onset of die-offs usually is sudden: larval populations at a pond may appear normal on one day, and show massive casualties two days later; duration of iridoviral die-offs ranges from five days to as much as six weeks; longer die-offs tend to involve multiple amphibian species; die-offs affecting only one species generally produce casualties for 5 to 14 days with >90% reduction of the larval population.

Four distinct fungal diseases are documented. Two fungi (Ichthyophonus and Dermocystidium), which for many decades have had uncertain taxonomic status, have been placed in the newly erected clade, Mesomycetozoa.[24] It is proposed that a third amphibian fungal organism, known as *Dermosporidium penneri*,[14,25] also belongs in the clade, Mesomycetozoa. Dermosporidiosis was documented in three morbidity events involving adult, breeding age, American toads (*Bufo americanus*), and one larval spring salamander (*Gyrinophilus porphyriticus*); no deaths were associated with these cases. However, extensive casualties occurred in association with a previously unreported systemic disease caused by an organism resembling Dermocystidium or rosette agent of fish;[26,27] these mortality events were limited to ranid tadpoles; casualties were not observed in recent metamorphs and adult amphibians. Ichthyophonus—the second fungal organism in the clade, Mesomycetozoa—was the cause of two mortality events of unknown extent and one morbidity event. The morbidity event in recent metamorphs was characterized by frogs with a marked swelling of muscles and soft tissues around the urostyle similar to those previously reported in adult newts;[28,29] however, the swelling at the rump and urostyle was absent in adult frogs in the two mortality events, which suggests larvae and adults have different disease courses when infected by Ichthyophonus. Subclinical and nonlethal infections by Ichthyophonus were occasionally detected in other larvae, recent metamorphs, and adults (data not shown) and were interpreted as very mild incidental infections. Hence, the three Mesomycetozoa-like fungi caused three distinctive disease syndromes: Dermocystidium-like infection caused high mortality rates in ranid tadpoles only; Dermosporidium infections had low prevalences, no mortalities, and infections were limited to adult, breeding age toads and one larval salamander; infections by Ichthyophonus caused low mortality rates in adult ranids and intermediate prevalence rates with distinctive gross swellings of the rump region in recently metamorphosed ranids.

Chytrid fungal infections by the amphibian pathogen, *Batrachochytrium dendrobatidis*, caused mortalities only in postmetamorphic frogs and toads. Although chytrid fungal infections were observed in ranid tadpoles and salamander larvae, no mortalities and no die-offs attributed to chytrid infection were seen in salamanders and larval anurans. Mortality events due to chytrid fungal epizootics are insidious, persistent, and associated with serious and dramatic population declines in three western species: boreal toads, Wyoming toads, and mountain yellow-legged frogs. Because no more than one sick or dead amphibian was found at each survey of a site, chytrid fungal epizootics are considered an insidious mortality event that could easily be overlooked by experienced herpetologists; detection of chytrid mortality events usually requires repeated surveys of a site to detect just two casualties. Hence, chytrid fungal epizootics, because of their insidious nature, are a leading candidate for many additional unexplained amphibian population declines in the United States.

Intoxications associated with agrichemicals and other contaminants were not confirmed in any of 64 MME, but tissues from only a small number of amphibians were submitted for toxicological analyses. The only confirmed intoxications in this study were two die-offs of tiger salamanders in Idaho due to combined iridovirus infection and selenium poisoning. Both mortality events occurred in tailing ponds of phosphate mines, and it is not clear whether chronic selenosis impaired the immune systems of these populations and predisposed larvae to viral infections, or whether the iridovirus die-offs would have occurred in the absence of elevated tissue concentrations of selenium. Intoxications may have contributed to seven mortality events in which an etiology was not detected. Infectious diseases such as chytridiomycosis are just as likely to have contributed to these die-offs, because the submitted carcasses frequently were too decomposed for meaningful cultures and histological examinations.

An additional six distinct but general categories were used in morbidity events, including dermal metacercarial infections; skin nodules, pustules, or swellings; limb malformations; trauma; runting; and giantism. Although the metacercaria of multiple genera of trematodes infect the skin of amphibians, few genera produce nodules of sufficient size to be detected by the unaided eye in live amphibians. The most common dermal metacercaria to produce visible skin nodules is *Clinostomum* sp. Precise causes were not determined for some morbidity events, such as limb malformations, hypopigmentation, and giantism.

In summary, numerous infectious diseases are implicated in amphibian MME in the United States, but red leg disease was not found. While ranaviruses, chytrid fungi, and a newly recognized mesomycetozoan fungal infection were the cause of 77% of mortality events, it is not clear whether any of these pathogens are endemic diseases or newly introduced pathogens at each casualty site, because there are no data from health surveys of normal-appearing amphibian populations with which to make comparisons.

CONCLUSIONS

- Three distinct infectious diseases accounted for 77% of 44 mortality events: these pathogens are Ranavirus, chytrid fungus (*Batrachochytrium dendrobatidis*), and a previously unreported Dermocystidium-like mesomycetozoan fungus.

- Mortality events in American salamanders usually occur where populations are dense and usually are due to iridovirus infections.

- In the eastern United States, iridovirus die-offs involve both anurans and caudates. In the western United States, iridovirus die-offs involve only one species, usually the tiger salamander.

- Iridoviral mortality events affected predominantly larval amphibians, usually those in metamorphic climax. Accordingly, iridoviral mortality events are observed primarily during late spring and summer when a population of larval cohorts is in metamorphic climax.

- Iridoviral mortality events have a sudden onset, and casualties number in the scores to thousands of amphibians daily.

- Iridoviral epizootics have not been associated with DTE species, but few DTE species have been examined, and further studies are warranted.

- Chytrid epizootics are insidious with field casualties, usually numbering only one amphibian per two or three surveys of a site. Hence, it is likely that many chytrid epizootics are undetected.

- Amphibian mortalities due to chytrid fungal epizootics have been observed only in postmetamorphic anurans. Mortalities in larval amphibians and caudates have not been detected.

- Larval anurans and caudates may be infected by chytrid fungi, but such infections produce morbidities only and are limited to the oral discs of tadpoles and tips of digits of larval caudates.

- Chytrid epizootics in the western United States have features of an introduced, highly lethal infectious disease to which amphibian populations have no innate resistance.

- Chytrid fungal epizootics are the only infectious disease currently associated with population declines of multiple species.

- Mortality events associated with Dermocystidium-like organisms have occurred only in ranid larvae in states east of the 97th meridian.

- Insufficient MME associated with Dermosporidium, Ichthyophonus, and anchorworms have been observed to make any conclusions.

- Red leg disease, commonly attributed to infection by *Aeromonas hydrophila*, was not documented as a factor in any of 64 MME in amphibians, thus calling into question many published reports of die-offs due to this disease in the twentieth century.

ACKNOWLEDGMENTS

The authors gratefully acknowledge the diagnostic assistance of Douglas Docherty, Renee Long, Candace Cullen, and Tina Jaquish in virology; Mark Wolcott, Brenda Berlowski, and Heather Gutzman in bacteriology and mycology; and Rebecca Cole, Anindo Choudhury, and Connie Roderick in parasitology. The names of contributing biologists are too numerous to list, but we most gratefully thank the many federal herpetologists, park rangers, refuge scientists, state biologists, state ecologists and environmental protection officers, professors and graduate students, and NGO biologists who detected, collected, and contributed amphibians for diagnostic examinations.

REFERENCES

1. FELLERS, G.M. & C.A. DROST. 1993. Disappearance of the cascades frog *Rana cascadae* at the southern end of its range, California, USA. Biol. Conserv. **65:** 177–181.
2. DROST, C.A. & G.M. FELLERS. 1996. Collapse of a regional frog fauna in the Yosemite area of the California Sierra Nevada, USA. Conserv. Biol. **10:** 414–425.
3. FISHER, R.N. & H.B. SHAFFER. 1996. The decline of amphibians in California's Great Central Valley. Conserv. Biol. **10:** 1387–1397.
4. LAURANCE, W.F., K.R. MCDONALD & R. SPEARE. 1996. Epidemic disease and the catastrophic decline of Australian rain forest frogs. Conserv. Biol. **10:** 406–413.
5. CAREY, C., N. COHEN & L. ROLLINS-SMITH. 1999. Amphibian declines: an immunological perspective. Dev. Comp. Immunol. **23:** 459–472.
6. BRADFORD, D.F. 1991. Mass mortality and extinction in a high-elevation population of *Rana muscosa*. J. Herpetol. **25:** 174-177.
7. KAGARISE SHERMAN, C. & M.L. MORTON. 1993. Population declines of Yosemite toads in the eastern Sierra Nevada of California. J. Herpetol. **27:** 186-198.
8. LIPS, K.R. 1999. Mass mortality and population declines of anurans at an upland site in western Panama. Conserv. Biol. **13:** 117-125.
9. WOLF, K., G.L. BULLOCK, C.E. DUNBAR & M.C. QUIMBY. 1968. Tadpole edema virus: a viscerotropic pathogen for anuran amphibians. J. Infect. Dis. **118:** 253-262.
10. JANCOVICH, J.K. *et al.* 1997. Isolation of a lethal virus from the endangered tiger salamander *Ambyostoma tigrinum stebbinsi*. Dis. Aquatic Organisms **31:** 161–167.
11. CUNNINGHAM, A.A., T.E.S. LANGTON, P.M. BENNETT, *et al.* 1996. Pathological and microbiological findings from incidents of unusual mortality of the common frog (*Rana temporaria*). Phil. Trans. Roy. Soc. London **B351:** 1529–1557.
12. BERGER L., R. SPEARE, P. DASZAK, *et al.* 1998. Chytridiomycosis causes amphibian mortality associated with population declines in the rainforests of Australia and Central America. Proc. Natl. Acad. Sci. USA **95:** 9031–9036.

13. LONGCORE, J.E., A.P. PESSIER & D.K. NICHOLS. 1999. *Batrachochytrium dendrobatidis* gen. et sp. nov., a chytrid pathogenic to amphibians. Mycol. **91:** 219-227.
14. GREEN, D.E. & C. KAGARISE SHERMAN. 2001. Diagnostic histological findings in Yosemite toads (*Bufo canorus*) from a die-off in the 1970s. J. Herpetol. **35:** 92–103.
15. MILIUS, S. 1998. Fatal skin fungus found in U.S. frogs. Sci. News **154:** 7.
16. MILIUS, S. 2000. New frog-killing disease may not be so new. Sci. News **157:** 133.
17. FELLERS, G.M., D.E. GREEN & J.E. LONGCORE. 2001. Oral chytridiomycosis in mountain yellow-legged frogs (*Rana muscosa*). Copeia. In press.
18. CONVERSE, K.A., J. MATTSSON & L. EATON-POOLE. 2000. Field surveys of Midwestern and Northeastern fish and wildlife service lands for the presence of abnormal frogs and toads. J. Iowa Acad. Sci. **107:** 160–167.
19. GOSNER, K.L. 1960. A simplified table for staging anuran embryos and larvae with notes on identification. Herpetol. **16:** 183–190.
20. BOLLINGER, T.K., J. MAO, D. SCHOCK, *et al.* 1999. Pathology, isolation and preliminary molecular characterization of a novel iridovirus from tiger salamanders in Saskatchewan. J. Wildlf Dis. **35:** 413–429.
21. DASZAK, P., L. BERGER, A.A. CUNNINGHAM, *et al.* 1999. Emerging infectious diseases and amphibian population declines. Emerg. Infect. Dis. **5:** 735–748.
22. FIJAN, N., Z. MATASIN, Z. PETRINEC, *et al.* 1991. Isolation of an iridovirus-like agent from the green frog (*Rana esculenta* L). Vet. Arhiv [Zagreb] **61:** 151–158.
23. MCKINNELL, R.G. & V.L. ELLIS. 1972. Herpesviruses in tumors of postspawning *Rana pipiens*. Cancer Res. **32:** 1154–1159.
24. HERR, R.A., L. AJELLO, J.W. TAYLOR, *et al.* 1999. Phylogenetic analysis of *Rhinosporidium seeberi*'s 18S small-subunit ribosomal DNA groups this pathogen among members of the protoctistan Mesomycetozoa clade. J. Clin. Microb. **37:** 2750–2754.
25. JAY, J.M. & W.J. POHLEY. 1981. *Dermosporidium penneri* sp. n. from the skin of the American toad, *Bufo americanus* (Amphibia: Bufonidae). J. Parasit. **67:** 108-110.
26. HEDRICK, R.P., C.S. FRIEDMAN & J.C. MODIN. 1989. Systemic infection in Atlantic salmon *Salmo salar* with a *Dermocystidium*-like species. Dis. Aquat. Org. **7:** 171–177.
27. ARKUSH, K.D., S. FRASCA, JR. & R.P. HEDRICK. 1998. Pathology associated with the rosette agent, a systemic protist infecting salmonid fishes. J. Aquat. Anim. Health **10:** 1–11.
28. HERMAN, R.L. 1984. Ichthyophonus-like infection in newts (*Notophthalmus viridescens* Rafinesque). J. Wildlf. Dis. **20:** 55–56.
29. GREEN, D.E. *et al.* 1995.

Immunolocalization of Vesicular Stomatitis Virus in Black Flies (*Simulium vittatum*)

ELIZABETH W. HOWERTH,[a] DANIEL G. MEAD,[b]
AND DAVID E. STALLKNECHT[c]

[a]*Department of Pathology,* [b]*Southeastern Cooperative Wildlife Disease Study,*
[c]*Department of Microbiology, College of Veterinary Medicine,*
University of Georgia, Athens, Georgia 30605 USA

ABSTRACT: Vesicular stomatitis, a disease of cattle, horses, and swine, is caused
by either vesicular stomatitis virus, New Jersey serotype (VSV-NJ), or vesicular stomatitis virus, Indiana serotype, which are related viruses in the genus *Vesiculovirus*, family Rhabdoviridae. Although recognized for at least 160 years,
the epidemiology and pathogenesis of this disease remains undefined. Black
flies have been suggested as a vector for VSV-NJ. In this study we infected
three- to four-week-old female black flies with VSV-NJ via feeding of virus-
spiked ox blood or intrathoracic inoculation, and demonstrated the location of
virus by immunohistochemistry. These preliminary findings suggest that
VSV-NJ initially infects the gut in the natural situation but that subsequent
spread to the salivary gland may be blocked in older flies, decreasing their ability to transmit the virus. The pattern of staining was different in intrathoracic
inoculated flies. In these flies, salivary gland involvement was more likely, and
extensive staining of eye, brain, and hemolymph suggested a more generalized
infection that apparently circumvented the gut. We conclude that intrathoracic
inoculation may be an inappropriate method of infection for determining vector competence and that the age of the vector should be considered when conducting competency studies.

KEYWORDS: vesicular stomatitis; black flies; salivary gland

Vesicular stomatitis is a disease of cattle, horses, and swine caused by two related
vesiculoviruses: vesicular stomatitis virus, New Jersey serotype (VSV-NJ) and vesicular stomatitis, Indiana serotype. As the name implies, the disease is characterized by vesicular lesions, particularly in the oral cavity, along the coronary bands,
and on the teats, and can be confused with economically important diseases, such as
foot and mouth disease. Although recognized for at least 160 years, factors involved
in the maintenance and transmission of vesicular stomatitis virus are unclear. Field[1]
and laboratory[2,3] data suggest that black flies are a possible vector of VSV-NJ. In
this study, we used immunohistochemistry (IHC) to examine the spatial distribution
of VSV-NJ antigen in three- to four-week-old female black flies (*Simulium vittatum*)

Address for correspondence: Dr. Elizabeth W. Howerth, Department of Pathology, College of
Veterinary Medicine, University of Georgia, Athens, Georgia 30605. Voice: 706-542-5833; fax:
706-542-5828.
ehowerth@vet.uga.edu

Ann. N.Y. Acad. Sci. 969: 340–345 (2002). © 2002 New York Academy of Sciences.

infected via feeding of virus-spiked cattle blood or intrathoracic inoculation. These findings coupled with virus isolation results suggested that vector competency diminishes with age.

MATERIALS AND METHODS

VSV-NJ used in this study was isolated from *Culicoides* sp. collected along the Rio Grande River near Belen, New Mexico. Virus was plaque purified and passed twice in Vero-M cells. Three to four-week-old *Simulium vittatum* females (IS-7 cytotype) were obtained from a continuous laboratory colony.[4]

Black flies were inoculated either intrathoracically or *per os.* Three flies were titrated immediately following injection or blood feeding to determine the baseline infection titer using a previously described plaquing method.[5] For intrathoracic inoculations, flies were injected with one μL of virus suspension per fly (initial titer of inoculum, $10^{6.7}$ plaque-forming units of VSV-NJ per milliliter (pfu/mL)).[6] After eight days, saliva was collected as described.[6] Virus isolation was then attempted from two flies, and seven were placed in 10% buffered formalin for IHC. For *per os* inoculations, flies were fed cattle blood containing $10^{6.2}$ pfu VSV-NJ/mL using a membrane feeding system.[4] Infected flies were held for 7 or 11 days postfeeding before saliva was collected for virus isolation. Whole flies (2 on postinoculation day (PID) 11) were then evaluated for presence of virus by virus isolation or IHC (12 on PID 7; 9 on PID 11). Flies found dead on PID 1 and 2 were fixed in 10% buffered formalin and examined by IHC.

Saliva samples were evaluated for presence of virus by direct observation of cytopathic effects on confluent Vero cell culture monolayers. Virus titers in whole flies were determined using a previously described plaque assay.[5]

For immunohistochemistry, formalin fixed flies were oriented in 3% agar to obtain whole body longitudinal sections, embedded in paraffin, sectioned at 3 μm, and stained using a streptavidin-biotin alkaline phosphatase IHC method. Deparaffinized and rehydrated sections were microwaved for 7 min in 0.01 M citrate pH 6, and then incubated with 0.03 HCl for 7 min at room temperature (RT) followed by incubation with HistoMark Blue (Kirkegaard & Perry) for 10 min at RT to block endogenous phosphatase. Sections were then blocked with Dako Protein Block for 8 min at RT, incubated with a 1:1500 dilution of anti–VSV-NJ hyperimmune mouse ascitic fluid for 1 h at RT, and subsequently incubated with streptavidin-labeled anti-mouse antibody (Biogenex), alkaline phosphatase-conjugated biotin (Biogenex), and fast red (Dako) as the chromagen. Sections were counterstained with hematoxylin. The positive control was a skin vesicle from a VSV-NJ–infected pig. Negative controls included the same vesicle but replacing the primary antibody with a commercially available mouse antibody control (Biogenex) and an uninfected fly that received the anti–VSV-NJ antibody.

RESULTS

Baseline virus titers for flies infected by intrathoracic injection and *per os* were $10^{3.7}$ and $10^{3.1}$ pfu/fly, respectively. Following incubation, virus was detected in the

TABLE 1. Virus isolation from saliva, immunohistochemical distribution of virus antigen, and intensity of staining in selected tissues

Treatment group	Virus Isolation	Immunohistochemistry					
	Saliva	Salivary gland & duct	Gut	Eye	Brain	Hemolymph	Ovary
Intrathoracic	9/9 (100%)[a]	3/3 (100%)[b]	1/2 (50%)	4/4 (100%)	4/4 (100%)	4/4 (100%)	0/4 (0%)
PID 8		+++[c]	+++	+++	+++	+++	
Per os	0/12(0%)	0/7 (0%)	5/10(50%)	0/9(0%)	0/9(0%)	0/12(0%)	0/9(0%)
PID 7			+++				
Per os	0/9 (0%)	0/3 (0%)	1/8 (12.5%)	0/3(0%)	0/6(0%)	0/9(0%)	0/8(0%)
PID 11			+				

[a] Number of flies with positive saliva/number of flies examined. Percentage in parentheses.
[b] Number of flies with positive tissue/number of flies with specific tissue identified in sections. Percentage in parentheses.
[c] Intensity of IHC staining (+=weak to +++=strong).

saliva of all flies infected by intrathoracic inoculation (TABLE 1). The average whole body virus titer of the two flies sampled on PID 8 was $10^{4.3}$ pfu/fly. Virus was not detected in the saliva of the *per os*–infected flies, even though virus was recovered from both of the flies sampled on PID 11 (TABLE 1). The average whole body virus titer was $10^{4.7}$ pfu/fly.

Immunohistochemical staining results of specific tissues are given in TABLE 1. Similar tissues were not observed in sections of each fly. This was particularly true for the salivary gland and duct, which were small and often missed in sectioning. In intrathoracic-inoculated flies, there was generalized intense staining of all structures in the thorax and head. Hemolymph throughout the body stained positive for viral antigen. Staining in the salivary gland and duct epithelium (FIG. 1D), eye (FIG. 1F), and brain (FIG. 1F) was diffuse and intense. Immunoreactivity in the gut epithelium of one fly was intense but focal. One fly with extensive staining of the head, salivary gland/duct, and hemolymph had no evidence of viral antigen in the gut. The generalized immunoreactivity seen in the thorax and head of the intrathoracic group was not observed in flies inoculated *per os*. Flies inoculated orally that died on PID 1 and

FIGURE 1. (A) Gut from orally inoculated fly on PID 7. Note focal immunoreactivity for VSV-NJ antigen in epithelial cells (*arrow*) surrounded by negative nonstained epithelium (*arrowheads*). (B) Gut from orally inoculated fly on PID 7. Note diffuse and intense staining of the gut epithelium (*arrow*) with adjacent negatively stained epithelium (*arrowhead*). (C) Orally inoculated fly, PID 7. Note lack of immunoreactivity to VSV-NJ antigen in epithelium of salivary gland and duct. (D) Fly inoculated intrathoracically, PID 8. Note diffuse positive staining in epithelium of salivary gland and duct. (E) Head of orally inoculated fly, PID 7. Note lack of staining in eye (E) and brain (B). (F) Head of fly inoculated intrathroacically, PID 8. Note diffuse positive staining for VSV-NJ antigen in eye and brain. Fast red chromagen.

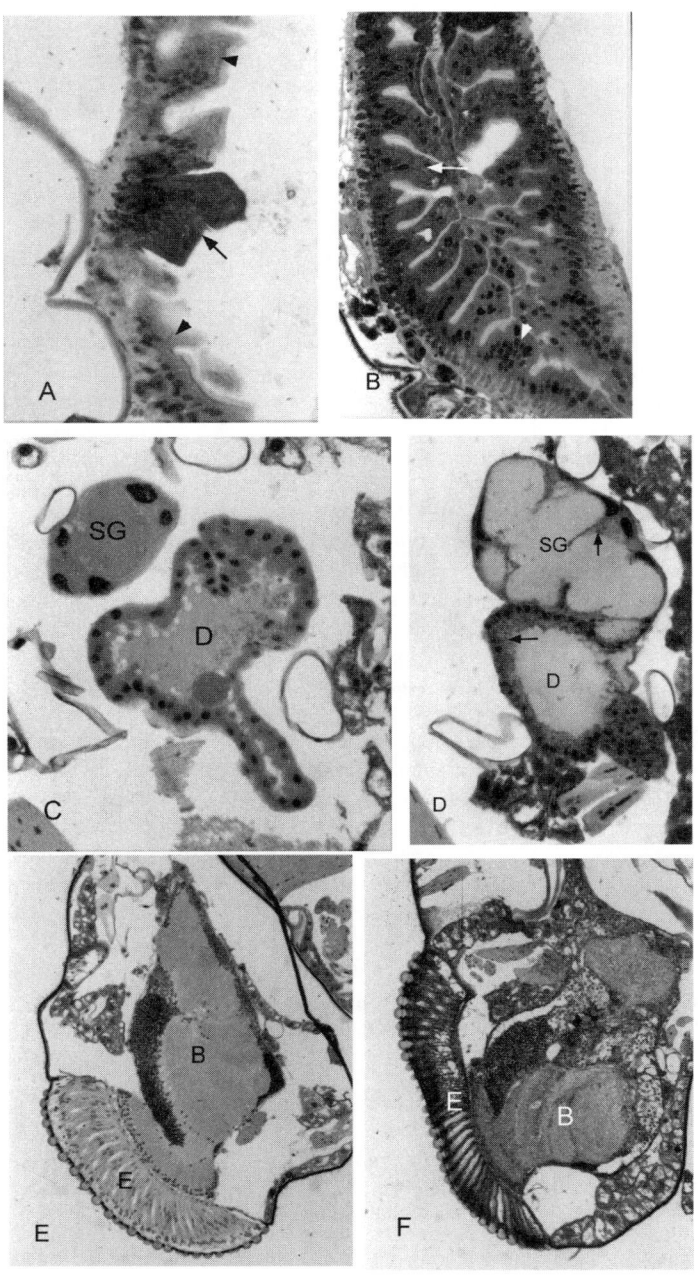

FIGURE 1. *See preceding page for legend.*

2 had either bacterial or fungal infection, but one fly had staining for VSV-NJ antigen in the gut epithelium. At PID 7 and 11, immunoreactivity for VSV-NJ antigen in the gut epithelium of orally inoculated flies varied from focal (FIG. 1A) to diffuse (FIG. 1B) but, in general, was more obvious than that seen in the intrathoracic group. Virus antigen was not detected in salivary gland or duct (FIG. 1C), brain (FIG. 1E), or eye (FIG. 1E) of orally inoculated flies.

DISCUSSION

In our study, three- to four-week-old female *S. vittatum* did not appear to be competent vectors of VSV-NJ. Although virus was found in gut by IHC and in whole ground bodies by virus isolation in orally inoculated flies, virus was not found in salivary gland by IHC or in saliva by virus isolation in these flies. This indicates that, although older flies can be infected with VSV-NJ, this age fly would not be capable of transmitting virus. In contrast, Cupp *et al.*[2] isolated virus from saliva of female *S. vittatum* orally inoculated with VSV-NJ (Camp Verde strain) at 1–2 days of age, demonstrating that very young female *S. vittatum* are competent vectors of VSV-NJ. Thus, while all ages of *S. vittatum* probably can be naturally infected with VSV-NJ via a blood meal, subsequent spread to salivary gland may be blocked in older flies, decreasing their ability to transmit virus. The VSV-NJ strain used in this study differed from the Cupp *et al.*[2] study, and possible strain differences need to be considered as a possible cause of salivary gland blockage.

By IHC, fewer flies inoculated *per os* had detectable virus antigen in the gut on PID 11 (12.5%) than on PID 7 (50%). Thus, with time, flies may clear the virus.

The distribution of viral antigen, as detected by IHC, in intrathoracic inoculated flies was different from those inoculated *per os*. In these flies, salivary gland/duct was more likely than gut to contain viral antigen, and there was extensive staining of eye, brain, and hemolymph not seen in flies inoculated *per os*. This suggested a more generalized infection, which apparently circumvented the gut in flies inoculated intrathoracically. IHC detection of virus antigen in salivary gland/duct and virus isolation from saliva in flies inoculated intrathoracically indicate that these flies could be used in transmission studies. However, because spread to the salivary gland and subsequent release in the saliva could not be demonstrated in flies inoculated *per os*, a more natural method of infection, intrathoracic inoculation, is probably not an appropriate method for determining vector competency.

REFERENCES

1. FRANCY, D.B., C.G. MOORE, *et al.* 1988. Epizootic vesicular stomatitis in Colorado, 1982: isolation of virus from insects collected along the northern Colorado Rocky Mountain front range. J. Med. Entomol. **24:** 343–347.
2. CUPP, E.W., C.J. MARE, *et al.* 1992. Biological transmission of vesicular stomatitis virus (New Jersey) by *Simulium vittatum* (Dipteria: Simuliidae). J. Med. Entomol. **29:** 137–140.
3. MEAD, D.G, C.J. MARE, *et al.* 1997. Vector competence of select black fly species for vesicular stomatitis virus (New Jersey serotype). Am. J. Trop. Med. Hyg. **57:** 42–48.

4. BERNARDO, M.J. & E.W. CUPP. 1986. Rearing black flies (Diptera: Simuliidae) in the laboratory: mass-scale in vitro membrane feeding and its application to collection of saliva and to parasitological and repellent studies. J. Med. Entomol. **23:** 666–679.
5. MARÉ, C.J. & S.L. GRAHAM. 1973. Falcon herpesvirus, the etiologic agent of inclusion body disease of falcons. Infect. Immun. **8:** 118–126.
6. MULLER, M.J. 1987. Transmission and *in vitro* excretion of bluetongue virus serotype 1 by inoculated *Culicoides brevitarsis* (Diptera: Ceratopogonidae). J. Med. Entomol. **24:** 206–211.

Intestinal Parasites Found in the Research Group of Mountain Gorillas in Bwindi Impenetrable National Park, Uganda

Preliminary Results

JESSICA M. ROTHMAN,[a] DWIGHT D. BOWMAN,[a] MARK L. EBERHARD,[b] AND ALICE N. PELL[a]

[a]Cornell University, Ithaca New York 14853, USA

[b]Centers for Disease Control and Prevention, Atlanta, Georgia 30341, USA

ABSTRACT: Mountain gorillas *(Gorilla gorilla beringei)* are critically endangered, remaining only in two isolated populations in Central Africa. The objective of this study was to determine the prevalence and intensity of intestinal parasites in a single group of mountain gorillas in Bwindi Impenetrable National Park, Uganda over 7 weeks from June to August 2000. Fecal samples were collected from night nests and transported in formalin for examination at Cornell University and the Centers for Disease Control. All fecal samples were examined microscopically for parasitic larvae, cysts, and eggs. The following were found: strongylid eggs, *Probstymaria* sp. larvae, and two parasitic nematode larvae that were not identified. Additional examination techniques will be used to further examine the fecal material specifically for protozoan cysts. An increasing threat to this group of gorillas is the presence of local field assistants and researchers. We found no evidence of human parasites in the fecal samples from this gorilla group.

KEYWORDS: mountain gorillas; Uganda; intestinal parasites; fecal material; Strongylid eggs; *Probstymaria* sp. larvae

Highly endangered mountain gorillas (*Gorilla gorilla beringei*) are found in two small populations: the Bwindi Impenetrable National Park in southwest Uganda and the Virunga Volcano region within the borders of Rwanda, Uganda, and the Democratic Republic of Congo. Both areas are surrounded by some of the most densely populated and intensively cultivated areas in Africa. Approximately 620 mountain gorillas remain, their population split almost equally between the two parks. While mountain gorillas in the Virunga Volcanoes have been extensively studied for the past 30 years, those in the Bwindi Impenetrable National Park are virtually unknown scientifically. Basic data on habitat use, population dynamics, health, behavior, and

Address for correspondence: Jessica M. Rothman, Cornell University, Ithaca, New York 14853.
jmr12@cornell.edu

Ann. N.Y. Acad. Sci. 969: 346–349 (2002). © 2002 New York Academy of Sciences.

diet of the Bwindi gorilla population are not yet available. This information is critical to the conservation of Bwindi gorillas and the management of their habitat.

Little is known about the parasites of mountain gorillas. The first descriptions of the gastrointestinal parasites of mountain gorillas in the Virunga region gave descriptions of eggs and larvae that were found in mountain gorillas in 1976–1978.[1] A survey of the mountain gorillas in Rwanda and the Democratic Republic of Congo (formerly Zaire) found nine helminths, five protozoa, and no hemoparasites.[2] Another survey of the gastrointestinal parasites of the mountain gorillas in Rwanda found strongylid eggs, four helminths, protozoa, one trematode egg, and one ascarid egg.[3] The surveys of the intestinal parasites in the Bwindi population found strongyle eggs, *Oesophagostomum*, *Murshidia*, *Strongyloides fuelleborni* larvae, and larvae of a *Probstmayria* sp.[4,5] *Cryptosporidium* sp. and *Giardia* sp. were recently found in the feces of some gorilla groups in Bwindi.[6]

An increasing threat to the Bwindi mountain gorilla is their habituation to humans. Three groups of gorillas are habituated for tourism, and one group of gorillas is habituated for research. On a daily basis, trackers, guides, and porters guide the tourists into gorilla habitat for one hour of gorilla viewing. Several opportunities for disease transmission exist, including the infection of water and soil with human feces. The effects of tourism on mountain gorillas are not well understood and should be the subject of future research.[7] The habituated research group of gorillas is visited on a daily basis by approved researchers and local field assistants for approximately four hours per day. No studies have specifically examined the parasite load of the research group, but the group has been included in other surveys of the Bwindi gorilla population.

The objective of this study was to determine the prevalence and intensity of intestinal parasites in the research group of mountain gorillas habituated for research over a seven-week period. This was a short preliminary study in preparation for a larger, more comprehensive longitudinal study of the gastrointestinal parasites of the Bwindi research group of gorillas.

MATERIALS AND METHODS

Fecal samples ($N=73$) were collected from the night nests (<24 hours old) of the Kyaguriro research group of mountain gorillas in Bwindi Impenetrable National Park for seven weeks during June to August 2000. The samples were taken once weekly, with the exception of one week in June. The age-sex class of an individual was determined by the diameter of the dung and the placement of the nest.[8] At the time of the study, the research group contained one silverback, two blackbacks, five females, three juveniles, and three infants. During the study, the two blackbacks emigrated and their dung was not found. The color and consistency of the fecal matter was described. Fecal material was weighed, placed in 10% formalin, and transported for examination to the Department of Microbiology and Immunology, College of Veterinary Medicine, Cornell University, and to the Centers for Disease Control and Prevention, Atlanta, Georgia, USA. A concentrate of each fecal sample was made using the formalin/ethyl-acetate centrifugal sedimentation method. All fecal samples were examined microscopically for parasitic larvae, cysts, and eggs. When present, parasite stages were identified, counted, measured, and photographed. Results were statistically analyzed using Fisher's exact test and the Chi-squared test of independence with the help of SAS computer software.[9]

RESULTS AND DISCUSSION

This group of mountain gorillas had a low prevalence of gastrointestinal parasites. Strongylid eggs were found in 35% of the samples with a mean number of 640 eggs per gram of feces in positive samples collected repeatedly from members of the group. Strongylid egg prevalence varied significantly over the seven-week course of the study ($P < 0.01$). The mean egg count varied significantly over the seven-week period ($P < 0.01$) in all samples and in only positive samples. There were no significant differences between strongylid eggs counts of different age-sex classes ($P = 0.96$). Based on the results of other gastrointestinal parasite surveys in mountain gorillas, we speculate that these eggs probably represent species of *Trichostrongylus*, *Oesophagostomum*, *Hyostrongylus*, *Impalaia*, *Paralibyostrongylus* or *Murshidia*. An earlier survey of fecal samples from mountain gorillas in Bwindi found strongylid egg prevalence to be 100%.[4] Gorillas may reinfect themselves or other gorillas through the accidental ingestion of contaminated vegetation and/or soil.

The larvae of a *Probstmayria* species were found in 12% of the samples, with a mean number of 75 larvae per gram of feces in positive samples. An earlier survey found 100% prevalence in Bwindi gorillas.[4] *Probstmayria* is a 3 mm long pinworm that is transmitted through fecal contamination. *Probstmayria* is expected to pose a minimal if any health threat to the gorillas, especially when the intensity of infection is low.

There was no indication of any protozoa in fecal samples from the research group. This is in agreement with earlier surveys.[4,5] Nizeyi *et al.* did not find any evidence of *Cryptosporidium* sp. or *Giardia* sp. in the research group, although these protozoa were found in other groups of gorillas in Bwindi.[6] It is also possible that our identification techniques were not sensitive enough to detect protozoa. Additionally, no cestode or trematode eggs were found. Two parasitic nematode larvae were not identified. We suspect that these may be a species of Trichostrongylidae recently discovered in Bwindi gorillas.[10] We found no evidence of human parasites in this group of gorillas.

We plan a comprehensive longitudinal study of parasites found in this group of mountain gorillas. Understanding and monitoring the parasitological health of this endangered population is crucial to its management, conservation, and ultimate survival.

ACKNOWLEDGMENTS

We thank the Uganda Wildlife Authority, the Uganda Council for Science and Technology, and the Institute of Tropical Forest Conservation for their permission to conduct this study and logistical support. The field assistants of the Institute of Tropical Forest Conservation are especially thanked for their assistance with field work. We are grateful to the Centers for Disease Control and Prevention, USA for invaluable assistance in the preparation of this study. The Mario Einaudi Foundation at Cornell University provided financial support.

REFERENCES

1. REDMOND, I. 1983. Summary of parasitology research. *In* Gorillas in the Mist. D. Fossey, Ed.: 271–286. Hodder and Stoughton. London, UK.
2. HASTINGS, B.E., L.M. GIBBONS & J.E. WILLIAMS. 1992. Parasites of free ranging mountain gorillas: survey and epidemiological factors. *In* Proceedings of a joint meeting of the American Association of Zoo Veterinarians and the American Association of Wildlife Veterinarians, pp. 301–302.
3. SLEEMAN, J.M., L.L. MEADER, A.B. MUAKIKWA, *et al.* 2000. Gastrointestinal parasites of mountain gorillas *(Gorilla gorilla beringei)* in the Parc National des Volcans, Rwanda. J. Zoo Wildl. Med. **31:** 322–328.
4. ASHFORD, R.W., H. LAWSON, T.M. BUTYNSKI, *et al.* 1996. Patterns of intestinal parasitism in the mountain gorilla *(Gorilla gorilla)* in the Bwindi Impenetrable Forest, Uganda. J. Zool. (Lond.). **239:** 507–514.
5. ASHFORD, R.W., G.D.F. REID & T.M. BUTYNSKI. 1990. The intestinal faunas of man and mountain gorillas in a shared habitat. Ann. Trop. Med. Parasitol. **84:** 337–340.
6. NIZEYI, J.B., R. MWEBE, A. NANTEZA, *et al.* 1999. *Cryptosporidium* sp. and *Giardia* sp. infections in mountain gorillas *(Gorilla gorilla beringei)* of the Bwindi Impenetrable National Park, Uganda. J. Parasitol. **85:** 1084–1088
7. BUTYNKSI, T.M. & J. KALINA. 1998. Gorilla tourism: a critical look. *In* Conservation of Biological Resources. E.J. Milner-Gulland & R. Mace, Eds.: 294–313. Blackwell Science. London.
8. SCHALLER, G.B. 1963. The Mountain Gorilla: Ecology and Behavior. University of Chicago Press. Chicago, Illinois.
9. AGRESTI, A. 1996. An Introduction to Categorical Data Analysis. Wiley Series in Probability and Statistics. J. Wiley & Sons, Inc. New York.
10. DURRETTE-DESSET, M.C., A.G. CHAUBAUD, R.W. ASHFORD, *et al.* 1992. Two new species of the Trichostrongylidae (Nematoda: Tichostrongyloidea), parasitic in *Gorilla gorilla beringei* in Uganda. Syst. Parasitol. **23:** 159–166.

Causes of Mortality in the Florida Panther (*Felis concolor coryi*)

C. D. BUERGELT, B. L. HOMER, AND M. G. SPALDING

Department of Pathobiology, College of Veterinary Medicine, University of Florida, Gainesville, Forida 32610, USA

ABSTRACT: Panthers necropsied at the University of Florida ranged between 2 weeks and 14 years of age; there were 38 males and 17 females in the cohort. Main categories of causes of death included trauma inflicted from either vehicular collisions (43%) or territorial fights (16%). Specific endogenous diseases involved the respiratory system in 13%, the urinary system in 4%, and the central nervous system in 2%. Ostium secundum atrial septal defects (ASD) were diagnosed in 11% of the panthers necropsied. Seventeen (54%) of the 38 male panthers had either unilateral or bilateral cryptorchidism. Cause of death remained undetermined in 11% of the total cohort.

Keywords: Florida panther; panther mortality; genetic diversity

INTRODUCTION

The Florida panther (*Felis concolor coryi*) is a subspecies of the cougar (*Felis concolor*) that has adapted to the subtropical environment in Southern Florida. It is estimated that a population of between 50 and 70 adult free-ranging panthers is left in Florida, making it one of the most endangered species. Based on a contract between the Florida Fish and Game Commission and the University of Florida, panthers found dead in the field are submitted for necropsy to the College of Veterinary Medicine in Gainesville, Florida. Between 1988 and 2000, complete necropsies were performed on 55 panthers. Prior to 1988, 33 panthers were necropsied elsewhere. This paper summarizes the pathologic findings from 55 panthers.

MATERIALS AND METHODS

A complete necropsy was performed on all animals submitted. The procedure included measurements of external markings, total body determination, and weight and size determination of major internal organs. Whole-body radiographs were performed prior to necropsy when illegal hunting was suspected. Pieces of tissue were fixed in 10% neutral buffered formalin for microscopic examination; pieces of major

Address for correspondence: Dr. C.D. Buergelt, Department of Pathobiology, College of Veterinary Medicine, University of Florida, Box 110 880, Gainesville, FL 32610. Voice: 352-392-4700, Ext.3924; fax: 352-392-9704.
BuergeltC@mail.vetmed.ufl.edu

Ann. N.Y. Acad. Sci. 969: 350–353 (2002). © 2002 New York Academy of Sciences.

organs were collected and frozen for toxicologic analyses; gastrointestinal contents were screened for endoparasites; one half of the brain was subjected to rabies examination. Fur and skeleton were retained by the Florida State Museum, Gainesville, Florida. Tissues collected for histopathologic examination were embedded in paraffin and sectioned at 6 microns. All sections were stained with hematoxylin and eosin, and selected sections were stained with a Brown-Brenn gram stain for bacteria. Findings were recorded as a final necropsy report.

RESULTS

Trauma cases included vehicular collision and intraspecies aggression (TABLE 1). Vehicular collisions occurred in 24 or 43% of the animals necropsied, and often had direct hits to the head, spine, chest, or pelvis, resulting in multiple, severe disabling fractures, leading to the immediate demise of the animal. Severe internal bleeds in either the abdominal or thoracic cavities accompanied the fractures. Intraspecies aggression resulted from fights over territorial rights between an older and a younger male panther. An occasional female panther was involved in intraspecies aggression. This diagnosis was made in 9 or 16% of the cases. There are two distinct wound patterns. One was a bite to the head with penetration of the canine teeth through the skull into the brain; the other was bites to the distal limbs that become infected, leading to septicemia and death.

Most endogenous diseases involved the respiratory system (13%). There were three cases of diffuse acute hemorrhagic pneumonia, suggesting toxicosis from herbicides or pesticides, although none could be identified from routine panel asseys. Three cats had pleuritis and/or pyothorax, respectively, suggesting infection other than FIP or trauma-related events because of a failure to identify any visible trauma signs. One cat had severe noncardiogenic pulmonary edema. Two cats had evidence of interstitial nephritis and intratubular crystal casts suggestive of either infection or nephrotoxicosis. One panther was diagnosed with rabies. The most likely source for the infection was the consumption of a rabies-infected raccoon or wild hog.

Congenital diseases involved the heart in males and females and/or the male gonads. Six (3 males and 3 females), or 11% of the animals had evidence of an atrial septal defect large enough to have contributed to the demise of the animals. The

TABLE 1. Disease categories leading to mortality in 55 Florida panthers (*Felis concolor coryi*) (1988–2000)

Categories	Number of panthers (%)
Vehicular trauma	24 (43)
Aggression	9 (16)
Respiratory	7 (13)
Nervous (rabies)	1 (2)
Urinary	2 (4)
Cardiac	6 (11)
Undetermined	6 (11)

mean diameter of the clinically apparent defects was 9.0 mm; the largest was 15 mm. Histological examination of the lungs of the three affected panthers revealed edema with perivascular fibrosis, suggesting congestive heart failure. Cryptorchidism was present in 17 (45%) of the 38 male animals necropsied. Although the majority of the cryptorchidism was unilateral, a lowering impact on reproductive performance could have been expected in these animals.

The cause of death remained undetermined in 6 (11%) of the necropsies. This was partially because of severe decomposition of the submitted animals, but also in one fresh case despite detailed microscopic, microbiologic/virologic, and toxicologic screening.

DISCUSSION

Florida panthers may range over an area of 800 square kilometers.[1] Individual male panthers may travel 30 km overnight or may stay in the same area for a week or more. The size of the female's territory varies with her reproductive status. The territorial demand brings the Florida panther into conflict with the human habitat with increased human housing and road devevelopment and landscape changes. Most of the mortality is human-inflicted, with an increase during the winter months when tourism is high. The Florida panther is a secretive animal that avoids humans. There are no documented reports of a panther attacking a human. The opposite is the case in the majority of panther deaths. Road kills and habitat loss are detrimental to panther survival.[2,3] Human encroachment and activity are in conflict with the panther's lifestyle. Illegal shooting was listed as a human-related category in 9% of deaths prior to 1988.[3]

As a large carnivore—males weigh between 100 and 150 pounds; females between 65 and 100 pounds—the panther needs a substantial amount of food and is adapted to catch large prey, often bigger than itself. An adult panther eats about 35 to 50 deer-sized animals per year. It takes about 10 raccoons to equal the food value of one deer. Besides deer and raccoons, the Florida panther hunts wild hogs, rabbits, armadillos, cotton rats, and birds. Females give birth to one or two, less frequently to three, kittens in simple dens. Females become sexually mature at about 2.5 years of age; males at about three years of age.

It is of interest to note that the records state that the Florida panthers necropsied were in good body condition, suggesting that there was plenty of prey available.

Genetic analysis has determined that the Florida panther's DNA is 65% less diverse than that of the cougars in the western states.[4] Inbreeding due to the limited number makes the Florida panther even more vulnerable to genetic limitations. Known consequences from lack of genetic versatility are atrial septal defects in males and females,[5] cryptorchidism in males, and also kinks in the tail in both male and female panthers.

The outlook for panther survival in Florida is grave despite a surveying program that is successful in preventing endogenous diseases. First steps toward salvage should include acquisition of more habitat and reduction of highway kills. Several highway underpasses have been successfully used by crossing panthers. The increase of genetic diversity through outbreeding with Texas cougars will widen the gene pool. The introduction of seven sexually mature female Texas cougars between

1995 and 1998 has resulted in the production of 12 hybrid kittens and hope for genetic restoration. Captive breeding programs and the removal of all panthers from the wild have been suggested alternatives.

ACKNOWLEDGMENTS

Gratitude is extended to Drs. M. Roelke-Parker, S. Taylor, M. Dunbar, and M. Cunningham for their involvement in the field work and necropsy procedures.

REFERENCES

1. MAEHR, D.S., E.D. LAND & J.C. ROOF. 1991. Social ecology of the Florida panther. Natl. Geogr. Res. Explor. **7:** 414–431.
2. MAEHR, D.S. & M.E. ROELKE. 1991. Mortality pattern of panthers in southwest Florida. Proc. Souteast. Assoc. Fish Wildl. Agencies **45:** 201–207.
3. TAYLOR, S.K., C.D. BUERGELT, E.D. LAND, *et al.* 1997. A review of causes of mortality of the Florida panther (*Felis concolor coryi*), 1972–1997. Proc. Wildl. Dis. Conf.: 89. St. Petersburg, FL.
4. ROELKE, M.E., J.S. MARTEN & J. O'BRIEN. 1993. The consequence of demographic reduction and genetic depletion in the endangered Florida panther. Curr. Biol. **3:** 340–350
5. CUNNINGHAM, M.W., M.R. DUNBAR, C.D. BUERGELT, *et al.* 1999. Atrial septal defects in the Florida panthers. J. Wildl. Dis. **35:** 519–530.

Pathology of Avian Pox in Wild Red-Legged Partridges (*Alectoris rufa*) in Spain

C. GORTÁZAR,[a] J. MILLÁN,[a] U. HÖFLE,[a,b,c] F. J. BUENESTADO,[a] R. VILLAFUERTE,[a] AND E. F. KALETA[c]

[a]*Instituto de Investigación en Recursos Cinegéticos (IREC), Ronda de Toledo s.n., E-13005 Ciudad Real, Spain*

[b]*Centro de Estudios de Rapaces Ibéricas (CERI), 45671 Sevilleja de la Jara, Spain*

[c]*Institut für Geflügelkrankheiten, Justus-Liebig-Universität, 35392 Giessen, Germany*

ABSTRACT: The diagnosis and pathology of an avian pox outbreak in free-living red-legged partridges in Cádiz, Southern Spain, is described. Diagnosis of the disease was based on histopathology, ultrastructural examination of, and virus isolation from lesions of necropsied animals. Lesions were present mainly in juvenile partridges (41%), and were observed primarily on the dorsal part of the digits or on the hock joint. The lesions ranged from small wartlike nodules to large tumor-like lesions. The presence of acute lesions of any grade as opposed to absence of lesions or healed lesions adversely affected body condition of the partridges ($P < .01$). Further investigations on the epidemiology of the disease and on the relation of the isolated strains to other avian poxviruses are under way.

Keywords: *Alectoris rufa*; avian pox; red-legged partridges; Spain

INTRODUCTION

Members of the genus *Avipoxvirus* infect birds of all taxa, especially galliform and passerine species.[1] Avian pox is characterized by the development of wartlike cutaneous lesions or diphtheroid lesions in mucous membranes. An acute fatal form is more rare and occurs mostly in pet canaries.[2] On occasions some birds develop large tumor-like lesions.[3]

The cutaneous form that produces lesions mostly in nonfeathered regions of the skin, such as the legs, eyelids, and ceres, can be a self-limiting mild disease or result in a severe debilitating infection that contributes to mortality.[4,5] Secondary bacterial infections of the lesions may lead to a complication in the course of the disease.[6] Lesions on mucous membranes of the upper respiratory and digestive tract are observed in the diphtheric form of the disease. In mixed forms, diphtheric lesions are associated with higher mortality than the cutaneous ones.[1]

Address for correspondence: Dr. Christian Gortázar, Instituto de Investigación en Recursos Cinegéticos (IREC), P.O. Box 535, E-13080 Ciudad Real, Spain. Voice: +34-926-295450; fax: +34-926-295451.

gortazar@irec.uclm.es

Ann. N.Y. Acad. Sci. 969: 354–357 (2002). © 2002 New York Academy of Sciences.

Diagnosis of the disease is by histopathologic examination of the lesions in which large, eosinophilic cytoplasmic inclusions (Bollinger bodies) are evident. Brick-shaped virions can be demonstrated by electron microscopy (EM). Virus isolation can be attempted in embryonated specific pathogen-free chicken eggs and in chicken embryo fibroblast cultures.[7]

The genus *Avipoxvirus* consists at present of ten species.[8] Owing to a lack of molecular information on the existing isolates, clear species classification is difficult. Natural infection has been described in pheasants, partridges, and quail. The susceptibility of the red-legged partridge (*Alectoris rufa*) to the disease was proven experimentally,[9] but there are no reports of natural avian pox infections in the red-legged partridge. Avian pox is a common disease among red-legged partridges in Spain. Thus, we were interested in describing the pathology of naturally occurring avian pox in the birds observed during a radio-tracking study.

MATERIALS AND METHODS

During a radio-tracking study carried out from March to December 2000 in Medina Sidonia (Cádiz, Southern Spain, 05°58' W, 36°27' N), 26 chick, 46 juvenile, and 45 adult free-living red-legged partridges were captured and tagged with radio transmitters. Classification in age classes was based on plumage characteristics: still in chick plumage, less than 10 weeks old (chicks), almost full-grown partridges with adult plumage (juveniles), and born before 2000 (adults). On each capture or recapture, the birds were inspected for avian-pox-compatible lesions on the nonfeathered parts of the body. Additionally, 10 nontagged chicks or juveniles and 34 adults were found dead and necropsied, and 74 juveniles and 34 adults were inspected after a hunting drive in October.

Pox-compatible lesions were grouped into four categories: (1) absent or healed, (2) mild (less than three proliferative skin lesions of <3 mm), (3) moderate (more than three lesions or any lesion >3 mm), and (4) severe (many lesions, including several large ones and apparently affecting the bird's condition, that is, their movements or their vision). Also, body condition was defined as the residual of the regression between body weight and the cube of tarsus length.[10]

Tissue from the lesions of dead animals was fixed in 10% neutral buffered formalin, processed and examined microscopically. Tissue from foot lesions of two partridges was cut into 1-mm cubes, fixed in 3% glutaraldehyde, postfixed in 1% osmium tetroxide, and after dehydration embedded into Epon. Uranyl acetate and lead citrate stained ultrathin sections were examined under a transmission electron microscope (Siemens I). Also, lesion material was homogenized in Basal Medium Eagle (Seromed, Biochrom, Berlin, Germany), sonicated, and inoculated onto chicken embryo fibroblast (CEF) cultures. At the appearance of cytopathologic effects, the cultures were harvested and passaged in order to carry out virus identification. This included treatment of virus suspension with 10% chloroform prior to culturing, cultures with IUDR (5-iodo-2-desoxy-uridin), testing for hemagglutinating activity in cell culture supernatant, and examination of culture supernatant by scanning EM (Siemens II).

RESULTS

Gross lesions indicative of avian pox were observed in a total of 29 out of 70 (41.4%) young-of-the-year red-legged partridges captured for radio-tagging, and on 20 additional partridges found dead during the study period or shot at the beginning of the hunting season.

Of the individuals with macroscopic pox-compatible lesions ($n = 49$), 48 had proliferative skin lesions on the featherless parts of the legs (98%), and only 4 also had lesions on the head (8%), either on the eyelids ($n = 3$) and/or on the ceres ($n = 2$). Three birds presented moderate-to-severe conjunctivitis or keratoconjunctivitis, but in none of these were pox lesions present on the eyelids. Lesions on the third eyelid were not observed in any of the cases. Four birds had lesions on other parts of the body, including the radio-metacarpal joint of the wings (8%). Secondary infections were demonstrated histologically in lesions of 2/11 (18%) cases.

According to their severity, 31 cases were rated as mild (63%), 11 as moderate (22%), and 7 as severe (14%). Severe cases included a bird with a broken wing and another one with a completely deformed leg.

The only adult bird with lesions was a nontagged male that had severe proliferative lesions on the eyelids, ceres, and legs. Juvenile red-legged partridges with pox lesions had a poorer ($F_{1,104} = 8.67$, $P < .01$) body condition ($CI = -0.28 \pm 0.9$, $n = 32$) than those without or with healed lesions ($CI = 0.33 \pm 1.0$, $n = 74$). Six out of 46 radio-tagged juveniles (13%) showed severe pox-compatible lesions. None of them survived into the hunting season. In contrast, six birds that had mild-to-moderate lesions during their capture in July and August were found healed in autumn. Smooth scars were observed in the epidermis of these individuals, especially on the digits and hock joint.

In both foot and eyelid lesions, large eosinophilic intracytoplasmic inclusions were observed microscopically in the epithelial cells. Varying degrees of epidermal hyperplasia, ballooning degeneration, and in some cases moderate heterophilic infiltrations in the dermis could also be observed. Infiltrates were related to ulceration and the presence of coccoid and/or rod-shaped bacteria in the serocellular crust of the lesion in two of the examined partridges.

EM revealed numerous pox virions in the inclusion bodies. The isolated viruses could be identified as poxvirus by their biochemical properties, lack of hemagglutination, and by EM.

DISCUSSION

This is the first description of a natural avian pox infection in red-legged partridges. Due to the existence of a radio-tracking study in the area, animals of different age classes could be observed throughout the outbreak. The disease affected mostly juvenile birds, which is consistent with observations in California quail (*Callipepla californica*).[11]

The poorer body condition of the juvenile birds that showed pox-lesions could have had an influence on their survival due to an increased risk of predation or a higher susceptibility to other diseases. This was evident in birds with severe lesions that impaired their movements. Debilitation and mortality due to cutaneous pox have been reported in different species in which the lesions generally had a wide distribution or a tumor-like appearance.[4,5]

Although bacterial contamination of lesions present on digits could be observed histologically, the course of the disease did not seem to depend on the presence of secondary infections, since the virus was the primary pathogen responsible for the deterioration of the condition of the affected birds. In experimental infections, only mild lesions could be produced in red-legged partridges in contrast to other galliform birds,[9] but body condition of the infected birds was not assessed. In this outbreak a high proportion (36%) of the affected juveniles developed pronounced lesions. In this respect the origin of the strain that caused the outbreak is of interest, as is the immune status of the juveniles at infection. Further investigations are under way in order to determine the relationship of the partridge isolates to other avian poxviruses.

REFERENCES

1. BOLTE, A.L., J. MEURER & E.F. KALETA. 1999. Avian host spectrum of avipoxviruses. Avian Pathol. **28:** 415–432.
2. TRIPATHY, D.N. & W.M. REED. 1997. Pox. *In* Diseases of Poultry, 10th ed. B.W. Calnek *et al.*, Eds.: 643–659. Mosby-Wolfe. London.
3. ARAI, S. *et al.* 1991. Cutaneous tumour-like lesions in Chilean flamingos. J. Comp. Pathol. **104:** 439–441.
4. KREUDER, C. *et al.* 1999. Avian pox in Sanderlings from Florida. J. Wildl. Dis. **35:** 582–585.
5. OROS, J. *et al.* 1997. Debilitating cutaneous poxvirus infection in a Hodgson's grandala (*Grandala coelicolor*). Avian Dis. **41:** 481–483.
6. SAMOUR, J.H. & J.E. COOPER. 1993. Avian pox in birds of prey (order Falconiformes) in Bahrain. Vet. Rec. **132:** 343–345.
7. TRIPATHY, D.N. & W.M. REED. 1998. Pox. *In* A Laboratory Manual for the Isolation and Identification of Avian Pathogens. D. E. Swayne *et al.*, Eds.: 137–143. American Association of Avian Pathologists. New Bolton Center, PA.
8. VAN REGENMORTEL, M.H.V. *et al.*, Eds. 2000. Virus Taxonomy. 7th Report of the International Committee on Taxonomy of Viruses. Academic Press. New York.
9. MEIGNIER, B. *et al.* 1974. Etude de la contamination experimentale du gibier a plumes (faisans, perdrix rouges, perdrix grises) par le virus de la Variole aviaire. Rev. Méd. Vét. **128:** 83–94.
10. ANDERSSON, S. 1992. Female preference for long tails in lekking Jackson's widowbirds: experimental evidence. Anim. Behav. **43:** 379–388.
11. CRAWFORD J.A. 1986. Differential prevalence of avian pox in adult and immature California quail. J. Wildl. Dis. **22:** 564–566.

Elk Restoration in Ontario, Canada

Infectious Disease Management Strategy, 1998–2001

R. ROSATTE,[a] J. HAMR,[b] B. RANTA,[c] J. YOUNG,[d] AND N. COOL[e]

[a]Ontario Ministry of Natural Resources, P.O. Box 4840, Peterborough, Ontario, Canada, K9J 8N8

[b]Cambrian College, 1440 Barrydowne Road, Sudbury, Ontario, Canada, P3A 3V8

[c]Ontario Ministry of Natural Resources, Kenora, Ontario, Canada, P9N 3X9

[d]24 Karen Drive, Lindsay, Ontario, Canada, K9V 5V5

[e]Parks Canada, Elk Island National Park, Fort Saskatchewan, Alberta, Canada, T8L 2N7

ABSTRACT: Ontario has embarked upon a program to restore elk (*Cervus elaphus*) that were once native to that province. A comprehensive disease-management strategy has ensured that elk are free of infectious diseases such as brucellosis and tuberculosis prior to shipment to Ontario. Postmortem analysis occurs on elk mortalities in Ontario to ensure that elk are not infected with diseases such as chronic wasting disease and tuberculosis. Between 1998 and 2001, a total of 443 elk were transported from Elk Island National Park, Alberta, and released in four different areas of Ontario. Cumulative mortality for elk in all areas was 26% from 1998 to January 2001. The primary causes of mortality were post-release stress-induced emaciation (21%), wolf predation (20%), transport/handling injuries (10%), bacterial infections (10%), and drowning (7%). Female calves had the highest mortality rates (37%) compared to the other sex and age cohorts (23–24%). Preliminary findings suggest an inverse correlation between the length of time elk are held in enclosures prior to release and the distance they disperse from the release site. The 2001 estimated population of elk in Ontario is about 400 individuals.

KEYWORDS: elk; Ontario; chronic wasting disease; tuberculosis

THE ONTARIO ELK RESTORATION PROGRAM

Once native to the province of Ontario, elk (*Cervus elaphus*) were extirpated by the late 1800s as a result of several factors including unregulated hunting, market hunting, and loss of habitat because of human settlement. There have been several attempts to restore elk to the province, the most recent ones made in the 1930s and 1940s.[1] Unfortunately, most of these animals were subsequently killed because of unfounded concerns that they were infecting cattle with the giant liver fluke (*Fascioloides magna*). However, two small herds of elk managed to survive in the

Address for correspondence: Dr. R. Rosatte, Ontario Ministry of Natural Resources, P.O. Box 4840, Peterborough, Ontario, Canada, K9J 8N8. Voice: 705-755-2280.
rick.rosatte@mnr.gov.on.ca

Ann. N.Y. Acad. Sci. 969: 358–363 (2002). © 2002 New York Academy of Sciences.

Burwash/French River area. The objective of the current elk restoration program is to supplement the Burwash/French River herd as well as to restore elk to other areas of Ontario.

Ontario's elk restoration initiative involves partnership among 14 agencies and postsecondary institutions, as well as many volunteers. The partners provide guidance to the initiative through participation on the Provincial Elk Restoration Advisory Committee (PERAC). Local Implementation Committees (LICs) have been established in the four areas where elk restoration programs are under way. The Plan for the Restoration of Elk in Ontario was prepared and approved by the Ontario Ministry of Natural Resources (OMNR) in 1997 and provides overall direction to Ontario's elk restoration efforts.[2] The Plan identifies six broad geographic areas as offering suitable elk habitat.

ELK ACQUISITION, PROCESSING, TRANSPORTATION, RELEASE, AND MONITORING

Elk Island National Park (EINP) near Edmonton, Alberta is the source of elk for Ontario's restoration efforts. It operates one of the most rigorous disease-management programs in North America, in cooperation with the Canadian Food Inspection Agency (CFIA).[3] The Park's boundary is completely fenced, thereby minimizing the chances of transmission of infectious diseases from animals outside of the park. The primary focus of the processing of elk at EINP was to ensure that the animals were free of infectious disease. That included injecting bovine and avian tuberculosis (TB) antigen in the midcervical region of each elk on the first day of processing. The animals were also weighed, sexed, aged, and a blood sample (10–20 mL) collected from the jugular vein of each animal for disease testing (brucellosis) and DNA analysis. The animals were then ear-tagged and treated orally with Fascinex (10% triclabendazole) to control liver-fluke infestation. The dosage for the first drenching of Fascinex was 170 mL for adults and 100 mL for yearlings and calves. All elk were also given a subcutaneous injection of ivermectin as a general antiparasitic agent (10 mg/50kg body weight). To limit the effects of capture myopathy, all elk were also given a subcutaneous injection of Dystosel (1 mL/45kg body weight). Three days after being injected with TB antigen, the elk were again processed to determine whether there was any reaction at the site of inoculation. Animals in prime condition that were negative for both TB reactions were selected for the Ontario elk shipment. Most of those animals were fitted with large mammal VHF or GPS radio-collars. The animals were also given a second drenching of Fascinex. Any elk dying at EINP were screened for chronic wasting disease (CWD)—all have been negative to date.

Between February 1998 and February 2001, 460 elk (245 cows, 84 bulls, 60 male calves, and 70 female calves) were transported from Alberta to Ontario. Seventeen died (primarily from bacterial infections) or were euthanized (because of injuries/infections) prior to release. Upon arrival in Ontario, the elk were placed in holding pens to recuperate from the trip as well as to get accustomed to their new surroundings. The length of the holding period varied from an unplanned immediate release (hard release), to 4–10 days (semi-soft release), to 6–15 weeks (soft release) (TABLE 1). Following release, attempts were made to locate each animal every one

TABLE 1. Length of holding period and dispersion of cow elk following release in four areas of Ontario during 1998–2000[a]

Area (ERA)	Release date	Days held in pen	Mean (SD) distance moved (km)	Shortest distance moved (km)	Greatest distance moved (km)[b]	Elk moving > 50 km (n)	Elk moving < 5 km (n)	Total elk	Mortality from release to 9/2000 (%)
LNFR	3/27/98	27	16.7 (20.5)	1.0	84	1	10	23	8.6
LNFR	1/15/99	4	27.8 (24)	2.5	120	3	3	31	45.6
LNFR	3/31/00	43	5.1 (9.2)	0.5	50	0	29	32	11.1
BNH	1/09/00	0	31.7 (33.3)	4.0	140	6	2	37	20
LOW	1/29/00	10	37.7 (53.9)	1.0	200	5	5	14	7.1

[a]LNFR, Lake Nipissing/French River; BNH, Bancroft/North Hastings; LOW, Lake of the Woods.

[b]Calculations include movements from the date of release to September of the release year.

[c]Elk group composition includes 1998 LNFR: 23 cows (2+ years old); 1999 LNFR: 30 cows, 1 yearling cow; 2000 LNFR: 13 cows, 19 yearling cows; 2000 BNH: 32 cows, 5 yearling cows; 2000 LOW: 13 cows, 1 yearling cow.

TABLE 2. Causes of mortality of elk released in four areas of Ontario during 1998–January 31, 2001

Area[a] (ERA)	Year	Total Mortality % (n)	Emaciation (n)	Wolf Predation (n)	Injury (n)	Shot (n)	Drowning (n)	Road Kill (n)	Bacterial Infection (n)	Other[b] (n)
LNFR	1998	**40** (19/47)	0	4	5	1	1	0	7	1
LNFR	1999	**48** (33/69)	14	12	0	1	2	0	1	3
LNFR	2000	**15** (6/40)	1	1	0	0	3	1	0	0
BNH	2000	**24** (17/70)	3	0	3	2	0	3	0	6
LOW	2000	**13** (8/60)	0	0	0	3	0	0	0	5
LHNS	2000	**6** (3/50)	0	0	1	0	0	0	1	1
ALL 98/01[c] % (n)		**26** (86/336)	**21** (18)	**20** (17)	**10** (9)	**8** (7)	7 (6)	**5** (4)	**10** (9)	**19** (16)

[a]LNFR=Lake Nipissing/French River; BNH=Bancroft/North Hastings; LOW=Lake of the Woods; LHNS=Lake Huron North Shore; ERA=Elk Release Area.

[b]Other sources of mortality include bear predation (1), accident (fell over cliff) (1), unknown (7), suspected predation (2), train (1), tumor (1), hypothermia (1), capture myopathy (1).

[c]% (n) refers to the row of mortality causes.

to two weeks using radiotelemetry. As of July 2001, elk have been released within four of the six areas identified in the Plan to Restore Elk in Ontario[2]: Lake Nipissing–French River (LNFR), Bancroft/North Hastings (BNH), Lake of the Woods (LOW), and Lake Huron North Shore (LHNS).

ELK DISPERSION, MORTALITY AND PRODUCTIVITY FOLLOWING RELEASE IN ONTARIO

Cow elk dispersion following release from the holding pens appears to be related to the length of time they were held prior to release (TABLE 1). Elk that were held for six weeks, as during the 2000 LNFR release, tended to remain in the vicinity of the holding pens (TABLE 1). In fact, most of those elk remained within 5 km of the release site for at least six months after release. Elk that experienced a hard release (as in the 2000 BNH release) tended to disperse over a much wider area (TABLE 1). In fact, by December 31, 2000, the BNH 2000 elk released were spread over a 10,000 km^2 area. Only about 50% of the remaining 53 elk were within 20 km of the release site at that time.

Some animals (about 10) moved 100–140 km from the release site. Four elk from the 2000 LOW release (held for 3 or 10 days) ventured into Minnesota (about 70–90 km from the release site) and at least six elk dispersed to the Ft. Francis/Rainy River area (about 40–60 km from the release site); however, most of the elk are ranging only as far as about 20 km from the release site. Elk movements (2) of up to 160 km (to Algoma Mills and to Parry Sound) have been noted (1.5 years after release) for the 1998 and 1999 LNFR–introduced animals (held for 26 and 4 days, respectively). The longest movement of a 2000 LNFR animal (held for 6 weeks) was 50 km, but one of the 2000 LOW elk moved 200 km to Minnesota. It must be emphasized that these data are only preliminary and that experiments with the length of time elk are held in the release pen will need to be replicated before concrete conclusions can be made.

As part of the disease-management strategy, elk that died in Ontario were sent to the Canadian Cooperative Wildlife Health Centre (CCWHC) in Guelph, Ontario for postmortem analysis. There they were screened for several diseases including CWD—all have been negative for CWD to date as of July 2001. Total accumulated mortality among the 336 elk that were transported to Ontario between January 1998 and December 2000 was 26% (TABLE 2). Mortality was high following the 1998 LNFR shipment, possibly due to a two-day stop in Manitoba because of a blizzard. Wolf predation was also high at the LNFR release area during 1999 (TABLE 2). Seven of the 1998 LNFR elk died or were euthanized prior to release from the pen. Most of these mortalities were thought to be stress related (i.e., pneumonia, etc.). Calf mortality during 1999 in LNFR was exceptionally high (84%). Accumulated calf mortality averaged 31% for all years and all areas (TABLE 3). Although mortality for bull and cow elk was similar for all years and areas (24% and 23%, respectively), there were yearly differences as well as those among areas (TABLE 3).

Elk productivity in Ontario has been variable. In the winters of 1999 and 2000, only 10–20% of the adult cows introduced to the LNFR area in 1998 and 1999 were accompanied by calves. That included sightings of six calves during 1999 and 12 calves during 2000. A December 2000/January 2001 calf survey showed that over

TABLE 3. Cumulative mortality per sex and age class of elk at the four Elk Restoration Areas in Ontario during 1998–January 31, 2001[a]

Area[b] (ERA)	Year	Adult males % (n)	Adult females % (n)	Male calves % (n)	Female calves % (n)
LNFR	1998	29 (4/14)	45 (15/33)	NA	NA
LNFR	1999	0 (0/7)	41 (17/42)	100 (6/6)	77 (10/13)
LNFR	2000	NA	25 (5/20)	0 (0/7)	8 (1/13)
BNH	2000	29 (4/14)	14 (5/36)	30 (3/10)	50 (5/10)
LOW	2000	39 (5/13)	9 (3/33)	0 (0/8)	0 (0/6)
LHNS	2000	0 (0/7)	7 (2/31)	0 (0/7)	25 (1/4)
ALL	1998–2001	**23** (13/56)	**24** (47/194)	**24** (9/38)	**37** (17/46)

[a]Actual mortality may have been higher during the 1999 and 2000 LNFR program because 3 of the 1999 calves and 5 of the 2000 cows did not have radio-collars. Similarly, during the 2000 LOW program, 18 cows, 4 calves, and 8 bulls did not have radio-collars; however, visual observations were made on 4 of the calves.
[b]LNFR, Lake Nipissing/French River; BNH, Bancroft/North Hastings; LOW, Lake of the Woods; LHNS, Lake Huron North Shore; ERA, Elk Release Area. Any known mortalities among uncollared animals are included this table.

30% of the adult cows in the LNFR elk population (both resident and restored elk) had calves (22 in total). However, only 2 calves/22 cows could be spotted during a repeat survey in March 2001. Only four calves were noted in the Lake of the Woods area during 2000; however, 40% (10/25) of the cows observed in the BNH area during February 2001 had calves. EINP biologists estimate that about 60–70% of the cows are with calves during each winter. This suggests that calf mortality in Ontario may be high.

A number of graduate research programs focusing on elk productivity, habitat selection, diseases, and competition have been initiated at several universities in Ontario. However, the key to a successful elk restoration program in Ontario will be the continuation of the stringent disease-management guidelines in the provinces of both Alberta and Ontario.

ACKNOWLEDGMENTS

The Ontario Elk Restoration Program was directed by PERAC co-chairs Ivan Filion (Cambrian College) and Dan Elliott (OMNR). Special thanks go to the staff at EINP, CFIA, and CCWHC for all their cooperation in assisting with the Ontario elk program and to all the LIC and Elk Research Network members, graduate students at Trent University, Lakehead University, University of Guelph, and Laurentian University, drivers, and volunteers who made the Ontario Elk Restoration program possible.

REFERENCES

1. RANTA, W., H. MERRIAM & J. WEGNER. 1982. Winter habitat use by wapiti, *Cervus elaphus*, in Ontario woodlands. Can. Field Nat. **96:** 421–430.
2. BELLHOUSE, T. & J. BROADFOOT. 1996. Plan for the restoration of elk in Ontario. Ontario Ministry of Natural Resources internal report, Ontario, Canada, 55pp.
3. ROSATTE, R., J. HAMR, B. RANTA & J. YOUNG. 2001. Ontario elk restoration program summary, 1998–2001. Ontario Ministry of Natural Resources internal report, Ontario, Canada, 13 pp.

Appendix 1

Resolution by the Wildlife Disease Association and
the Society for Tropical Veterinary Medicine Calling for
International Donor Community Recognition of
Animal Health Sciences as Critical for the Design and Management of
Sustainable Wildlife and/or Livestock-Based Programs

Whereas, contact and resource competition between wildlife and livestock continuously expand as more and more land comes under some form of human use;

whereas, wild and domestic animals have many diseases in common and both groups can and do play different roles in disease epidemiology, and recognizing that these interrelationships can have significant implications for disease prevention or control schemes;

whereas, livestock-based and wildlife-based activities are undertaken separately as well as jointly as primary modes of sustenance, economic betterment and support of rural livelihoods, with the sustainability thereof inextricably linked to ecologically appropriate land-use choices;

whereas, the sustainable management of livestock as well as the conservation of wildlife require ground-level stewardship, including disease surveillance, by those communities closest to and most dependent on these resources;

whereas, numerous governmental and non-governmental organizations worldwide provide financial resources, incentives, leadership, and advice targeted at boosting productivity and sustainability of the livestock and/or natural resource management sectors without always recognizing concomitant disease implications, which can be significant and complex;

whereas, limited funding streams for wildlife and/or livestock initiatives require prudent use;

whereas, donor organizations seldom possess sufficient internal expertise regarding the myriad disease issues implicit in ensuring the success of wildlife and/or livestock-based programs; and

whereas, the Wildlife Disease Association and the Society for Tropical Veterinary Medicine, along with other local, national, and international organizations, represent professionals who possess unique skills, knowledge, and experience with wild and domestic animal diseases and their underlying causes, ecological relationships, and economic implications.

Now, therefore, be it resolved that, the Wildlife Disease Association and the Society for Tropical Veterinary Medicine urge those organizations contemplating the funding and implementation of programs involving wildlife or livestock resources to:

Ann. N.Y. Acad. Sci. 969: 364–366 (2002). © 2002 New York Academy of Sciences.

encourage projects that foster integrative approaches to livestock production, food security, human health, economic growth, democracy and governance, biodiversity conservation, and natural resource management in order to build upon synergies among these sectors while precluding conflicting policies and/or negative impacts on either livestock or wildlife health;

formalize steps in their project design, environmental impact assessment, and implementation processes which address wildlife, livestock, and rangeland health issues and their implications for sustainability and thus success, recognizing that these projects may alter fundamental relationships between animal hosts and potential pathogens and parasites;

when contemplating projects involving domestic and/or wild animals, establish relationships with appropriate wildlife and domestic animal health-oriented organizations and recognized local, national, regional, and international experts, thereby identifying an appropriate pool of professionals who can assist in ensuring the inclusion of timely, science-based advice in planning, implementation, and monitoring processes; and

put a premium on local human capacity-building to address the long-term technical needs of development activities that require expertise in domestic animal health and wildlife health by building adequate support into project design and implementation so as to engage local expertise and to foster capacity-building at professional as well as community levels as a first-tier priority within and beyond the life-spans of such programs.

Index of Contributors